Introduction to Sound

Acoustics for the Hearing
and Speech Sciences

Introduction to Sound

Acoustics for the Hearing and Speech Sciences

Charles E. Speaks, Ph.D.

Professor
Department of Communication Disorders
University of Minnesota
Minneapolis, Minnesota

CHAPMAN & HALL
London · New York · Tokyo · Melbourne · Madras

Published by Chapman & Hall, 2–6 Boundary Row, London SE1 8HN

Chapman & Hall, 2–6 Boundary Row, London SE1 8HN, UK

Chapman & Hall, 29 West 35th Street, New York NY 10001, USA

Chapman & Hall Japan, Thomson Publishing Japan, Hirakawacho Nemoto Building, 6F, 1-7-11 Hirakawa-cho, Chiyoda-ku, Tokyo 102, Japan

Chapman & Hall Australia, Thomas Nelson Australia, 102 Dodds Street, South Melbourne, Victoria 3205, Australia

Chapman & Hall India, R. Seshadri, 32 Second Main Road, CIT East, Madras 600 035, India

This edition not for sale in North America and Australia; orders from these regions should be referred to Singular Publishing Group, Inc., 4284 41st Street, San Diego, CA 92105, USA.

Typeset in 10/12 Trump Mediaeval by CFW Graphics
Printed in the U.S.A. by McNaughton & Gunn

ISBN 0 412 48760 8

A catalogue record for this book is available from the British Library

Library of Congress Cataloging-in-Publication data available

To Nancy, Brandon, and Jeffrey

Contents

Preface

This book was written to *teach* the fundamental concepts of acoustics, particularly to those who are interested in the discipline of the speech-language-hearing sciences. Readers who are thoroughly grounded in mathematics and physics should be able to move through the various topics quickly. Those who are less comfortable with basic concepts of physics, or with mathematics beyond elementary algebra, will require more careful study of some of the concepts, but ultimately the concepts should be understood.

Students of the speech-language-hearing sciences must have a thorough understanding of the elements of acoustics before they can successfully embark on more advanced study of both normal and disordered human communication. At the University of Minnesota, for example, students in the Department of Communication Disorders who pursue an undergraduate degree must complete a five-credit course in acoustics, which is *prerequisite* to registration in more advanced courses such as Speech Science, Hearing Science, Hearing Loss and Audiometry, Noise and Humankind, Cleft Palate: Oral-Facial Anomalies and Speech, and Voice Disorders. Treatment of the fundamental concepts of acoustics with two or three weeks of lectures in the context of a broader course such as "speech and hearing science" or "introduction to audiology" cannot, in our opinion, do justice to the topic or serve students well.

There are many aspects of sound that might interest readers other than students in the speech-language-hearing sciences. Why is a "sonic boom" created when an airplane exceeds the speed of sound? Why is a foghorn designed to emit a low-pitched sound instead of a high-pitched whistle? If you are hunting in the woods, why is your distant prey more likely to hear you if it is downwind from you? How do "whispering galleries" work? In what ways do echoes off a canyon wall behave like billiard balls bouncing off rails on the billiard table? When you contemplate purchasing a stereo system, what does the salesperson mean by terms such as frequency response, noise floor, dynamic range, signal-to-noise ratio, decibels, percentage harmonic distortion, and so on? The answers to these and other questions are sprinkled throughout the text.

In the opening sentence, the word "teach" was emphasized because the fundamental goal is to *teach* the important elements of acoustics, not just present the topics. Two examples should suffice. First, some readers will not know, or will have forgotten, what is meant by "antilog$_{10}$ 2." However, everyone will certainly know that $10^2 = 100$. To understand the *concept* of antilogarithms, then, one needs only to realize that "antilog$_{10}$ 2 = ?" is exactly the same as asking "what is 10^2?"

Once the concept is understood, all that remains is to learn the simple steps for solving antilog problems that are computationally, but not conceptually, more difficult. Second, learning of several concepts in acoustics, the decibel for example, can be enhanced by solving problems. For that reason, the book includes nearly 400 practice problems that are followed by *answers and explanations* of how the correct answers were obtained.

The organization of the topics in the book reflects a combination of both logic and personal preference. For example, the concepts of antilogarithms and logarithms must be understood before one can study decibels, and it is difficult to imagine how one can understand complex sound waves without first mastering the concept of sinusoidal wave motion. The location of other topics within the book reflects the author's preference for teaching. Some might prefer, for example, to begin by reading about "fundamental and derived physical quantities" and "proportionality" from Chapter 1 and "scientific notation" from Chapter 3. Those topics, and some others, should be treated as free-standing modules to be addressed when the reader or teacher elects.

Acknowledgments

Any list of persons who should be acknowledged would be woefully incomplete, but the contributions of some must be recognized. One group is my own mentors, including Francis Flynn, Edward Penson, Robert Bilger, Gordon Peterson, Martin Schultz, and James Jerger. The second and equally important group is former students, both undergraduate and graduate.

I express my sincere appreciation to Bob Bilger, Dave Fabry, Larry Feth, Ted Glattke, Ray Kent, Dianne Van Tasell, and Dix Ward for their careful reading of an earlier version of the manuscript and for their excellent suggestions for improvement. I also wish to thank Tom Crain for his careful preparation of the illustrations and Tim Trine for his excellent help with preparation of the final draft. Finally, I wish to thank Nancy Niccum for her encouragement and patience, and Nancy, Brandon, and Jeffrey for the time that could not be devoted to them.

The Nature of Sound Waves

What is sound? One can hardly resist referring to a question that often is posed in high school science courses. "If a tree falls in a forest and no one is around to hear it, is there sound?" Put in more modern terms, "If the Muzak system in the elevator is turned on, but there are no passengers, is there sound?"

Albers (1970) stated that sound "in the strict sense, is a compressional wave that produces a sensation in the human ear" (p. 36). We need not worry for the moment what Albers meant by a "compressional wave," but his reference to producing a "sensation of hearing" deserves comment. When "sensation of hearing" is included in the definition of sound, we emphasize the *psychological* attributes of sound: pitch, loudness, and timbre. In other words, from a psychological point of view, "sound is what we hear."

We certainly are aware of the many "sounds" around us — sounds such as human speech, the barking of a dog, the crying of an infant, the cooing of the dove or of a "significant other," music of all forms, thunder, traffic noises, and the exhilarating roar of water cascading down the side of a mountain. A psychological approach to defining sound might have an intuitive appeal because it might seem that it would be easy to understand the *physical events* that characterize sound by reference to the psychological sensations or feelings that are associated with the myriad of sounds that we experience daily.

An alternative is to define sound from a *physical* perspective. In this case, sound is defined by reference to properties of the source of the event that we call "sound" and to properties of a "medium" in which, or along which, sound is transmitted. When *physical* properties of sound are emphasized, sound is considered to exist *even if the receiver is absent or is not functional*. In other words, sound does exist even if no one is in the forest or if the elevator is empty. To understand the nature of sound, we must identify and describe the physical characteristics of the events that take place among the trees or within the high-rise building.

Many things can serve as a source of sound: vocal folds; the strings of a piano, guitar, or violin; the membrane on a drum; the bar on the xylophone; the metal plates of the cymbals; the whistle; the tapping of heel and toe in dance; and so on. We shall see that there is one principal prerequisite for a body to be a source of sound — it must be able to vibrate. If a body is to be set into vibratory motion, it must have the physical properties of **mass** and **elasticity**, and all bodies in nature possess both of those two properties to some degree.

When something happens to those potential sources *that causes them to be set into vibratory motion or oscillation*, "a sound event" occurs, and the event can then be transmitted from the source through or along some medium. Air is probably the most common medium that we are likely to encounter. But, as we shall see, other molecular structures such as, for example, water, wires, strings, or steel rails also can transmit sound. Because all molecular structures have some finite **mass** and **elasticity**, all are capable of being both a source of sound and a medium for its transmission. Of course, some structures will be more effective sources or transmitters than others.

Although the properties that permit a structure to be a source of sound are essentially identical to the properties that permit a medium to transmit sound, it is convenient to describe the properties of the transmitting medium and the properties of the source separately.

■ PROPERTIES OF THE TRANSMITTING MEDIUM

Consider the medium of air. Air consists of approximately 400 billion billion (4×10^{20}) molecules per cubic inch (in.). In the quiescent state (before a source of sound has been energized), the molecules are in random motion and are moving at speeds that average nearly 940 miles per hour (MPH), which corresponds to 1,500 kilometers per hour (KPH). During that random motion they maintain some *average distance* from one another, which allows us to envision the molecules as being distributed fairly evenly throughout the air space.

The billions upon billions of molecules exert a pressure on whatever they come in contact with. When, for example, the random motion causes the air molecules to impinge on the human ear drum (or any other structure), a pressure is exerted on the drum. Interestingly, as we shall see later, that does not produce a sensation of "hearing" sound. At sea level that pressure, which also is called "atmospheric pressure," amounts to about 14.7 pounds (lb) per square in., and 14.7 lb/in.^{2} in the English measurement system is equivalent to approximately 100,000 newtons (Nt) per square meter (Nt/m^2) or 1,000,000 dynes per square centimeter (dynes/cm^2) in the metric system. The Nt/m^2 and dyne/cm^2 as measures of pressure will be defined later when the concepts of both pressure and force are developed more fully.

To conceptualize the pressure in air, consider the cylindrical tube shown in Figure 1–1, which has a cross-sectional area equal to 1 in.^{2} and extends from sea level to a height of 25 miles above sea level. At sea level, in the quiescent state, there is a pressure acting downward that amounts to approximately 14.7 lb/in.^{2} At 10 miles above sea level, the pressure is reduced to about 1.57 lb/in.^{2}, and at the height of 25 miles it is only a negligible 0.039 lb/in.^{2}

Air, and all other bodies that can serve to transmit sound, is characterized by two important physical properties: **mass** and **elasticity**.

Mass

By mass we mean *the amount of matter that is present.* Air, of course, is gaseous matter, but the definition of mass also holds for the two other forms of matter: liquids and solids.

Mass Contrasted With Weight

Mass is often confused with **weight**, and it is important to distinguish between them. Whereas mass refers to the quantity of matter

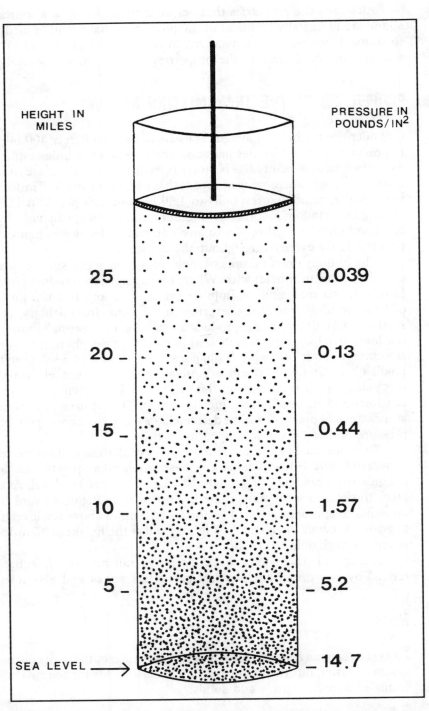

Figure 1–1. A cylindrical tube with a cross-sectional area of 1 in.² that reflects how pressure and density in an air medium vary with height above sea level.

present, weight refers to the *attractive gravitational force exerted on a mass by the earth.* For example, a person is said to weigh 160 lb because the earth attracts the person with a force of 160 lb. However, if the person is flown to the moon, the same amount of matter will be present, but because of the lessened gravitational pull, the weight will only amount to about 27 lb because the force of gravity is only about one-sixth as great on the moon as it is on earth. The weight of an object is directly proportional to its mass, but weight and mass are simply different concepts. Weight is a force, whereas mass is the quantity of matter present.

Although it might be hard to imagine, air has weight as well as mass. In fact, a cubic meter of air weighs about 1.3 kilograms (kg), and the air in a classroom with the dimensions of 9 × 12 × 4 m weighs about 560 kg. For those who are not yet comfortable with meters and kilograms, a cubic yard (yd) of air weighs 35.1 ounces (oz), and the air in a classroom with the dimensions of 30 × 40 × 12 feet (ft) weighs about 1,170 lb. From that we might conclude that professors who deliver long lectures in a classroom of that size are truly "throwing a lot of weight around."

Mass and Density

It is also useful to distinguish between mass and **density**. Look again at the cylindrical tube filled with air in Figure 1–1. Notice that the air molecules are shown to be crowded together very closely near the bottom of the tube, whereas they are rather far apart in the higher regions of the tube. This occurs because of the pull of gravity.

Because of the force of gravity, the molecules of the atmosphere accumulate near the surface of the earth. There exists, therefore, a downward force or pressure (the distinction between force and pressure will be made subsequently) and the molecules are compressed into a smaller volume. The volume near the bottom of the tube is more densely packed, and when a greater number of molecules is compressed into a volume of a certain size, the density is increased.

Density (ρ) is *the amount of mass per unit volume.* For example, if we could exert a force that would cause a volume of 1 cubic in. of air to contain 800 billion billion (8×10^{20}) molecules instead of 400 billion billion (4×10^{20}), the density — the mass per unit volume — will have doubled. It is easy to see in Figure 1–1 that the amount of mass per unit volume in the cylinder decreases with increasing height above sea level.

It might be difficult to imagine the different densities associated with the invisible molecules in volumes of air, but there are more visible examples that should serve to make the distinction between mass and density clear. Imagine a grocery bag with a volume 0.06 cubic meters [about 2 cubic ft ($2 \ ft^3$)] that is filled with 50 loosely crumpled sheets of newspaper. If you now pack the paper more tightly until the same amount of paper (50 sheets) occupies only half of the bag's volume [0.03 cubic meters ($0.03 \ m^3$); about 1 cubic ft ($1 \ ft^3$)], the same amount of matter is present — the **mass** — but the matter will be packed into a smaller volume. After compression, the amount of mass per cubic meter — the **density** — will have doubled.

With respect to the first property of a transmitting medium, it is useful to refer to both the **mass** of a medium and to the **density** of a medium, a quantity derived from mass. We shall subsequently explain more explicitly what is meant by "a quantity that is *derived* from another quantity."

Elasticity (E)

The second property of a transmitting medium is **elasticity**. All matter, whether it be gaseous, liquid, or solid, undergoes distortion of either shape or volume or both when a force is applied to it. Moreover, all matter is characterized by the tendency to "recover" from that distortion. The property that enables recovery from distortion to either shape or volume is called **elasticity**.

Imagine a weight attached to a spring that is suspended from the ceiling. When the spring is stretched and then released, it will return to its original unstretched position (and beyond, but that will be the subject of a later topic), unless it has been "overloaded." By "overloaded" we mean that the original stretching of the spring was sufficient to exceed what is called its **elastic limit**.

A portable radio has a spring that holds the battery in place. If you remove the spring, you can verify that it is relatively easy to stretch it so far that it will not "spring back" when released. Its elastic limit was exceeded. In some forms of matter, the elastic limit is very small. In other forms of matter, such as tempered steel, the elastic limit is very large. The elastic limit of air is so very large that it need not concern us.

With air, the concept of elasticity can mean *the tendency of a volume of air to return to its former volume after compression.* Return again to the air-filled cylinder in Figure 1-1. We know that air molecules are present, that they are in random motion, that — on the average — they are equidistant from one another, and that the density of the air is greater near the bottom of the tube.

Suppose we now insert a plunger into the top of the cylinder and push downward. All of the molecules that are present in the full length of the tube will now be crowded into a smaller space; the **density** is increased. When the plunger is removed, the air molecules return to their former "position," or more appropriately, the air volume resumes the density that existed before compression. The density of the air is said to be *restored,* and the restoring force is called **elasticity**.

■ PROPERTIES OF THE SOUND SOURCE

Let us turn now from a discussion of transmitting media to a consideration of bodies that can serve as a source of sound. We will be concerned with the same two properties that characterized the transmitting medium: **mass** (or density) and **elasticity**.

Vibratory Motion of a Tuning Fork

One object that can serve as a source of sound is a tuning fork, as shown in Figure 1–2. The tuning fork is a U-shaped metal bar. The prongs, or tines, of the fork have the property of **mass** (a quantity of matter is present) and they also possess the restoring force of **elasticity**. Because of their elasticity, the tines of the fork will return to their former position after they have been displaced. This can be best illustrated by striking the fork gently with a soft hammer. The tines will be set into **vibration**, which takes the form of each tine moving back and forth — the two tines will always move in opposite directions.[1]

Displacement From Equilibrium

Imagine a microscopic view of the pattern of vibration of the two tines. The position of the fork before a force is applied is called its *equilibrium position,* and equilibrium for the fork is shown by the heavy solid lines labeled **X** in Figure 1–2. When the hammer strikes the fork, a force is applied that causes the tines to be displaced from equilibrium. The force causes both tines to move inward toward positions **Y**, which are shown with the thin solid lines.

The amplitude of displacement is proportional to the magnitude of force applied. In other words, the harder we strike the fork with the hammer, the greater the amplitude of displacement. The magnitude of force applied determines how far the tines are displaced. Upon reaching maximum points of displacement, the tines' motion is momentarily halted, and then, because of the restoring force of elasticity, the tines return toward equilibrium, **X**. Motion does not cease after the tines have returned to positions **X** by the restoring force of elasticity. The tines continue to move through equilibrium toward maximum displacement in the opposite direction, which is shown by the dashed lines labeled **Z**.

Newton's First Law of Motion: Inertia

The reason that the tines continue to move beyond equilibrium to a maximum outward displacement (**Z**) is explained by the first of Sir Isaac Newton's three laws of motion: *All bodies remain at rest or in a state of uniform motion unless another force acts in opposition.* In other words, no force is required to keep the tines (and stem) moving through and beyond the positions of equilibrium, but rather, a reaction force will be required to *stop* such a motion. The property that Newton's first law addressed is called **inertia**, and his first law can be stated

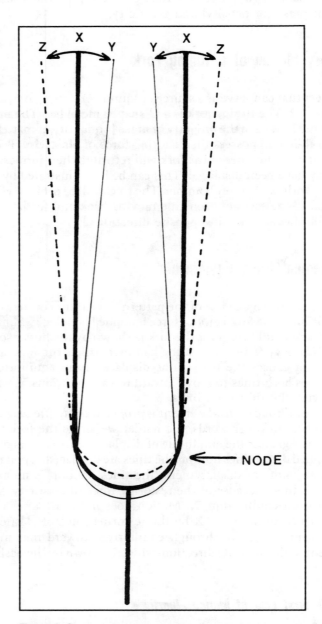

Figure 1–2. The vibratory pattern of a tuning fork, a U-shaped metal bar with the properties of **mass** and **elasticity**. Once struck, the tines move from **X** (equilibrium) to **Y** (maximum displacement in one direction), back to **X**, to **Z** (maximum displacement in the other direction), and back to **X** to complete one cycle of vibration.

differently as *the tendency of a body in motion to remain in motion, and the tendency of a body at rest to stay at rest.*

The amount of **inertia** that an object has is directly proportional to the **mass** of the object. In fact, we may think of mass, the quantity of matter present, as a *measure of inertia.* Thus, a massive object such as a steel ball with a circumference of 1 meter has considerable inertia in comparison with the more negligible mass and inertia of a ping-pong ball. Because of the large inertia of the steel ball, a large force is required to start it in motion, to stop its motion, or to change the direction of its motion. In contrast, a ping-pong ball can easily be set into motion, its motion can easily be stopped, and the direction of its motion can easily be changed.

Vibratory Motion

We have seen, then, that the fork was displaced (toward **Y**) by application of an external force, and that the magnitude of displacement was proportional to the force of application. Next, we saw that the restoring force of **elasticity** caused the tines to return toward equilibrium (**X**), and an **inertial** force caused the tines to move *through equilibrium* toward maximum displacements in the opposite direction (**Z**). The process continues as the restoring force of elasticity returns the tines back toward equilibrium (**X**), the force of inertia causes the tines to be displaced beyond equilibrium (**Y**), and so on.

Because of the interaction of the two opposing forces, **elasticity** and **inertia**, the tines of the fork continue to move to and fro, and the fork is said to have been set into **vibration**. It is convenient to refer to displacement in one direction as positive (+) and displacement in the opposite direction as negative (−); the designation of which direction is positive and which is negative is arbitrary.

Vibratory motion consists of back and forth movement of a body that has the properties of mass and elasticity, and because all bodies are characterized by some finite amount of mass and elasticity, all are capable of being set into vibratory motion. The back and forth motion occurs as the result of two opposing forces: **inertia** and **elasticity**.

Newton's Third Law of Motion: Reaction Forces

The fact that two forces are operating rather than one is consistent with Newton's third law of motion, which states: *with every force there must be associated an equal reaction force of opposite direction.* A hammer, on striking a nail, exerts a force on the nail. The nail exerts an equal, but opposite, force on the hammer to cause a rapid deceleration of its movement.

Another example of a reaction force can be observed by pushing your hand against the edge of a desk. You are exerting a force on the desk. You should notice, though, that the shape of your hand has been distorted, and that distortion occurs because of the reaction force exerted on your hand by the desk. The reaction force exerted on your hand occurs because the desk is elastic. All solid materials possess some degree of elasticity, and because of their elasticity they can exert forces on other objects.

Newton's third law tells us that a force cannot exist alone, which is why it is impossible to have a one-person tug of war. A more familiar, but distressing, analogy for those who live in regions of the frozen tundra is to consider why a car gets stuck in the snow. Because of the slippery snow, we cannot develop sufficient frictional force to "push the car out." It is stuck, and even a powerful engine might not alter that unhappy state. Instead, we must develop sufficient traction by spreading a substance, such as sand, or by digging down to the earth to allow the "push of the ground" to allow the car to move.

In terms of the tuning fork, after the original force was applied that caused the tines to be displaced, the tines moved in one direction due to the force of inertia, and the movement continued in that direction until the inertial force was overcome by the elastic restoring force. In other words, *elasticity serves as the "reaction force" to inertia.*

An important feature of the vibratory motion of the tuning fork (and of other sources of sound) is that we do not need constant reapplication of the external force that produced the initial displacement from equilibrium. The opposing forces of inertia and elasticity sustain the movement of the fork much as one push of a child's swing in the park is sufficient to keep the child swinging for quite a while. The movement of the tines from equilibrium to maximum displacement in one direction, back to equilibrium, to maximum displacement in the opposite direction, and finally back to equilibrium is called one **cycle** of vibration. Many such cycles of vibration will occur before the vibratory motion is finally stopped, and then we must strike it again to achieve additional vibration.

■ SOUND SOURCE ACTING ON A MEDIUM

We have seen that **mass** and **elasticity** are the two critical properties of both the source of sound and of the medium that transmits sound. Next, let us place the tuning fork in a medium such as air, apply an external force to cause the tines to be displaced, and see how the moving tines affect the surrounding air medium.

Those effects are illustrated in Figure 1–3. The rows, from top to bottom, represent discrete positions of the tines of the tuning fork and of individual air molecules at various moments in time during vibratory movement: equilibrium, maximum displacement (+), equilibrium, maximum displacement in the opposite direction (−), equilibrium, and so on. Each column, from left to right, shows the position of a single air molecule.

Movement of Air Particles

In the top row the molecules are shown to be equidistant from one another before they are energized by the moving tines. Imagine, then,

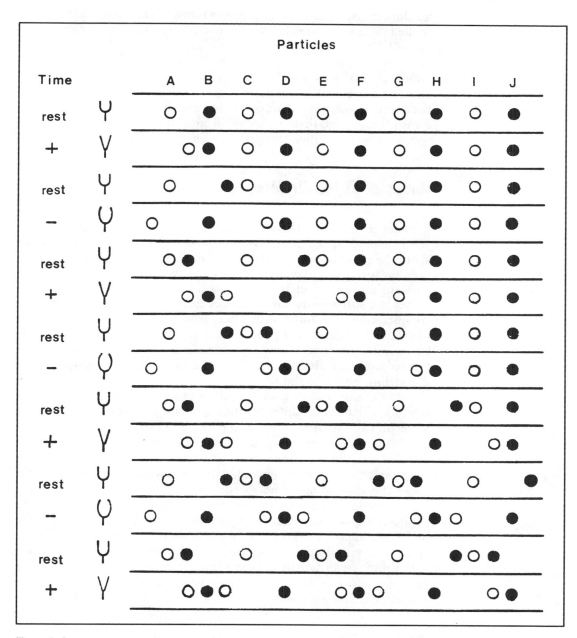

Figure 1–3. Displacement of individual air particles due to the vibratory motion of a tuning fork. Each particle moves back and forth over an infinitesimally small distance about its average position.

that the tuning fork has been vibrating to and fro for some time and that, with considerable license, it is possible for us to visualize the effects of the moving tines on air molecules, one by one, over time.

The vibratory motion of the fork exerts a force on molecule **A**. In Row 2, we see that molecule **A** is displaced from equilibrium to some maximum displacement that is proportional to the magnitude of force applied. The molecule also has been set into vibratory motion and it moves back and forth (from row to row) about its position of equilibrium — because of the opposing forces of inertia and elasticity — in the same way that was described for tuning fork tines.

The movement of molecule **A**, in turn, exerts a force on molecule **B**, causing it to begin vibratory motion, and this application of forces is spread from molecule to molecule (from column to column) much as you see when you flick the first of a long row of standing dominoes.

Movement of the Air Mass

Remember that in air there are approximately 400 billion billion (4×10^{20}) molecules per cubic in., and it therefore makes more sense to talk about the effect of tine movement on the surrounding **air mass** rather than on just a single molecule. This is illustrated in Figure 1–4. The outward movement of the tines toward a positive (+) displacement causes the surrounding air molecules to be crowded, or condensed, or compressed as the force of displacement is passed from molecule to molecule. In other words, there is an increase in **density** of the air because the force of the moving tines causes the molecules to be compressed into a smaller volume. This is called the **compression**, or **condensation**, phase of sound.

As the tines return toward equilibrium because of the elasticity of the fork, the force on the surrounding medium is relieved, and the air molecules also return toward their position of equilibrium. This results in a thinning of the molecules in the sense that they are now less crowded and the medium is therefore characterized by less density. This thinning, or decreased density, is called the **rarefaction** phase of sound because the volume of air has been "rarefied."

As we look at the air mass at points farther and farther from the tuning fork, we see that there are alternate regions in which the molecules are crowded together with an increase in density of the air space (**compression**) and regions in which the molecules are thinned with a decrease in density of the air space (**rarefaction**). These alternate regions of compression and rarefaction are caused by the effects of the moving tines being passed from region to region of the air.

Displacement of the Air Medium and Wave Motion

It is important to emphasize that the *medium is not displaced over any appreciable distance during this process.* An individual molecule is displaced only over a very small distance. What is moving through the air space is referred to as a "wave of disturbance." Alternate regions of increased and decreased density move through the air medium. If we could take a microscopic look at just one region of the air to see how its

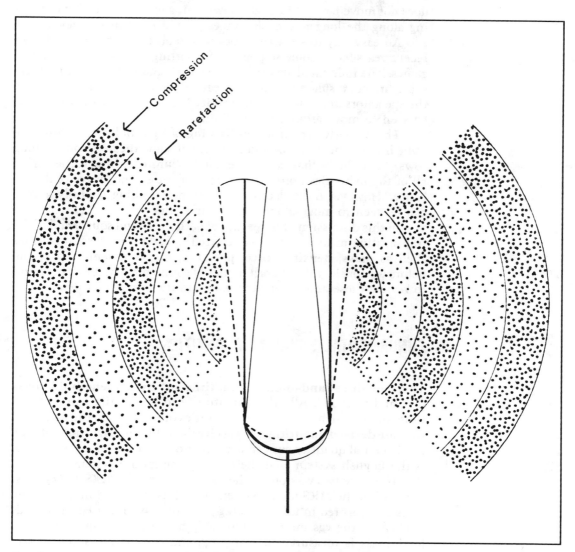

Figure 1–4. Alternate regions of **compression (condensation)** and **rarefaction** move outward through an air mass because of the vibratory motion of a tuning fork.

density changes over time, we would see that its volume is characterized by alternately increased and decreased density. The increased density of one region, in turn, is followed by an increased density of the next region, and so on. Thus, a region characterized by compression in Figure 1–4 at one moment in time will be characterized by rarefaction a brief moment later in time.

In a very elastic medium, such as air, sound is characterized by the *propagation of density changes*. Although changes in density are propagated through the medium, the individual molecules are not permanently displaced. Think again of the domino analogy. A single domino does not move far — it just falls down. But a wave of disturbance moving along the long row of dominoes should be clearly visible.

An easy way to see wave motion is to observe "the wave" that in recent years has become so popular at sporting events such as football games. The individual spectators move back and forth and, if properly sober, are not displaced from their seats. However, if the movements of the spectators are properly synchronized, a "wave of disturbance" can be seen to move around the stadium.

The properly synchronized flashing of light bulbs can create the same image. The entrance and marquee of some theaters contain long rows of light bulbs that can be alternately illuminated and turned off. If all of the lights flash on and off together, we see no "wave of disturbance." However, if the electrician times their flashing carefully, a wave can be seen to move along the row of lights.

In this discussion of properties of both the sound source and of the transmitting medium, we have referred to certain physical quantities such as **mass, density, force, pressure, displacement,** and so on. Before we consider the characteristics of sound further, it will be useful to review these and other physical quantities in greater detail.

■ FUNDAMENTAL PHYSICAL QUANTITIES

There are three **fundamental quantities** in physics: **length (L), mass (M),** and **time (T).** All other quantities can be described in terms of those three, which is to say that quantities other than length, mass, and time are **derived quantities.** To specify the value, or magnitude, of each fundamental quantity, we can use either of two units of measure. One is the English system, and the other is the metric system.

There are two versions of the metric system: the **MKS** and **cgs** systems. With the **MKS** metric system, length is measured in meters (m), mass is measured in kilograms (kg), and time is measured in seconds (sec). With the **cgs** metric system, length is measured in centimeters (cm), mass is measured in grams (g), and time is measured in seconds (sec).

The English system, sometimes called the **fps** system, is more cumbersome. With this system, length is measured in feet (f), mass is measured in pounds (p) — although the pound is actually a measure of gravitational force rather than mass — and time is still measured in seconds (sec).

We will describe the three fundamental quantities and their derivatives primarily by reference to the metric system. The **MKS** metric system has become the system of choice in physics. However, the **cgs** system appears in much of the literature that has been written over the decades and we must, therefore, be familiar with both systems and be able to move back and forth between them. Both metric systems will be used throughout this text, but the emphasis will be on the **MKS** system. Only on rare occasions will we persist with reference to the **fps** system.

Length

Length is simply a measure of distance, which is *the extent of spatial separation between any two points*. To determine the magnitude of distance, we select a unit of measure such as the meter (the **MKS** system), and through the process of measurement, we determine how many times this unit (the meter) is contained in a given distance. To measure the length of a board, we select a meterstick (or a yardstick in the **fps** system) and determine how many times the meterstick can be contained over the length of the board.

For many years the meter was defined arbitrarily. In the late 1700s, for example, the meter was defined as 1/10,000,000 of the distance from the equator to the north pole along the surface of the earth. But confirming that distance proved to be virtually impossible as well as hazardous. New definitions emerged in 1889 and again in 1960. Finally, in 1983 the 46-member General Conference on Weights and Measures met in Paris and agreed to define the meter relative to another of the three fundamental physical quantities — **time**. The speed of light is 299,792,458 meters per second (m/sec), and one meter is now defined as the distance traveled by light in a vacuum during 1/299,792,458 of a second.

When we compare the old definition with the new one by showing the relation between meters and inches, it might seem that the change in definition is trivial; 1 m used to equal *about* 39.37 in., but as of 1983, 1 m equals *exactly* 39.37007874 in.; all additional decimal values beyond the 8th decimal equal zero. This seemingly small difference actually is fairly important, at least to the physicist. Previously, 1 in. equaled *approximately* 2.54 cm, but now 1 in. corresponds to *exactly* 2.54 cm and 1 ft now equals exactly 0.3048 m. More importantly, the new definition accomplishes a goal that physicists had sought for a long time; the physical quantity **time**, which is the most accurately measured of the three fundamental quantities, is now used to define another physical quantity, **length**.

The metric system, either **MKS** or **cgs**, is very convenient for describing multiples or submultiples of the standard unit of length. All are expressed as multiples of 10 (.001, .01, .1, 1, 10, 100, 1,000, and so on). A centimeter (cm) is 1 one-hundredth (.01) of a meter (m), a millimeter (mm) is 1 one-thousandth (.001) of a meter and one-tenth (0.1) of a centimeter, and a kilometer (km) corresponds to 1,000 m. That is why the metric system is less cumbersome than the English system where you must divide by 12 to convert inches to feet; by 3 to convert feet to yards; by 5,280 to convert feet to miles; by 1,760 to convert yards to miles; and so on. Only the submultiples of the inch (¼, ⅛, ¹⁄₁₆, ¹⁄₃₂, ¹⁄₆₄, and so on) possess reasonable regularity.

Mass

Mass, as we discussed previously, is a property of all matter and can be defined as the quantity of matter present. When we use the word "quantity," we mean simply that there is an observable property that can be measured or in some way specified numerically. Recall, also, that it is important to distinguish between **mass** and **weight**. The unit of measure of mass is the kilogram in the **MKS** system and the gram in the **cgs** system. A kilogram is defined as the mass of a cylinder of platinum housed at the International Bureau of Weights and Measures, and a gram is 1/1,000 of a kilogram.

The concept of **mass** is tied inextricably to the concept of **inertia** and the word, mass, is sometimes used to refer to how much inertia a body has. The greater the mass of an object, the greater its inertia.

Time

Time might be the physical quantity that is most easily and accurately measured, but it is also a quantity that is difficult to define in a way that has any intuitive appeal. Daniloff, Schuckers, and Feth (1980), for example, said:

> It is difficult to define *time* without saying that it is that quantity we measure in seconds, minutes, or hours. Any physical event that recurs on a regular basis can be used to mark off equal intervals of time. Thus, the period required for one complete revolution of the earth is identified as one day. (p. 75)

Because a solar day is divided into 24 hours (hr), an hour into 60 min, and a minute into 60 sec, each day has 86,400 sec. That led to the concept that the second is 1/86,400 of a solar day.

■ DERIVED PHYSICAL QUANTITIES

By a **derived quantity** we simply mean a quantity that is expressed as either a quotient, or a product, of the fundamental quantities. For example, length is a fundamental physical quantity. On the other hand, the *area* of a rectangle is given by the product of two measures of length (usually referred to as the "length" times the "width"), and area, therefore, is a derived physical quantity. Derived quantities of interest in the study of sound include **displacement (x)**, **velocity (c)**, **acceleration (a)**, **force (F)**, and **pressure (P)**.

Displacement (x)

Displacement (x) is defined as *a change in position,* and it is specified by calculating the distance from a reference, or starting position, to a new, or ending position. It is important to note that displacement actually involves two concepts: **distance** and **direction**. A body moves over a certain **distance**, and, for a given distance, the body moves in one of any number of **directions**. Thus, *to specify displacement we must account for both the direction moved and the distance moved.*

Quantities that are specified by both *magnitude and direction* are called **vector quantities**, or just **vectors**. Consider the examples shown in Figure 1–5. Starting points are shown by an **x** and ending points by an **o**. The length of the line represents the magnitude of distance moved, and the direction the arrow points represents the direction moved. Thus, **A** and **B** have different displacements, because the movement has occurred in different directions, even though both are shown to have moved the same distance. Correspondingly, **A** and **C** have different displacements because they have occurred over different distances even though the movements occurred in the same direction. Finally, **B** and **C** have different displacements because their movements are characterized both by different directions and different distances.

Quantities such as mass, time, energy, and so forth are specified only by reference to magnitude; they have no direction associated with them. They are called **scalar quantities**, or just **scalars**. The distinction between scalars and vectors is particularly important when we wish to add or subtract the values of some particular quantity. When the quantities are scalars, simple algebraic addition or subtraction is sufficient. **Time** is a scalar. If the time required to travel from point **a** to point **b** is 1 sec, and the time required to travel from point **b** to point **c** is 1.5 sec, then algebraic addition tells us that the time required to travel from **a** to **c** must be 2.5 sec. However, when the quantities are vectors, we must use methods of vector analysis rather than algebraic addition or subtraction.

Velocity (c)

Velocity (c), from the Latin word "celeritas," refers *to the amount of displacement per unit time.* Velocity also is a vector quantity because

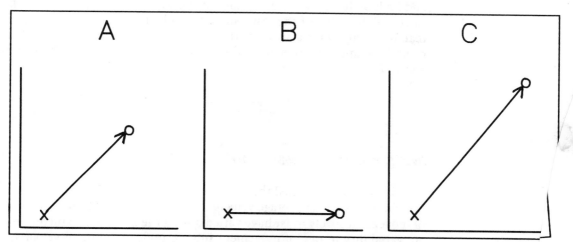

Figure 1–5. Explanation of vector quantities in which the length of each line represents the **magnitude of displacement** (distance moved) and the direction of the arrow represents the **direction of displacement**.

specification of displacement per unit time must incorporate a specification of both the distance moved and the direction moved. Thus, displacement is accomplished during some period of time. If we divide displacement by the time required to complete the displacement, we obtain what is called the **average velocity** of the body that was displaced.

If a motorcycle travels in a northwesterly direction for a distance of 180 kilometers (km), or 112 mi, in 2 hr, the average velocity of travel is 90 KPH (56 MPH). We are accustomed to think of **speed** rather than velocity in such cases, but the two are not always equal. Speed corresponds to velocity *when direction is not considered;* speed has only magnitude, whereas velocity has both magnitude and direction.

It is easy to see the difference between speed and velocity if you imagine the task of paddling a canoe across a lake. As you cross over the lake, suppose there is virtually no wind and the surface of the water is glassy. You simply aim toward your desired destination and paddle. By the time you are ready to return, suppose a strong wind has come up that is blowing at right angles to your intended path. Now it will be necessary to compensate for the wind by aiming your canoe in a direction different from where you want to end up.

Figure 1–6 illustrates the difference between the speed and velocity of the canoe during the windy condition. Let x be the starting point. The length of the line S_1 shows the speed with which the canoe is moving in one direction, and the length of the line S_2 shows the speed with which the canoe is moving at right angles to the first direction because of the wind. Each of those speeds is given by the simple formula:

Equation 1.1
$$s = \frac{d}{t,}$$

where s = average speed, d = distance, and t = time.

The dashed line c represents what is called the **resultant velocity**, and its length is greater than either of the two speeds alone. We could calculate the value of the resultant velocity by the use of the Pythagorean theorem, which states that the square of the hypotenuse in a right triangle is equal to the sum of the squares of the two sides of the triangle. Thus,

Equation 1.2
$$c_{resultant} = \sqrt{S_1^2 + S_2^2}.$$

Average and Instantaneous Velocity

We previously mentioned the concept of **average velocity**. The motorcycle moved with an average velocity of 90 KPH (56 MPH), but the rate of movement surely must have varied during the 2-hr trip. To incorporate variability in rate of movement into an understanding of velocity, we distinguish between average velocity and **instantaneous velocity**. Instantaneous velocity is the velocity that is measured over an infini-

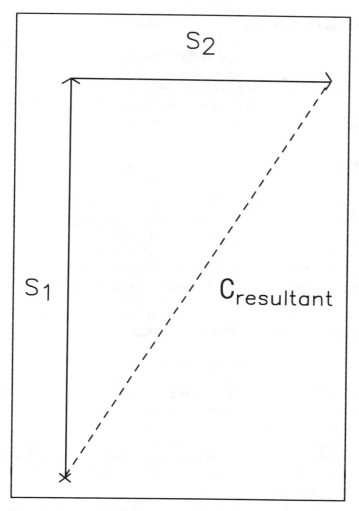

Figure 1-6. Velocity (c), the amount of displacement per unit time, is shown as a vector quantity in relation to the speed of movement (S_1 and S_2) in two directions at right angles to each other.

tesimally small time interval, an interval perhaps as small as a millionth or billionth of a second.

The distinction between **average velocity** and **instantaneous velocity** applies also to **speed**. For example, if a car is driven 80 km (approximately 50 mi) in 1 hr, its **average speed** is 80 KPH. However, during the period of travel, the **instantaneous speed**, the speed measured for such a small interval of time that the speed can be considered to be a constant during the interval, might vary over a considerable range.

Summary of Velocity

Velocity (either average or instantaneous), then, is displacement per unit time and it can be expressed in a myriad of ways: meters per second (**MKS** system), centimeters per second (**cgs** system), miles per hour, feet per day, or whatever (**fps** system). We simply calculate the ratio of the measure of displacement to the measure of time.

Acceleration (a)

Velocity was defined as the amount of displacement per unit time. That is the same as saying that velocity is the *time-rate of displacement*. Just as velocity is the time-rate of displacement, **acceleration (a)** is the *time-rate change in velocity*. Acceleration also is a vector quantity, because a change of velocity in one direction is not the same as a change of velocity in another direction. The magnitude might change, the direction might change, or both might change.

Although it might at first seem strange, an automobile traveling at a constant **speed** around a circular path is undergoing acceleration. If we think about it for a moment, though, it makes sense. The speed might not vary, but the *direction* of motion is constantly changing. If the direction is changing, the velocity must also be changing because the concept of velocity incorporates both speed and direction. Finally, then, if the velocity changes, acceleration must have occurred, because acceleration is the time-rate change in velocity.

If velocity increases, acceleration is said to be "positive," and if velocity decreases, acceleration is said to be "negative." Negative acceleration, of course, is commonly called *deceleration*. Acceleration (**a**) is given by:

Equation 1.3
$$a = \frac{\Delta c}{t,}$$

where $\Delta c = c_2 - c_1$.

If a car travels at a velocity of 10 m per sec (c_1) and then is accelerated to a velocity of 30 m per sec (c_2), and if that change is accomplished in 5 sec, acceleration equals 4 m per sec per sec, which usually is written as 4 m/sec²:

$$a = \frac{(30 - 10)}{5} = 4 \text{ m/sec/sec} = 4 \text{ m/sec}^2.$$

Force (F)

Force (F), which in simple terms is a *push* or a *pull*, is defined as *the product of* **mass (m)** and **acceleration (a)**:

Equation 1.4
$$F = ma.$$

Equation 1.4 is Newton's second law of motion, although his law originally was stated as: *The acceleration of an object is directly proportional to the net force applied to the object and inversely proportional to the object's mass.* Thus, Newton's second law expressed symbolically was $a = F/m$. When both sides of Newton's original equation are multiplied by the mass (m), we obtain Equation 1.4, which is the more familiar form of Newton's second law.

An equally correct way to state Newton's second law of motion is that *the net force applied is equal to the mass of an object multiplied by its acceleration.* A force is required to accelerate an object because the object has **mass**, and the object therefore has **inertia**. The inertia of the object serves to oppose a change in motion, and therefore a **force** must be applied to overcome the **inertia**.

Consequences of Applying a Force

Force can produce two consequences that are particularly important with respect to gaining an understanding of both sound sources and sound transmission. First, a force can cause matter to be *distorted*. If a wire spring is stretched by a pulling force or compressed by a pushing force, the spring is distorted. When the force that produced the distortion is removed, the spring will return to its original condition because of elasticity unless, of course, the force that caused the distortion was sufficiently large that the "elastic limit" of the spring was exceeded. Second, a force also can cause matter to be *accelerated*. Therefore, we can define **force** not only as a *push* or a *pull*, but also as *that which imparts acceleration to a mass.*

Force as a Vector Quantity

Force, like velocity, also is a vector quantity, and in order to define it completely we must specify not only the *magnitude* of force but also the *direction* of force. In other words, it *does* matter whether the force is acting to the left or the right or upward or downward in space. Almost without exception, a force of some magnitude pushing from a southerly direction on some body produces absolutely no effect in an easterly direction.

Because force is a vector quantity, we must be careful when we speak of the "addition of forces." If we have two forces of exactly the same magnitude acting on the same body, the resultant force will not necessarily have twice the magnitude of one of the forces alone. The resultant force could, in fact, be zero if the equal forces acted from exactly opposite directions, and in that case the body is said to be in equilibrium. If two people simultaneously apply equal forces to a swinging door, but from opposite directions, the door will not move.

With respect to hearing, you might have reasoned that there is a pressure (the distinction between pressure and force will be made in a moment) of 100,000 Nt/m^2 (1,000,000 dynes/cm^2) impinging on your ear drums. Fortunately, your ear drums will not "cave in" under this pressure because there is an equal air pressure in your middle ear cavity that produces a force from the opposite direction. That works well, of course, until something happens to reduce the pressure on the outside of the drum such as when you are in an airplane that climbs to 40,000 ft or so. When you feel the pain that results from the differential pressure on the two sides of the ear drum, you might elect to yawn or chew gum. That opens a tube that leads from the back of your mouth to the middle ear cavity and restores the pressure to the same value that exists outside the drum.

It is important to remember that a resultant force is not simply the algebraic sum of the two forces. Force is a vector quantity, and vector summation is required to calculate the resultant force. If the two forces operate at right angles to one another, the resultant force could be solved by use of the Pythagorean theorem in the same way that it was used for determining the resultant velocity in Figure 1–6.

Units of Measure for Force

With the **MKS** system, the unit of measure of force is called the **newton (Nt)** in honor of Sir Isaac Newton who first defined force in his second law of motion (Equation 1.4). One **newton** is defined as *the force required to accelerate a mass of 1 kg from a velocity of 0 m per sec to a velocity of 1 m per sec in 1 sec of time.* In other words, when the mass of 1 kg is stationary, it has a velocity of 0 m/sec. If you wish to accelerate that mass so that it will move with a velocity of 1 m/sec, and if you wish to accomplish that change in velocity in 1 sec, a force must be applied, and the value of that force is defined as 1 Nt.

With the **cgs** system, the unit of measure of force is the **dyne**. The definition of force in the **cgs** system is equivalent to that described above for the **MKS** system, but the units are changed from kilograms to grams and from meters to centimeters. Thus, one **dyne** is defined as *the force required to accelerate a mass of 1 gram (g) from a velocity of 0 cm per sec to a velocity of 1 cm per sec in 1 sec of time.* One newton (**MKS**) corresponds to 100,000 dynes (**cgs**).

Pressure

In the study of sound we will not be particularly concerned with measuring, for example, the force exerted by one molecule on another. However, we will want to determine the sum of many such small forces that act upon some surface — the ear drum — for example. To do this we will concern ourselves with the *amount of force per unit area*, which is called the **pressure (P)**, as shown in Equation 1.5:

Equation 1.5
$$P = \frac{F}{A,}$$

where **F** = the force applied and **A** = area.

Suppose we have a force of 1 Nt acting uniformly upon a surface that is 10 m² (100 square meters) such as is shown in Figure 1–7. We

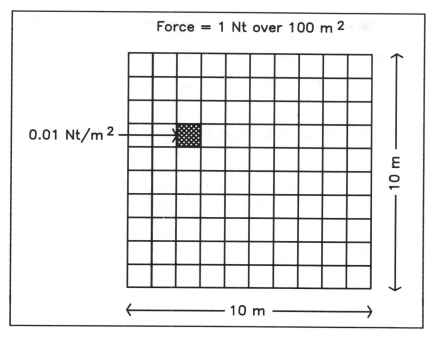

Figure 1–7. A **force** of 1 newton (Nt) distributed uniformly over an area of 100 m² produces a **pressure**, the amount of force per unit area, of 0.01 Nt/m².

could calculate with Equation 1.5 that the pressure, the amount of force per unit area, is 0.01 Nt/m².

Units of Measure for Pressure

Because force is measured in **newtons (MKS)** or **dynes (cgs)**, and because pressure is the amount of force per unit area, the unit of measure of pressure is the **newton per square meter (Nt/m²)** in the **MKS** system and the **dyne per square centimeter (dyne/cm²)** in the **cgs** system. A pressure of 1 Nt/m² in the **MKS** system corresponds to how many dynes/cm² in the **cgs** system?

$$1 \text{ Nt} = 100{,}000 \text{ dynes}$$

and

$$1 \text{ m} = 100 \text{ cm.}$$

Therefore, $1 \text{ Nt/m}^2 = 100{,}000 \text{ dynes/m}^2$

$$= 100{,}000 \text{ dynes/10{,}000 cm}^2.$$

And, $1 \text{ Nt/m}^2 = 10 \text{ dynes/cm}^2.$ **Equation 1.6**

An alternative to the newton per square meter with the **MKS** system is a unit called the **pascal (Pa)**. The relations among these various units of measure for pressure are shown below:

Equation 1.7

$$1 \text{ Pa} = 1 \text{ Nt/m}^2 = 10 \text{ dynes/cm}^2.$$

■ VIBRATORY MOTION OF A SPRING–MASS SYSTEM

Now that the fundamental and derived physical quantities have been defined, we can examine the nature of vibratory motion in a different, but more complete, way through reference to the spring–mass system shown in Figure 1–8. One end of a spring is attached to a rigid structure such as a wall, and the other end is attached to a mass that lies on a nearly frictionless surface. An arrow points toward what we will call a "displacement scale." In panel A of the figure, the arrow points to "0" (equilibrium) on the scale; the mass is at equilibrium because the net force acting on the spring–mass system is zero. Hence, there is no motion.

Characteristics of a Spring

A spring is a highly elastic object. Because of its elasticity, the spring can be displaced from equilibrium either by moving the mass to the left, which *compresses* the spring, or by moving the mass to the right, which *extends, or stretches,* the spring. When the spring is compressed, as is shown in panel B of Figure 1–8, the mass is displaced from equilibrium and the arrow in panel B points toward "−" on the displacement scale. When the spring is stretched, the mass is displaced from equilibrium in the opposite direction, and the arrow in panel C points toward "+" on the displacement scale.

Regardless of whether the spring is compressed or extended, the restoring force of elasticity will *oppose* the force that acts to deform the spring. Thus, the more the spring is compressed, the greater will be the force required to accomplish additional compression because of the restoring force of elasticity. Stated differently, the magnitude of the restoring force (**F**) of elasticity is directly proportional to the magnitude of the spring's displacement (**x**), which is called Hooke's law in honor of Robert Hooke who published his observation in the late 1600s. Hooke's law is expressed as:

Equation 1.8

$$F = -kx,$$

where **F** is the restoring force of elasticity,

x is the magnitude of displacement of the spring, and

k is a spring constant.

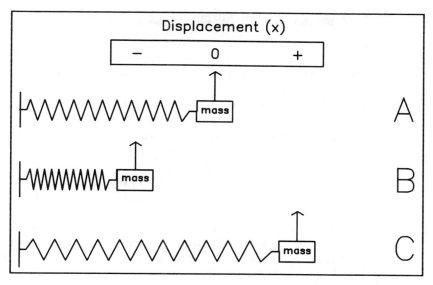

Figure 1-8. A spring–mass system with one end of the spring attached to a rigid structure. In panel A, the spring is in equilibrium, which corresponds to "0" on the displacement scale. In panel B, the spring is compressed, and the mass has moved to "−" on the displacement scale. In panel C, the spring is stretched (extended), and the mass has moved to "+" on the displacement scale.

The minus sign in Equation 1.8 serves to remind us that the direction of the restoring force is opposite the direction of the displacement.

Stiffness

Although all springs are elastic, some springs will require a greater force than others to be either compressed or extended because of differences among springs in what is called **stiffness**. **Stiffness** is the spring constant (**k**) in Equation 1.8. In other words, the stiffer the spring, the greater the value of **k**, and the greater the force that will be required to compress or stretch the spring some given distance.

Compliance

The elasticity of a spring also can be quantified by a measure of a spring's **compliance**. **Compliance** is inversely related to stiffness, which means that springs that have relatively little stiffness are characterized by a relatively large compliance. As compliance increases, the force required to compress or stretch the spring decreases. Hence, compliant springs can be displaced from equilibrium more easily than stiff springs.

Vibratory Motion of the Spring–Mass System

If the mass in Figure 1–8 is moved to the right and then released, *the system will be set into vibration*. Its motion will be similar in most respects to that of the tuning fork that was illustrated in Figure 1–2. The arrow will pass through equilibrium toward a maximum displacement to the left ("−" on the displacement scale) as the spring becomes progressively more compressed. When the restoring force of elasticity overcomes the inertial force, the direction of motion of the system will be reversed. The system then will return once again to equilibrium and beyond toward a maximum displacement to the right ("+" on the displacement scale) as the spring becomes progressively more stretched, and so on.

We shall see in Chapter 2 that the spring–mass system, the tuning fork, and any vibrating system for which the magnitude of the restoring force is directly proportional to the displacement ($\mathbf{F} \propto \mathbf{x}$) is engaged in what is called **simple harmonic motion**, or **sinusoidal motion**.

■ THE PENDULUM: AN EXAMPLE OF SLOW-MOTION VIBRATION

We are now in a position to incorporate an understanding of both the fundamental and derived quantities in physics to the study of sound. We previously discussed the vibratory motion of the tuning fork and the vibratory motion of air molecules that was occasioned by the motion of the fork. Because the movement of the fork is too rapid to see — and, of course, we certainly cannot see the air molecules, let alone discern how rapidly they are moving — the concept of vibratory motion might be difficult to grasp. However, we can achieve a more intuitive understanding of vibratory motion by examining the characteristics of a slow-moving vibratory system such as the pendulum shown in Figure 1–9.

The pendulum is shown to be in equilibrium when the bob is at point **X**. Next, let us displace the pendulum to point **Y** and then release it. The pendulum, of course, will return to equilibrium **X**. It does not stop when it reaches equilibrium, but rather it continues on toward a maximal displacement in the other direction **Z**. Upon reaching maximal displacement, it will again return toward and beyond the position of equilibrium **X**, and so on. In other words, the motion of the pendulum appears to be very similar to what we saw previously for the tuning fork. In fact, both are characterized by *vibratory motion*.

In essence, the same kinds of opposing forces that governed the motion of the tuning fork are responsible for the motion of the pendulum, with one important exception. When the pendulum or tuning fork tines are maximally displaced in either direction, they return toward equilibrium because of a **restoring force**. With the tuning fork in Figure 1–2 and the spring–mass system in Figure 1–8, the restoring

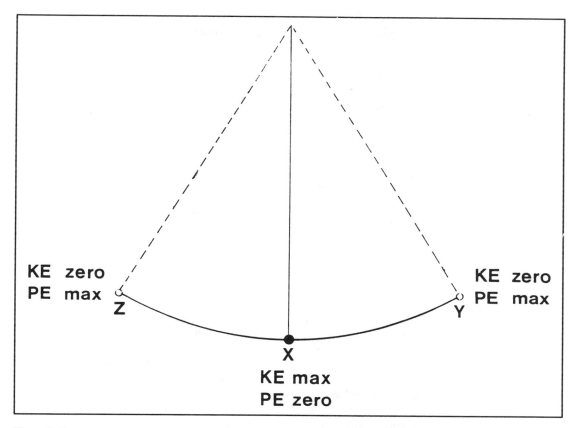

Figure 1–9. Vibratory motion of a pendulum moving from maximum displacement in one direction (where **potential energy** is maximal and **kinetic energy** is zero), through equilibrium (where kinetic energy is maximal and potential energy is zero), to maximum displacement in the opposite direction, and back to equilibrium.

force is **elasticity**. With the pendulum, the restoring force is **gravity**. With this exception in mind, we see that the pendulum is restored to equilibrium from maximal displacement because of the restoring force of gravity, and it moves beyond its position of equilibrium toward maximal displacement because of **inertia**.

Stated somewhat differently, the pendulum continues to move toward a maximal displacement until the restoring force of gravity overcomes the force of inertia. At the point of maximal displacement, the inertial value is zero and the force of gravity is maximal. As the pendulum moves back toward equilibrium, the restoring force of gravity diminishes and the force of inertia increases. When the pendulum reaches equilibrium, the net force of gravity on the motion is zero and the force of inertia is maximal, which results in the continuation of motion toward a new displacement.

When the concept of **force** as a derived physical quantity was introduced earlier, we stated that "almost without exception, a force pushing from a southerly direction on some body produces absolutely no effect in an easterly direction." The vibratory motion of the pendulum provides us with an exception. We will consider the downward-acting gravitational force to be in a "southerly" direction, and the path of excursion of the pendulum, therefore, to be in an "easterly/westerly" direction. In this circumstance, it is clear that the force of gravity in a southerly direction *does affect* the vibratory motion that takes place in an easterly/westerly direction.

Momentum

As we continue to think of the opposing forces that result in vibratory motion, it will be convenient to substitute the effect of **momentum** for the force of **inertia**. **Momentum (M)** is defined as *the product of mass (m) and velocity (c)*, as shown in Equation 1.9:

Equation 1.9 $$M = mc.$$

Thus, **momentum** is directly proportional to both the **mass** (the amount of matter present) and the **velocity** (the time-rate of displacement); as either mass or velocity increases, momentum increases. A large car traveling with the same velocity as a smaller car will have greater momentum because of its greater **mass**. Similarly, if two cars have identical mass, momentum will be greater for the car traveling with the greater **velocity**. With respect to the moving pendulum, we say simply that momentum is maximal and the net force acting on the pendulum is zero when the pendulum is at (passing through) the position of equilibrium. At maximal displacement, the force of momentum is zero and the force of gravity is maximal.

Why does the pendulum gain momentum as it moves toward equilibrium? In Equation 1.9, examine the two quantities that are known to determine momentum, and then recall the discussion of fundamental and derived physical quantities. Momentum of the pendulum does not change because of a change in **mass** — the quantity of matter present must remain the same. It follows, therefore, that the momentum must change because of a change in **velocity**. In other words, as the pendulum moves from maximum displacement toward equilibrium, momentum increases because the velocity of motion increases, and if the velocity increases, there must be **acceleration**.

The Energy Principle

The movement of the pendulum, as well as that of other matter set into vibratory motion, also can be described by what can be called the **energy principle**. According to the **law of conservation of energy**, any system that can do work (such as the pendulum, the tuning fork, the spring–mass system, or any other body that can be set into vibratory motion) must receive a supply of energy from somewhere.

What is energy? **Energy** is an abstract concept that refers to something that can produce a *change* in matter such as, for example, displacement of a mass, distortion of the shape of solid matter, expansion of gases, and so forth. When a change in matter occurs, **work** has been done, and **energy** is a *measure of the capacity to do work*. One way to distinguish between energy and work is to realize that **energy** is something that a body *possesses*, whereas **work** is something that a body *does*.

Work

Work is accomplished only when *a* **force** *succeeds in moving the body that the force acts upon,* and the quantity of work that is accomplished is given by *the product of the magnitude of force applied and the distance moved*:

$$W = Fd,$$

Equation 1.10

where **F** = the force applied and **d** = the distance moved.

If a force does not give rise to motion, no work has been done. The act of pushing against a cement wall with a force of 50 Nt accomplishes no work unless, miraculously, the wall is moved through some distance.

With the **MKS** system, force is expressed in newtons and distance is expressed in meters. The unit of measure of **work** in the **MKS** system is the **joule**. One joule of work is accomplished if a force of 1 Nt acts through a distance of 1 m (1 joule = 1 Nt × 1 m). In the **cgs** system, the unit of measure of **work** is the **erg** (1 erg = 1 dyne × 1 cm). To relate the two units of measure of **work**, 1 joule = 10,000,000 ergs.

Transformation of Energy

As we stated before, energy cannot be depleted, but rather it is transformed from one form to another, or it is transferred from one place to another. If you wind the spring on an old fashioned clock, the spring gains energy as it is wound. In turn, it loses energy as it does work on the clock. If you pull the trigger on a rifle, exploding gases do work on the bullet, which gives energy to the bullet. When the bullet strikes an object, it does work on the object and loses energy.

Let us now return to the pendulum shown in Figure 1–9 and discuss energy a little further. When the pendulum is raised from equilibrium to maximum displacement, the pendulum is said to have **potential energy (PE)**, which is a form of *stored energy*. In the case of the pendulum, the potential energy can be thought of as an energy of position, and it sometimes is referred to as **gravitational potential energy**; it has potential energy because of the gravitational attraction of the earth.

The potential energy associated with the pendulum in its raised position is transferred, or converted, into an energy of motion when released, which is called **kinetic energy** (**KE**). When the pendulum reaches the equilibrium position, potential energy is zero and kinetic energy is maximal. As the pendulum continues to move beyond equilibrium to a position of maximum displacement, kinetic energy is converted into potential energy, and at maximum displacement, kinetic energy will be zero and potential energy will be at a maximum.

At all points during the excursion, the sum of **PE** and **KE** *remains constant,* and that defines the **total energy** in accordance with the **law of conservation of energy**. According to that law, energy can be transformed from one kind to another, but energy is never created or destroyed — the total energy remains a constant.

Frictional Resistance

In the case of the pendulum, the tuning fork, and the spring–mass system discussed earlier, we have proceeded as if vibratory motion will continue indefinitely. Actually, that is not the case because of *opposition to motion by the force of **friction***. Because **friction** opposes, or resists, motion, it serves to limit the velocity of motion. As the pendulum swings along its path, friction at the point of suspension and friction on the bob of the pendulum because of air resistance, causes energy to be transformed from **kinetic energy** to **thermal energy** (heat). As a consequence of the opposing force of friction, the amplitude of each excursion of the pendulum will be less than the amplitude of the previous excursion.

In Chapter 2 we will refer to this circumstances as **damping** or as **damped vibration**. The resistance to motion attributable to friction, which sometimes is called **frictional resistance**, or just **resistance**, is analogous to electrical resistance, which serves to oppose or impede the flow of electrical current in any electrical circuit. We will return to the concept of **transfer of energy** shortly when we discuss sound wave propagation.

Characteristics of Pendular Motion

There are two important characteristics of the vibratory motion of the pendulum, **amplitude** and **frequency**.

Amplitude

The first characteristic is **amplitude** of displacement. Amplitude of displacement, a derived physical quantity, is a *vector quantity that specifies distance displaced and direction of displacement.* The amplitude of displacement of the pendulum is proportional to the force applied to it.

Frequency

The second characteristic is called the **frequency** of vibratory motion. We noted earlier that when the tines of a tuning fork move from equilibrium to maximum displacement (+), back through equilibrium (0), to maximum displacement in the opposite direction (−), and finally back to equilibrium (0), we have completed what is called one **cycle** of vibration. The same is true with the pendulum. Movement from **X** to **Y** to **X** to **Z** and back to **X** in Figure 1–9 defines one cycle of pendular vibration. **Frequency (f)** refers to *the rate at which the vibratory motion occurs, that is, the number of cycles completed per second* (**cps**). Thus, if the pendulum completes four cycles each second, the frequency is described as 4 cps. If the rate of motion were increased so that 25 cycles are completed each second, f = 25 cps.

The unit of measure for frequency has been changed from **cycles per second** (**cps**) to **hertz** (**Hz**) to honor a German physicist. The conversion between **cps** and **Hz** is simple: 1 **Hz** = 1 **cps**. Thus, for the two examples just mentioned, f = 4 cps and 4 Hz and f = 25 cps and 25 Hz.

Frequency is the number of *cycles per second.* We also can calculate the number of *seconds per cycle*, that is, *the amount of time required to complete just one cycle*. That is called the **period (T)**. Thus, if the pendulum completes four cycles of vibration in 1 sec (f = 4 Hz), then one cycle must be completed in 1/4 sec. Similarly, if f = 25 Hz, one cycle must be completed in 1/25 sec. For those two examples, we say that the period (T) was 1/4 (.25) sec and 1/25 (.04) sec.

You might already have noticed that the conversion from frequency to period or from period to frequency is fairly simple:

$$T = \frac{1}{f}$$

Equation 1.11

and

$$f = \frac{1}{T}.$$

Equation 1.12

Thus, if f = 4, T = 1/4 (.25), and if T = .25, f = 1/.25 = 4. When we divide 1 by some number, we are *taking the reciprocal of that number.* Thus, we say that period is the reciprocal of frequency and that frequency is the reciprocal of period.

Frequency and **amplitude** are independent characteristics of pendular motion (the value of one does not depend on the value of the other), but **frequency** and **period** are not independent.[2] The value of one completely determines the value of the other.

Determinants of Frequency of Vibration for a Pendulum

What properties of the pendulum determine the **period** and **frequency** of vibration? It is tempting to think that you might increase the frequency (and thereby decrease the period) if a greater force were applied. Recall, however, that the magnitude of force applied determines the magnitude of displacement and, hence, the amplitude of vibration.

If you recall the child's swing, you should remember that no matter how hard you pushed, the swing moved at the same rate. It was displaced farther in response to a greater force, but it did not move at a greater frequency. However, the more experienced child learns that you can swing faster (with greater vibratory frequency) by looping the rope around the supporting stanchion a few times. When that is done, the swing (or pendulum) is shorter, and it turns out that the *length* of the pendulum is the principal determinant of the frequency of pendular vibration.

The equation for the period (T) of the pendulum is:

Equation 1.13
$$T = 2\pi \sqrt{\frac{L}{G,}}$$

where **L** = length and **G** = gravitational force.

From Equation 1.13 we can see that the period of vibration is *directly proportional to the square root of the length,* which means that as length increases, period increases, and as length decreases, period decreases. But, because we know that frequency and period are inversely related, we should conclude that frequency is *inversely* related to the square root of the length. That, of course, is what we learned from the child who shortened the length of the rope in order to "swing" more rapidly.

The dependence of frequency of vibration of a pendulum on length was first discovered by Galileo who observed the swing of lamps hanging in the cathedral at Pisa. The frequency of swing of the lamps never changed. Gravity, of course, is a constant in the equation with a value of 9.8 m/sec^2 or 980 (more precisely, 981.456) cm/sec^2. Those values are the metric equivalents of 32.2 ft per sec per sec (32.2 ft/sec^2) in the **fps** system of measurement.

We have discussed two principal characteristics of pendular vibration. The first is **amplitude**, which is directly proportional to the force applied. The second is **frequency**, which is inversely proportional to the length of the pendulum, and frequency is the reciprocal of the period. We shall see that the concepts of amplitude and frequency will be used to help define characteristics of vibratory motion in general, not just the movement of the pendulum.

■ PROPORTIONALITY

It might be helpful to elaborate on what is meant by **inversely proportional** and **directly proportional**. When two things are inversely proportional, as one decreases the other increases and, conversely, as one increases the other decreases. An inverse relation can be stated simply as:

$$A \propto \frac{1}{B,}$$

Equation 1.14

which means that **A** is inversely proportional to **B**.

Equations 1.11 and 1.12 that specified the relation of frequency and period were of the form shown in Equation 1.14, which means that frequency and period are inversely related.

Direct proportionality can be described in the form:

$$A \propto B,$$

Equation 1.15

which means **A** is directly proportional to **B**.

Consider Equation 1.13 for the period of a pendulum. **L** appeared in the numerator, which means that period and length are directly related, and as we saw previously, period is directly proportional to the square root of length. It is easy to inspect an equation and know if you are dealing with an inverse or direct relation.

To determine if **A** is directly or inversely related to **B**, look at **B** in the equation. If **B** appears in the denominator of the ratio, **A** is inversely related to **B**. If **B** appears in the numerator of the ratio, **A** is directly related to **B**. What if there is no ratio? If there *appears* to be no ratio because there is no denominator (actually, the denominator has a value of "1"), the proportional relation takes the form shown in Equation 1.15, $A \propto B$. An example appeared in Equation 1.9 where we saw that momentum (**M**) was directly proportional to both mass (**m**) and velocity (**c**).

■ SOUND WAVE PROPAGATION

Let us return now to a sound wave that results from the vibratory motion of some mass. Suppose a source of sound is energized — a tuning fork, for example, is struck. The action produces a wave of compression, as shown in Figure 1–4, that moves through the air medium. As we learned earlier, the individual air molecules are caused to move back and forth relative to their average position of equilibrium, *but they do not move over a great distance.* Because of the force that was applied to them, the movement of those particles produces alternate regions of increased density (**condensation**) and decreased density (**rarefaction**), and it is that disturbance that is propagated through the medium.

In our previous discussion of vibratory motion, we considered the pendulum (an example of slow-motion vibration) because the vibratory movements of the tuning fork are too rapid to see. It might also be helpful to think of waves of compression that can be seen. Imagine that you are sitting on the dock over a lake on a day with the wind so calm that the surface of the water is glassy — the water medium is "in equilibrium."

Now, dip a stick in and out of the water one time. What happens? You will see a disturbance (a wave of disturbance) move out from where the stick entered the water. Do it again, but this time dip the stick in and out of the water repeatedly at regular intervals, say once every 2 sec. Now the wave of disturbance will be repeated, and you will see a series of concentric circles of larger and larger diameter moving away from the center. The water wave is reasonably analogous to the propagation of a sound wave in air, except that the water wave that we see is moving along a two-dimensional surface.

We should agree, then, that there is a wave of disturbance that moves along the surface of the water. But, are the water molecules displaced over any great distance? Place a small cork on the surface of the water and imagine it to represent a "water particle." As the wave of disturbance moves outward, the cork will be seen to bob (approximately) up and down. The cork moves over a relatively small distance, but a *wave of disturbance* is propagated through the medium for a considerable distance. The same is true of the propagation of sound in air — the propagation of density changes through an elastic medium.

Two events occur at some certain *rate* during sound wave propagation. One is the *rate of vibratory movement* of the air particles (**frequency** of vibratory motion). The second is the *rate with which the disturbance is propagated* through the medium (the **speed** of sound).

Frequency of Vibratory Motion (f)

The rate at which the source of sound vibrates in hertz (**Hz**) is called the **frequency (f)**. What determines the frequency with which the tuning fork, or any other sound source, will vibrate? *The frequency of vibration of the source of sound is determined by properties of the source.* It does not matter whether the sound wave that results will be propagated through air or water or along a steel rail, and it does not matter what force is applied to the source.

In the case of the tuning fork, the principal factors that determine the frequency of vibration are the density of the metal and the length of the bar. Thus, a single tuning fork that is always characterized by some constant density and length will always vibrate with the same frequency when it is struck. With the pendulum, we learned that length was the principal factor that determined frequency of vibration. We shall see later that the frequency of vibrating strings such as on a piano or guitar will depend on the length, mass, and tension of the strings. But, it is important to remember that as long as nothing happens to alter those characteristics of the source, the frequency of vibration will be the same.

What about the frequency of vibration, to and fro, of the air molecules in response to the vibration of the source? Their frequency depends on, and is the same as, the frequency of vibration of the source. Thus, if the tuning fork vibrates with a frequency of 125 Hz, the air molecules in the medium also vibrate with a frequency of 125 Hz. If we select a new fork that, because of a different density of the metal and/or a different length of the bar, vibrates with a frequency of 250 Hz, the frequency of air particle vibration also will be 250 Hz.

Speed of Sound

The vibration of either tuning fork mentioned above, the one with f = 125 Hz or the one with f = 250 Hz, results in a wave of compression that is propagated through the medium. How fast will the disturbance be propagated? In other words, what will determine the **speed** of sound wave propagation?

Whereas the frequency, or rate, of vibration of the source is dependent on characteristics of the source, *the speed of sound wave propagation is dependent on characteristics of the medium.* Thus, the waves of compression that result from the two forks vibrating with different frequencies move through the medium with the same speed.

We understand from common experience that some amount of time is required for a sound wave to reach our ears. We can see the ball leave the tee from a distant golfer before we hear the "crack" of the ball; we can see the conductor's hands signal the celebrity to commence singing the national anthem at the World Series before we hear the first words; and we can see the flash of lightning long before (we hope) we hear the crash of thunder.

These differences between how soon we "see something" and how soon we "hear something" occur because light and sound travel at different speeds. The speed of light is 299,728,377 km per sec (186, 282.397 mi per sec; a slight change from the value of 186,282.423 that was accepted before the General Conference on Weights and Measures met in Paris in 1983). The speed of sound in air at sea level with a temperature of 0° Centigrade (C) is only 331 m per sec (1,085.96 ft per sec). Thus, the speed of light is almost 1 million times faster than the speed of sound.

The speed of sound in air is given by:

$$s = \sqrt{\frac{E}{\rho,}}$$

Equation 1.16

where **E** refers to elasticity and ρ refers to density.

Thus, speed is directly proportional to the square root of the **elasticity (E)** of the medium, which is measured in Nt/m^2 (**MKS**) or dynes/cm^2 (**cgs**), and inversely proportional to the square root of the **density** (ρ) of the medium, which normally is measured in kilograms per cubic meter (kg/m^3), but sometimes in grams per cubic centimeter (g/cm^3). The relation between these two alternative expressions is given by:

$$1 \text{ g/cm}^3 = 0.001 \text{ kg/0.01m}^3 = 1,000 \text{ kg/m}^3.$$

We generally will be interested in the speed of sound waves traveling in air that is warmer than 0° C, and changes in air temperature do affect the speed of sound wave propagation. As the medium warms, the ambient pressure of the medium remains constant, but the expanding gases cause the density of the medium to decrease.

We can reason from Equation 1.16 that the speed of sound increases as temperature increases because an increase in temperature produces a decrease in density, and s $\propto$ 1/ρ. More specifically, the speed of sound increases approximately 0.61 m/sec (61 cm/sec or 2 ft/sec) for each 1° C increase in temperature. For example, if the speed of sound is 331 m/sec (33,101 cm/sec; 1,086 ft/sec) at 0° C, it will increase to 343 m/sec (34,320 cm/sec; 1,126 ft/sec) if the temperature rises to 20° C (68° Fahrenheit).

From Equation 1.16 it is obvious that the speed of sound in air is independent of the frequency of vibration of the source, because only characteristics of the medium are included in the equation. Thus, the speeds of two sound waves, one with f = 125 Hz and one with f = 250 Hz, will be identical when the waves travel in the same medium.

If also follows that the sound wave that results from a tuning fork vibrating with a frequency of, for example, 500 Hz will be propagated at different speeds in different sound transmission media. In air, the disturbance will travel with a speed of about 331 m/sec (1,086 ft/sec). In water with the temperature of 0° C (if it has not yet frozen), the disturbance from the same vibrating fork travels much faster, about 1,433 m/sec (4,702 ft/sec). On a steel rail the speed will be even greater, about 4,704 m/sec (15,434 ft/sec).

Does the contrast of speed along steel and speed through air make sense from Equation 1.16? Steel is a little more than 6,000 times as dense as air. If we ignore elasticity, we might conclude that the speed of sound would therefore be less in steel because speed and density are inversely proportional. However, we cannot ignore elasticity. In fact, steel is about 1,230,000 times more elastic than air. Thus, counter to our sometimes common intuition, **elasticity** can be thought of as the ability to *resist deformation,* and steel certainly offers a greater resistance to deformation than does water. The contribution of the difference in elasticity between air and steel far outweighs the difference in density. As a result, the speed of sound is approximately 14 times greater in steel than in air.

■ TYPES OF WAVE MOTION

We have talked about the nature of wave motion that occurs with a sound wave, and we then drew the analogy of wave motion on the surface of water. Now we wish to describe the characteristics of all wave motion in a little more detail. We say "all wave motion" because wave motion certainly is not confined to sound. The vibrations, or tremors, of buildings or of bridges also are examples of wave motion. Another is the pattern that you see if you flick one end of a stretched rope that is fastened at one end to a wall.

The types of waves that result from vibratory motion are classified according to *the direction of vibration of the medium relative to the direction in which the wave is moving.* That sounds more complicated than it actually is, and a few examples should serve to clear up any confusion. There are two types of wave motion: **transverse** and **longitudinal**.

Transverse Wave Motion

One type of wave motion is called a **transverse wave**. Consider a stretched rope such as that shown in Figure 1–10 with its two ends extending to infinity so that no "reflections" will occur. We have "painted" several open dots along the rope at equal intervals that, with considerable license, we will refer to as "rope particles." Next, we will flick the rope and, with the aid of a fast camera, we will periodically "stop the

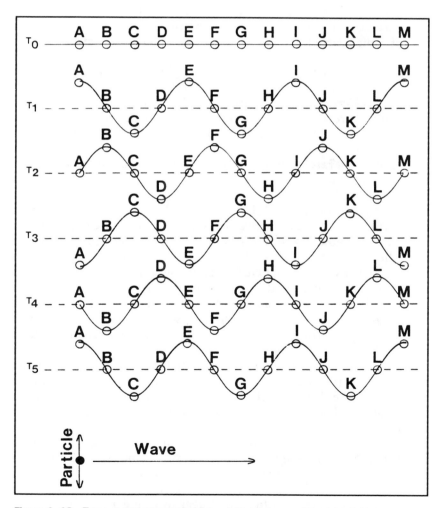

Figure 1–10. Transverse wave motion of a stretched rope. "Particles" (A through M) painted on the rope move alternately up and down over time (from T_0 through T_5) at right angles to the direction of wave motion from left to right.

action" and examine the position of each of the particles at different moments in time. If we take a series of such pictures at regular intervals, we will be able to see the course of movement of each of the rope particles from moment to moment. Time progresses from t_0 at the top of the figure to t_5 at the bottom.

The first picture, taken at time zero (t_0), shows the rope stretched — it is at equilibrium. In the second picture (t_1), taken a fraction of a second later, we see that particle **A** moved upward, **B** stayed in place, **C** moved downward, **D** stayed in place, **E** moved upward, **F** stayed in place, and so on. As you move down the rows of the figure, you see that, over time, each particle is moving up and down. Furthermore, each particle is moving up and down *with exactly the same frequency* as every other particle. Consider one cycle of vibration for particle **A**: Movement from equilibrium at time zero (t_0) to maximal displacement upward (t_1), to equilibrium (t_2), to maximal displacement downward (t_3), and back to equilibrium (t_4). Every other particle completes one cycle of vibration in exactly the same amount of time. Particle **B**, for example, completes one cycle between t_1 and t_5.

Look again at the position of the particles along the rope and you will see peaks occurring at regular intervals from left to right. At t_1 the peaks correspond to particles **A, E, I,** and **M.** Those peaks are analogous to regions of **condensation** or **high density** for sound transmitted through air. We also can see valleys from left to right that correspond to points **C, G,** and **K.** Those valleys are analogous to regions of **rarefaction** or **low density** for sound in air.

As we move through time by looking down the rows, you should note that the locations of the peaks move from left to right. At t_1, the first peak appeared at **A**, but at t_2 particle **A** has moved downward and particle **B** has moved upward. As a result, the peak that formerly (t_1) was at **A** now has moved toward the right to correspond to point **B**. The same is true for all of the other peaks, and so at t_2 the peaks are located at **B, F,** and **J.** Over time, as you move down through time t_5, the peaks have moved from left to right. For now, we won't concern ourselves with what happens when the peak finally moves far enough to the right to reach the imaginary surface to which the rope is attached (at infinity), but that concept will be introduced in Chapter 8.

With the type of wave motion that occurs with the rope in Figure 1–10, the direction of wave movement is from left to right in contrast to the direction of particle movement, which is up and down. That is called transverse wave movement, and a **transverse wave** is defined as one in which *the direction of vibration of the medium is at right angles (90°) to the direction of the wave that is propagated through the medium.* Transverse wave motion is the type of motion that happens, for example, when you pluck the string of a guitar. Another example of (almost) transverse wave motion occurs when you throw a pebble into a pond near to where a cork lies motionless (in equilibrium). A wave of disturbance with peaks and valleys will move out away from where the pebble struck the water. As the wave moves outward, the cork (and the water medium) will bob approximately up and down at right angles to the wave movement.

Longitudinal Wave Motion

The second type of wave motion is called a **longitudinal wave**, which is illustrated in Figure 1–11 by a spring–mass system that is lying on a frictionless surface. As with the stretched rope, the "individual particles" of the spring are identified with painted solid dots and are labeled from **A** through **H**. Time progresses from t_0 at the top of the figure to t_8 at the bottom.

When the spring is in equilibrium (t_0), the dots are spaced at equal intervals. In the next picture (t_1), a short segment of the spring has been compressed and then released. Particle **A** has moved leftward. From t_0 through t_8, particle **A** — and the mass attached to the spring — can be seen to move leftward and rightward (back and forth) through two complete cycles of vibration. Each new picture shows the position of the spring particles at progressively later moments in time, and ultimately each of the particles **B** through **H** undergoes exactly the same motion that was seen for particle **A**. That is to say, each particle vibrates back and forth with exactly the same amplitude and frequency as particle **A**.

Compressions, or **condensations**, are shown by the dots being crowded together and (high density) **rarefactions** are shown when the

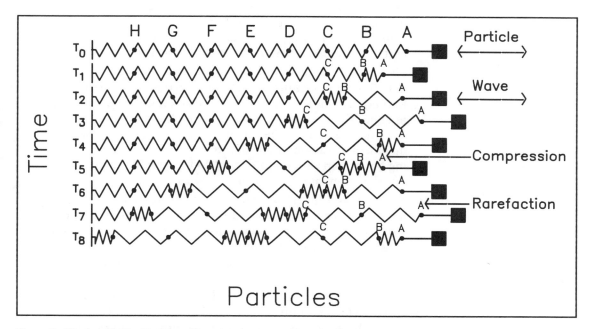

Figure 1–11. Longitudinal wave motion of a spring–mass system lying on a frictionless surface. "Particles" (A through H) painted on the spring move alternately back and forth from left to right over time (from T_0 through T_8) in the same plane as the wave movement from right to left.

dots appear far apart (low density). From picture to picture the particles of the spring move back and forth, and the compressions and rarefactions move in the same plane as the particles. This leads us, then, to the definition of a **longitudinal** wave. A **longitudinal wave** is one in which *the direction of particle movement is parallel to the direction of wave propagation.*

■ SOUND WAVES

How should sound waves be classified? Sound waves in air are **longitudinal waves;** *the direction of air particle movement is parallel to the direction of wave movement.* In fact, it is not unreasonable to think of the air molecules as small elements of matter attached to each other by springs. This is illustrated in Figure 1–3 in which 10 individual particles are in the columns from left to right and "frozen moments" in time are in the rows from top to bottom. The source of sound is the tuning fork. The first row shows the fork and the medium in equilibrium. Three and one-quarter cycles of vibration are shown. By way of review, we should be able to identify the following aspects of vibratory motion.

1. The tuning fork in Figure 1–3 moves through 3¼ cycles of vibration after it is struck by moving from equilibrium, to maximal displacement (+), through equilibrium, to maximal displacement in the opposite direction (−), and back to equilibrium during each cycle.

2. Each particle vibrates back and forth relative to its average position of equilibrium, which is shown in the top row of Figure 1–3. The **amplitude** and **period** of vibration of each particle is the same as for every other particle.

3. The individual particles do not vibrate together. That is to say, not all of them simultaneously move to the left or to the right. Rather, they move in a progressive fashion just as we observed in Figure 1–10 for the dots on the stretched rope and in Figure 1–11 for the dots on the spring–mass system. If the dots were members of a marching band, we would say they are "marching out of step with one another." In Chapter 2 we will learn to say that they are "out of phase" with one another.

4. The back and forth movement of the air particles produces a movement, or propagation, of the condensations (higher density) and rarefactions (lower density) from left to right in Figure 1–3. During the condensation phase, the particles are moving to the right, and during the rarefaction phase, the particles are moving to the left.

5. The individual particles are envisioned to be connected by a spring, which is equivalent to an **elastic bond**, and each particle can be viewed as *exerting a force on the one to the right of it.* By that we mean, during condensation, each spring pushes

the particle to its right forward, whereas during rarefaction, the springs or elastic bonds are stretched, which pulls the particle backward.

6. Each particle is doing **work** on the particle in front (to the right) of it. This results in a **transfer of energy** through the medium in the direction in which the wave is traveling.

■ TRANSFER OF ENERGY

We learned previously that the medium itself is not transferred during sound wave propagation; each particle is displaced from its position of equilibrium over only a very small distance. However, **energy** is transferred through the medium in the direction in which the wave is propagated as each particle does work on the one next in line.

The transfer of energy during transmission of sound is exactly the same as in the discussion of the pendulum. In other words, potential energy is greatest and kinetic energy is least when the molecule is at maximal displacement; and as the particle returns toward equilibrium, potential energy is transformed to kinetic energy. At the position of equilibrium, kinetic energy is maximal and potential energy is zero.

Previously, sound in air was said to be characterized as *the propagation of density changes through an elastic medium*. It is more correct to *define* sound as *the transfer of energy through an elastic medium*. We learned previously in our discussion of pendular vibration that **friction** serves to limit the velocity of pendular motion. The same thing occurs when sound energy is transferred through a medium such as air. The air mass offers a resistance, and some of the kinetic energy will be transformed into thermal energy (heat). When that transformation is complete, the sound energy will have been dissipated — which means that no more useful work can be accomplished because of friction.

The sound waves that we have discussed to this point have come from the vibratory motion of tuning forks, the pendulum, a stretched rope or string, and a spring–mass system. Each of those examples produces the same pattern of wave motion, which is called **simple harmonic motion**. The characteristics of simple harmonic motion will be described in the next chapter.

■ NOTES

1. The stem of the fork will also be set into vibration, but it will move up and down as the tines move back and forth. The fork also has two points located near to where the metal bars are bent at which no vibration occurs. Points of no vibration are called **nodes**.
2. Strictly speaking, the frequency of pendular vibration is independent of amplitude only if the amplitude is small. However, for our purposes, the influence of amplitude on frequency will be disregarded.

Simple Harmonic Motion

In this chapter the details of vibratory motion will be examined more closely. When we discussed the concept of transfer of energy in Chapter 1, the vibratory motion of air particles was simulated in Figure 1-11 by a spring–mass system. If the mass is pushed leftward to compress the spring, a rightward reaction force results, and if the mass is pulled rightward to extend the spring, a leftward reaction force results. In other words, there is always a restoring force to return the mass to its position of equilibrium, and the magnitude of the restoring force is proportional to the change in length of the spring, which we learned is **Hooke's Law** (Equation 1.8). That means that the *restoring force is proportional to the distance that the mass is displaced from the rest position.*

It follows, therefore, that during the course of the oscillatory motion of the spring–mass system, the magnitude of the restoring force changes over time because the magnitude of displacement changes. As the mass moves toward equilibrium, the restoring force diminishes, and as the mass moves away from equilibrium and toward a maximum displacement, the restoring force increases. Because of this buildup and decay of the restoring force, the mass is accelerated (toward equilibrium) and decelerated (away from equilibrium), which also means that the velocity of movement of the mass is constantly changing.

The result is called a **vibration**, or **oscillation**, of the mass backward and forward that simulates the to and fro vibratory, or oscillatory, motion of the air molecules. One cycle of vibration is defined just as it was previously: movement from equilibrium to maximal displacement (+), back through equilibrium, to maximal displacement in the opposite direction (−), and back to equilibrium again.

■ THE WAVEFORM

It is useful to study a graph that illustrates the nature of this simple vibratory motion by plotting changes in the magnitude, or amplitude, of displacement over time. Rather than designate the starting time as the moment when the mass was released, we will assume that the system has already been set into oscillation, and we will plot two cycles of oscillation that commence at the exact moment that the mass in Figure 1-11 passes through the position of equilibrium and heads in the opposite direction. That is analogous to the air molecules in Figure 1-3 being displaced from equilibrium to the right.

Such a plot is shown in Figure 2-1, which displays what is called the **time-domain waveform**, or just **waveform**. This is the kind of result you would obtain if, for example, the path of point **A** for the spring–mass system in Figure 1-11 were traced over time from t_0 to t_8. But, it is important to avoid a serious misinterpretation: The air mass *does not literally undergo an excursion of the type shown in Figure 2-1.* Instead, the air molecules move back and forth just as the spring–mass system moves back and forth, and the wave of disturbance moves through the medium in essentially a straight line. The curved line in the figure is simply a *graphic representation* (i.e., the **waveform**) of what is transpiring.

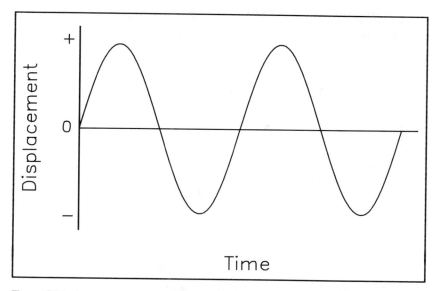

Figure 2–1. Graphic representation of the movement of the spring–mass system over time that was presented in Figure 1–11. The pattern of movement reflects **simple harmonic motion**, which also is called **sinusoidal motion**. This kind of representation is called the **waveform**.

In Figure 2–1, the waveform shows *displacement* as a function of time, but the concept of waveform is not restricted to a display of displacement. Many quantities (e.g., displacement, velocity, acceleration, force, pressure, momentum, and so on) can be shown as a function of time and properly be called waveforms.

■ THE CONCEPT OF SIMPLE HARMONIC MOTION

We can gain an understanding of why back and forth molecular movement can be represented by the kind of curve shown in Figure 2–1 by a study of **simple harmonic motion**. The type of motion that the spring–mass system (and the air molecule) undergoes is called **simple harmonic motion**, and we shall see subsequently why simple harmonic motion can also be called **sinusoidal motion**. Simple harmonic motion can be defined as *projected uniform circular motion*.

Uniform Circular Motion

What is meant by uniform circular motion? *Uniform circular motion occurs when a body moves around the circumference of a circle at a constant number of degrees of rotation per second.*

Figure 2–2 shows a wheel that is turning counterclockwise. The dot on the wheel moves at a *uniform* rate around the circumference. In

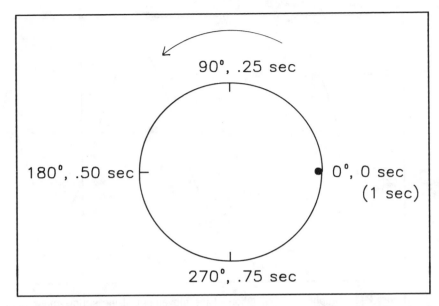

Figure 2–2. A dot moving at a uniform rate around the circumference of a wheel through 360° of rotation in 1 sec.

this example, one complete revolution of the wheel and, therefore, one complete revolution of the dot, is accomplished in 1 sec. Because the dot moves through 360° during one revolution, the wheel turns at a uniform rate of 1° per 1/360 sec.

We shall try to develop the concept that the back and forth movement of the mass, or the back and forth movement of the air molecules, is analogous to a point moving around the circumference of a circle at a constant rate. When that is accomplished, we will be able to say that the movement of the mass and of the air molecules are examples of **simple harmonic motion**. We will also be able to explain why straight-line back and forth motion, which is properly called **rectilinear motion**, can legitimately be pictured to have the curious pattern that is shown in Figure 2–1.

One of the best explanations was provided by Hirsh (1952), and Figure 2–3 is taken from his textbook. A person seated on a Ferris wheel is pointing a flashlight at a wall that is coated with a light-sensitive material. The Ferris wheel starts to move at a constant speed, which means that both the person and the flashlight will move around the circumference of the circle at a constant number of degrees of rotation per second. Thus, the rider undergoes **simple harmonic motion**.

What will the projected image look like when the wall is stationary? It will be a straight line. The upper limit will correspond to the moment in time when the person is at the top of the path of the wheel, the lower limit will correspond to the moment in time when the person is at the bottom of the path, and the midpoint of the line will correspond to the starting (rest) position. At this point, then, we can see that

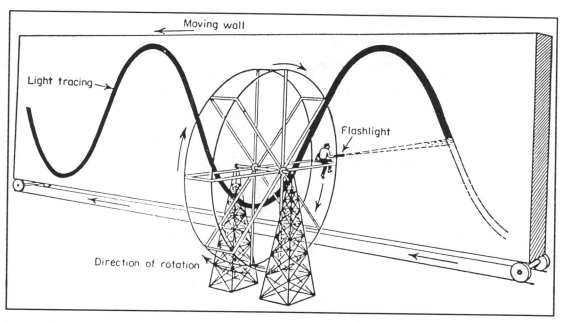

Figure 2–3. An illustration of how a sinusoid is created by the projection of uniform circular motion. From *The measurement of hearing* (p. 20) by I. J. Hirsh, 1952, New York, NY: McGraw-Hill Book Company, Inc. Copyright 1952 by the McGraw-Hill Book Company. Reproduced with permission.

circular motion can be projected as rectilinear (straight-line) motion. You can demonstrate this for yourself by pointing a flashlight at a wall and then moving the flashlight in a circular motion on a path perpendicular to the wall. The beam of light will move up and down in a straight line.

Next, suppose that the wall moves from right to left. The straight-line image that was observed when the wall was stationary will now take the form of the curved line that is shown in Figure 2–3. You can demonstrate this effect for yourself by pointing a flashlight toward a wall and attempting to walk along the wall from left to right at a constant speed as you rotate the flashlight as before. The curved image will result.

Projection of Uniform Circular Motion

In Figure 2–4 the projected circular motion — **simple harmonic motion** — is shown in more detail. The circle at the left of the figure represents the Ferris wheel with the passenger aboard. Point P_0 will be defined as the rest or starting position, and the rest or starting position is also labeled as 0°. The person then is set into counterclockwise motion around the circumference of the circle through points P_1, P_2, and so on until the person has moved completely around the circumference. The excursion around the circumference is marked at 45°

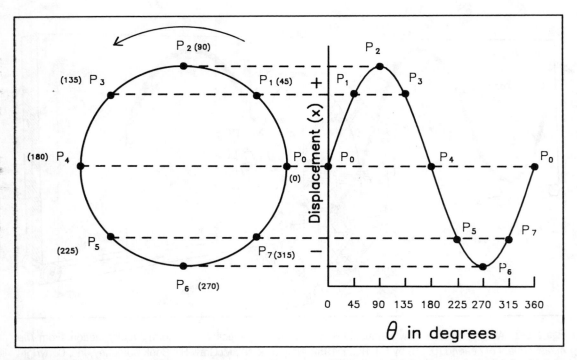

Figure 2–4. Projection of uniform circular motion. The points (P₀ through P₇) on the turning wheel, which is moving at a uniform rate and, hence, undergoing **simple harmonic motion**, are projected as corresponding points (also P₀ through P₇) on a sinusoidal function. Each point on the sinusoidal function shows the **magnitude of displacement** from the baseline corresponding to that angle of rotation.

intervals, and at the end of one complete rotation, the passenger will have passed through 360°.

At the right of Figure 2–4 we show the projection of that circular motion, just as the image of the flashlight beam was projected in Figure 2–3. In this case, the projection displays the **displacement waveform**. The only difference from what was shown in Figure 2–3 is that the "coated wall" has been rotated 90° relative to its position in Figure 2–3 so that the circle and the projection appear in the same two-dimensional plane. The projection (the **waveform**), of course, has exactly the same curved form that it did in Figure 2–3, where it resulted from a flashlight moving with the Ferris wheel.

The waveform in Figure 2–4 also is marked with dots at regular intervals labeled from **P₀** through **P₇**, and the precise location of each of those points on the projection corresponds to the location of the corresponding points on the turning wheel. It is worthwhile to examine the nature of the correspondence in detail, because the relation between circular motion and the form of its projection is fundamental to the understanding of simple harmonic motion in particular and to an understanding of sound in general.

When the passenger is at point **P₀**, the passenger is located on what we can call the "baseline," or reference line, and the projection of the beam also lies along the baseline. As the wheel begins to rotate counterclockwise, the passenger — and the projected beam — are displaced upward from the baseline. At 45° (P_1) of rotation, the horizontal (dashed) line indicates exactly where the projection would be at this point. That point on the projection is also labeled P_1, and it therefore corresponds to 45°. Between 45° and 90°, the passenger travels the same distance (through the same number of degrees) as between 0° and 45°, *but the magnitude of the linear displacement above the baseline is less between 45° and 90° than it was between 0° and 45°.* At 90°, of course, the height of the projected curve is at its maximum, which corresponds to the passenger being at the highest point above the baseline.

Between P_2 and P_6 the passenger is moving downward, and the projection also is moving in a downward or negative direction. At P_3 the height of the displacement is the same as at P_1, and in a similar vein, P_4 corresponds to P_0 and P_5 corresponds to P_7. The relation between the heights of displacement for P_2 and P_6 also should be apparent. P_2 corresponds to a maximal displacement above baseline (90°) and P_6 corresponds to a maximal and equal height of displacement below baseline (270°). From P_6 through P_0 the passenger is climbing back upward toward the baseline (and so is the projection) to complete one cycle of rotation, which corresponds to 360°.

Notice that the horizontal axis (abscissa) of Figure 2–4 is labeled in degrees. That allows us to specify exactly where the person (P) is in the excursion around the wheel at any given moment in time. Thus, the starting point P_0 corresponds to 0°, P_1 corresponds to 45°, P_2 to 90°, and so on until the passenger returns to the starting point, which corresponds to 360°.

When the passenger reaches the top of the circle, which corresponds to 90° of rotation (1/4 of a cycle), the projection has reached its maximal height in what can be called a *positive* direction of displacement. When the passenger has completed exactly half of the circle, which corresponds to 180° of rotation, the projected beam is in exactly the same position that it was at rest, or starting position. Maximal displacement of the beam in a *negative* direction occurs when the person has completed 270° of rotation, and finally, when movement around the circumference of the circle is complete, the person has returned to the starting point, which corresponds to 360° of rotation, and the projection is back to zero displacement.

One rotation of 360° is defined as a **cycle**, and that is identical to our previous definition: one cycle corresponds to displacement from equilibrium to maximum, back to equilibrium, to minimum, and back to equilibrium. Equilibrium corresponds to 0°, 180°, and 360°; maximal displacement corresponds to 90° (+) and 270° (−).

The projected graph of uniform circular motion, or simple harmonic motion, shows the magnitude of **displacement** (x) as a function of degrees of rotation. The abscissa also could have been labeled in units of time. Suppose the wheel rotates with a **frequency** (f) of one rotation per second. That means that the **period** of rotation — the time required to complete one cycle of rotation — is one second because T = 1/f and 1/1 = 1. Now we would see that 90° (1/4 of the cycle) corresponds to 0.25 sec (1/4 of 1 sec), 180° to 0.50 sec (1/2 of 1 sec), and so on. If we increase the frequency of rotation to two rotations per second, the period will equal 0.5 sec (the time required to complete one cycle of rotation). Now, 90° still corresponds to 1/4 of the excursion and to a maximal amplitude of displacement, but because of the increased frequency, it will correspond to 0.125 sec., which is 1/4 of 0.5 (the time required to complete one cycle).

The Sine Wave

Figure 2–5 is similar to Figure 2–4, but now the projections of three wheels of different sizes are shown. Look at the similarities and differences among the three projections. In all cases, one cycle corresponds to 360°, maximal displacement corresponds to 90° and 270°, and so on. Although maximal positive displacement corresponds to 90° for all

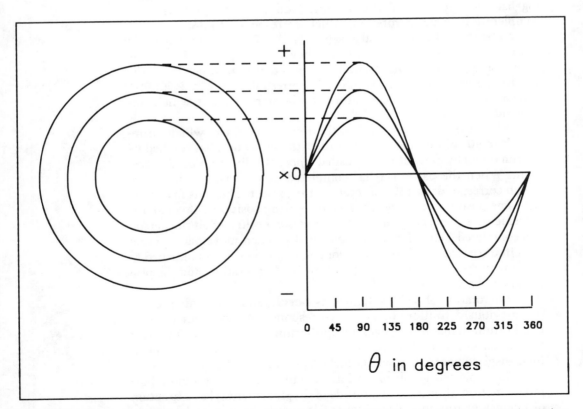

Figure 2–5. Projections of a rotating point on each of three wheels undergoing simple harmonic motion. Because the radius of each of the wheels is different, the magnitudes of displacement (**x**) of the projections of the three wheels also are different.

three wheels, it is obvious that the largest wheel results in the largest displacement of the projection.

Even though the magnitude of displacement (**x**) varies with the size of the wheel, the *general form or shape of the three projections (the three waveforms) is the same*. The next step, then, is to identify the constant feature that characterizes the three projections, which involves determining what is called the **sine of an angle**.

Consider the triangle shown in Figure 2–6. The angle is 45°, the side opposite the angle is labeled **x**, the base is labeled **b**, and the hypotenuse is labeled **r** because it equals the radius (**r**) of the circle. The sine of the angle, which is called **sin** θ, equals **x/r**. In other words, if we know the lengths of **x** and **r**, we divide **x** by **r** and the result is called the **sine**

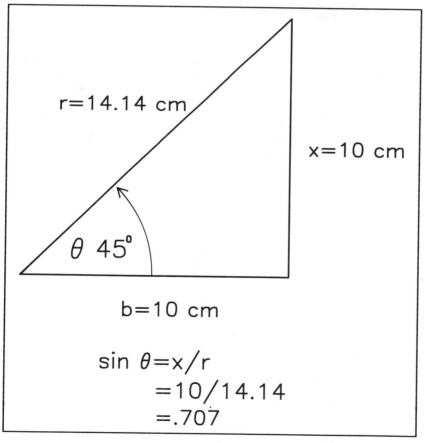

Figure 2–6. A triangle with an angle of 45°, hypotenuse **r**, base **b**, and side **x**. The ratio **x/r** is called the **sine of the angle** (sin θ), and the sine of any constant angle such as 45° is a constant, regardless of the absolute magnitudes of **x** and **r**. Thus, for a 45° angle, if **x** = 1.00, **r** must equal 1.414, and the sine of the angle is 0.707. If for the same angle, **x** = 2.0, **r** must equal 2.828, and the sine of the angle still is 0.707.

of the angle. With the example in the figure, the length of **x** is 10 cm, the length of **b** also is 10 cm, and the length of **r** is 14.14 cm. The ratio of **x** to **r**, **x/r**, is 10/14.14 = 0.707. That is the same as saying that the length of **x** is 70.7% of the length of **r**.

For any given angle, the ratio **x/r** (the sine of the angle) will also be a constant, but, of course, the constant ratio *for other angles* will not necessarily be 0.707. You will see later that $\sin \theta = 0.707$ only when the angle is 45° and 135° and −0.707 for 225° and 315°. The sine of other angles will be different from 0.707. For example, you can verify with your pocket calculator that the sine of 90° is 1.00, the sine of 270° is −1.00, the sine of 180° and 360° is 0.00, and so forth. However, in all cases, the fact remains that the sine of the angle is given by the ratio of **x** to **r**.

We could have formed other ratios for the triangle as well. For example, the ratio **b/r** is called the **cosine** of the angle, and the ratio **x/b** is called the **tangent** of the angle, and both of these are constants as well.

Figure 2–7 contains circles of the same three sizes that appeared in Figure 2–5, but in Figure 2–7 a triangle with an angle of 45° is placed within each circle. The radius (**r**) of each circle forms the hypotenuse for the triangle of each circle and, of course, the radius of each circle intersects the circumference of that circle. The length of **r** is different for each of the three circles.

The side of the triangle opposite the angle corresponds to the magnitude of displacement (**x**) just as it did in Figure 2–3 where a beam of light was projected from the Ferris wheel. And, finally, the length of

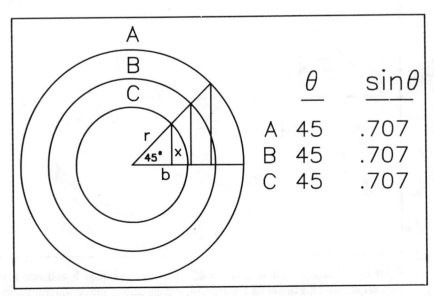

FIGURE 2–7. Three triangles inserted within the three wheels shown previously in Figure 2–5. Because the circumferences of the three circles are different, the absolute magnitudes of **x**, **b**, and **r** vary, but the sine of the 45° angle, **x/r**, is a constant 0.707 for all three triangles.

x and the length of the base (**b**) also are different for each of the three circles.

The important point to emphasize is that the *ratio of x/r, which is the **sine of the angle**, is identical for all three triangles* because the angle is constant. For each of the three triangles, **sin** θ = 0.707. In other words, it does not matter what the three lengths are; if the *angle* is 45°, the ratio of the length of **x** to the length of **r** will always be 0.707. As we stated previously, that is the same as saying that the length of **x** will always be 70.7% of the length of **r** when the angle is 45°. In other words, at 45°, the displacement *always* is 70.7% of the maximum displacement that will be achieved at 90°, regardless of the magnitude of the maximum displacement. Thus, for a constant angle, **sin** θ also is a constant.

Fortunately, we can use a pocket calculator or published trigonometric tables to find the sine (and cosine and tangent) of any angle rather than calculate it. For example, at 90°, **sin** θ = +1.00; at 135°, **sin** θ = 0.707 and it projects to the same height as at 45°; at 180° **sin** θ = 0.00; and at 270°, which projects to the same height (maximal displacement) as at 90°, but in the opposite direction, **sin** θ = −1.00.

Displacement (x) Represented by sin θ

In Figure 2–8 we have redrawn the three wheels from Figure 2–5, but in this case *the heights of the projections are shown by sin θ instead of x*. Now the three projections are superimposed upon one another, because for each angle throughout the cycle, the sine of the angle is a constant. In Figure 2–5 the same three circles produced projections that reached three different maximal heights of displacement. That is because we plotted "absolute displacement" above baseline in Figure 2–5, which was different for the three wheels of different sizes. However, in Figure 2–8 displacement is represented by **sin** θ, which is a constant for any constant angle. The result is three superimposed curves, which reveals that there is something constant about uniform circular motion even though that motion can occur along circumferences of different sizes.

Summary of Sinusoidal Motion

We have seen that the *common element* in all of the projections of simple harmonic motion, or uniform circular motion, is the **sine of the angle**. For any constant angle, regardless of the size of the triangle, the sine of that angle is the constant. In other words, each of the three wheels has achieved 38.3% of maximum displacement at 22.5° (sin 22.5° = 0.383), 70.7% at 45° (sin 45° = 0.707), 100% at 90° (sin 90° = 1.00), and so on. It is for that reason that **simple harmonic motion** also can be called **sinusoidal motion**, and the projection or graph of simple harmonic motion or sinusoidal motion is called a **sine wave**, a **sinusoidal wave**, or just a **sinusoid**.

Movement around the circumference of a circle at a constant number of degrees of rotation (uniform circular motion) per second is called

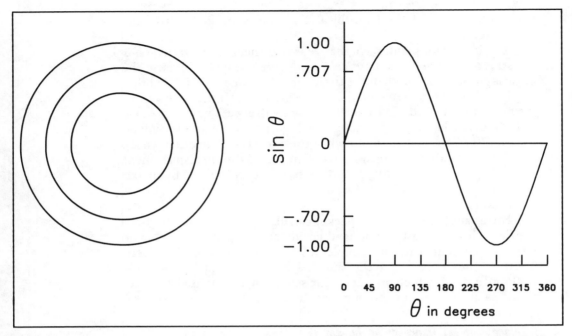

Figure 2-8. Projections of the same three rotating wheels shown previously in Figure 2-5. In Figure 2-5, magnitude of displacement was given by **x**. Now, however, the ordinate is the sine of the angle, sin θ, as the wheel moves through 360° of rotation. Because the sine of any constant angle is a constant regardless of the absolute magnitude of **x**, a single projection is common to all three wheels.

simple harmonic motion, or **sinusoidal motion**, and the projection or graph of sinusoidal motion is called a **sinusoidal wave**. You should notice, however, that movement of the spring–mass system in Figure 1–11 was rectilinear (back and forth in a straight line), not circular, and the movement of the air particles in Figure 1–3 also was back and forth, not circular. In spite of that seemingly significant difference, we still represented the back and forth motions as being sinusoidal in form in Figure 2–1, even though it was not labeled a sine wave at that time.

Rectilinear Motion Represented as Uniform Circular Motion

The task that remains, then, is to explain how back and forth motion of air particles can be *represented as uniform circular motion*. To do this we appeal again to a simple explanation provided by Hirsh (1952), which is illustrated in Figure 2–9. At the left of the figure is a wheel to which a rod is attached. The rod is connected to a piston, which is housed in a piston chamber in a way characteristic of the old-fashioned steam engine.

The point where the piston is attached to the wheel is labeled 0°, the starting or equilibrium point, and it corresponds to the starting

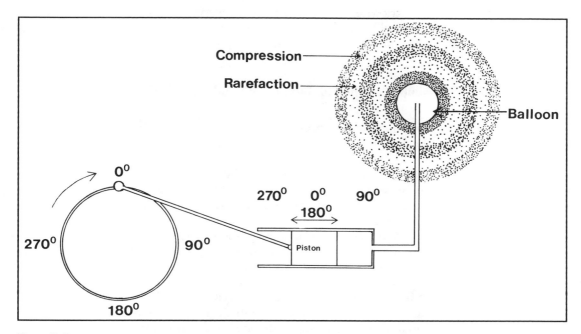

Figure 2–9. The relation between linear back and forth movement and uniform circular motion in the understanding of sinusoidal motion. The wheel, turning clockwise, causes the piston in the chamber to move *back and forth*. Each position of the piston can be identified in degrees that correspond to the angle of rotation of the wheel. The chamber is connected to a partially inflated balloon by a tube. Because of the changing air pressure in the chamber, tube, and balloon, the balloon acts as a pulsating sphere and produces a **spherical sound wave**. **Compressions** and **rarefactions** move outward through the medium in all directions as an increasingly larger sphere that, in a two-dimensional representation, appears as increasingly larger concentric circles. Adapted from *The measurement of hearing* (p. 22) by I. J. Hirsh, 1952, New York, NY: McGraw-Hill Book Company, Inc. Copyright 1952 by the McGraw-Hill Book Company, Inc. Printed with permission.

point of the person with the flashlight on the Ferris wheel in Figure 2–3. The wheel is now set into clockwise (it could be counterclockwise as well) rotation at a uniform rate, which also can be called **uniform angular velocity**. Thus, the point on the wheel where the piston rod is attached to the rim will undergo simple harmonic motion. What happens to the piston in the chamber? As the wheel turns, the piston rod will cause the piston in the chamber to move back and forth.

The position of the piston at the point of equilibrium is labeled 0°. When the wheel has rotated to the angle 90°, the piston will have moved maximally rightward and that position also is labeled 90°. When the wheel has reached 180°, the piston has returned to its position of equilibrium, which also is labeled 180°. The piston has been moved maximally leftward when the wheel reached 270°, and therefore maximal displacement of the piston to the left is labeled as 270°. Finally, when the wheel has completed one full cycle, the piston is returned to equilibrium (360°). The important point is that the wheel is engaged in uniform circular motion, but the piston is engaged in rectilinear (straight-line) motion. Thus, with a simple "mechanical translation," we are able to label points along a rectilinear excursion in degrees in a way that corresponds exactly to points along a circular excursion.

Simple Harmonic Motion and Sound Waves

To achieve sound from the motion observed in Figure 2–9, we rely on the rest of the apparatus that is shown. At the right of the piston chamber there is an opening to a tube that leads to a partially inflated balloon. The balloon acts as a pulsating sphere and produces a spherical wave — one in which the condensations and rarefactions move outward from the center of the source in all directions as increasingly larger concentric circles.

When the wheel and piston are motionless, the balloon remains partially inflated, which we shall call equilibrium. When the wheel moves clockwise to 90°, the piston will be displaced maximally to the right, which in turn will force air up the tube and cause the balloon to be inflated. As the wheel continues to turn, the piston will move back and forth, and alternately it will cause the balloon to move from inflated, to equilibrium, to deflated, to equilibrium, and so on.

One cycle of the wheel's movement corresponds to one cycle of the piston's movement, and each, in turn, corresponds to one cycle of movement of the balloon. Each cycle, whether it be that of the wheel in uniform circular motion or the piston in rectilinear motion, comprises 360°.

When the balloon surface expands outward because air is forced up the tube, a force is applied to the air molecules just as that which occurred with the movement of the tuning fork. Thus, the circular motion of the wheel and the straight-line movements of the piston cause the inward and outward movements of the balloon surface, which affect the air medium in the same way that occurred with the vibratory motion of the fork. The result is increases (condensation) and decreases (rarefaction) in density that are propagated through the elastic medium. Sound has been created, and one line of propagation of the sound wave that results from the pulsation of the sphere (balloon) is shown in the figure.

If the back and forth movements of the piston are simple translations of the circular motion of the wheel, then we also should be able to label the sound wave in degrees if we perform a simple translation. We know that 90° corresponds to the wheel having moved 1/4 of the way through its cycle and to the piston having moved 1/4 of the way through its cycle. When the piston has completed 1/4 of a cycle, it is maximally displaced, and air is forced up the tube to inflate the balloon. Thus, maximal outward displacement of the balloon also corresponds to 90°. Finally, maximal outward displacement of the balloon produces a condensation in the air medium, and maximal condensation, therefore, occurs at 90°. Similarly, maximal rarefaction corresponds to 270°.

■ DIMENSIONS OF THE SINE WAVE

When we previously discussed the vibratory motion of the tuning fork and the pendulum, factors such as the amplitude of displacement, frequency, and period were mentioned. Those are called "dimensions" of the sound wave. In this section, these, and other dimensions, will be considered in greater detail.

Amplitude

The first dimension is called the **amplitude**, which is a measure of the strength, or magnitude, of the sound wave. In most of the examples that will be cited, use of the term amplitude will refer specifically to the **sound pressure**. The top waveform in Figure 2–10, which is adapted from Hirsh (1952), represents the inward and outward movements of the balloon surface that were caused by the turning wheel and moving piston shown in Figure 2–9. The balloon surface is displaced sinusoidally over time, but of course our interest is in the sine wave (sound wave) that results, not the source of the wave (displacement of the balloon surface).

As the balloon moves outward, air molecules immediately adjacent to the balloon surface are pushed outward from their resting position. As more and more molecules are pushed outward, there is an increased number of molecules per unit of space — they are crowded together — which results in an increased density (condensation). As the balloon begins to deflate, the molecules move back toward their original position, but there are fewer molecules in the immediate surface area of the balloon. That, of course, is the region of decreased density (rarefaction).

In the second waveform of Figure 2–10 the movement or displacement of a single air molecule (particle displacement as a function of time) is shown. The individual particle is displaced sinusoidally over time. Stated differently, the **amplitude of displacement** varies sinusoidally over time. Maximum amplitude of displacement corresponds to 90° (+) and 270° (−). However, the magnitude of particle displacement would indeed be difficult to measure.

The difficulty of measurement can be overcome by considering some of the derived quantities that were described in Chapter 1. The particles can be said to move with some speed, but we also know that because the *direction* of movement is changing, the **velocity** of particle displacement must also be changing because the concept of velocity incorporates both magnitude of displacement and direction.

The third curve in Figure 2–10 shows the particle velocity waveform, and we can see that the magnitude of particle velocity also is changing sinusoidally over time. However, it is important to note that the particle velocity waveform is *shifted* relative to the particle displacement waveform. This can be understood by recalling the previous discussion on pendular oscillation.

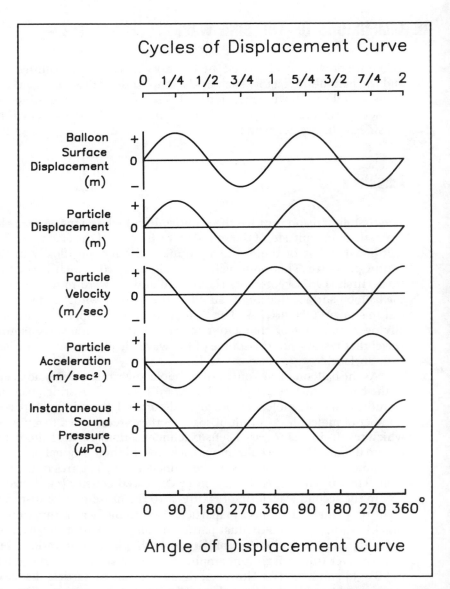

Figure 2–10. Sinusoidal functions that show the relations among **displacement, velocity, acceleration,** and **sound pressure** as measures of one dimension of sine waves: **amplitude.** Adapted from *The measurement of hearing* (p. 24) by I. J. Hirsh, 1952, New York, NY: McGraw-Hill Book Company, Inc. Copyright 1952 by McGraw-Hill Book Company, Inc. Printed with permission.

When displacement is maximal, velocity is zero. When displacement is zero (when the body is moving through equilibrium), velocity is maximal. This relation between displacement and velocity is preserved in Figure 2–10. Particle velocity is at maximum when particle displacement is zero, and particle velocity is zero when displacement is maximal (when displacement corresponds to 90 and 270°).[1] Thus, we see that the amplitude of simple harmonic motion can be described by reference to either particle displacement or to particle velocity.

If particle velocity is changing, then the particle must be undergoing acceleration, either positive or negative. The fourth curve in the figure shows the particle acceleration waveform. Acceleration is greatest *when velocity is undergoing the most rapid change,* which corresponds to maximum displacement in either direction because acceleration was defined in Chapter 1 as the *time-rate change in velocity.* The particle acceleration waveform in Figure 2-10 is shifted relative to both the particle displacement waveform and the particle velocity waveform.[2]

Recall that atmospheric pressure amounts to 100,000 Pa (Nt/m^2) at sea level. As the balloon surface moves outward and inward, the number of molecules per unit volume (density of the medium) changes over time, and **pressure** in the medium is related to the density of the medium. Thus, there will be changes in air pressure that also occur sinusoidally over time. Those changes in pressure take the form of alternate increases and decreases *relative to the resting pressure of 100,000 Pa.*

The pressure waveform is shown at the bottom of Figure 2-10. It reveals that the instantaneous sound pressures also vary sinusoidally. Moreover, we can see that the pressure waveform "mirrors" the particle velocity waveform, and that both are shifted by 90° relative to the particle displacement waveform.

Figure 2-11 shows two sinusoidal waveforms that display pressure as a function of time. The amplitude of wave **A** at 90° is 2 Pa and the amplitude of wave **B** at 90° is 4 Pa. It should be apparent that each sine wave's "pressure" is really many different values of instantaneous pressure that vary sinusoidally over time. In fact, the pressure is only 2 Pa for wave **A** when particle displacement is zero. (See Figure 2-10 for a review of that relationship.)

We will consider, therefore, various alternative metrics that can be used to express *the amplitude of the sine wave.* Although the same metrics will be used in Chapter 5 to express the amplitude of sound waves, such as speech or music, that are not sinusoidal, the equations that we will associate with each metric in this chapter *apply only to the sine wave.* Different equations will be required when we subsequently encounter "complex" waves — that is, waves that are not sinusoidal.

Instantaneous Amplitude (a)

By **instantaneous** amplitude (**a**) we simply mean *the amplitude of the waveform at some specified instant in time or at some specified angle of rotation.* Thus, at 0°, the amplitude of wave **A** is 0 Pa, at 90° it is 2 Pa, and as we shall see a little bit later, at 45° the amplitude is 1.414 Pa, because at 45° the displacement is always 70.7% of maximum (sin 45° = 0.707), and 70.7% of 2 = 1.414.

There are instances in which **instantaneous amplitude** is quite useful, but not generally so, and it never makes sense to specify the instantaneous amplitude without also specifying the corresponding

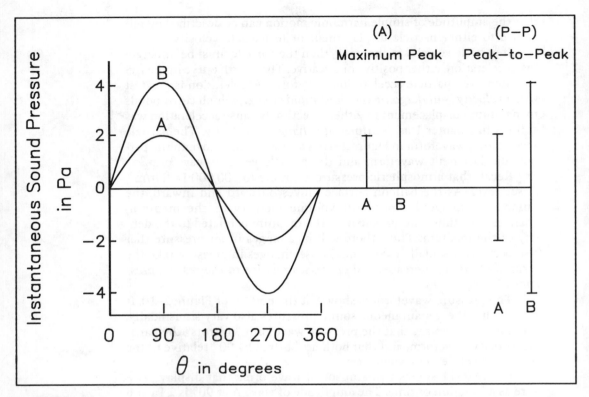

Figure 2–11. Sinusoidal distribution of instantaneous sound pressure for two sound waves of identical frequency that differ in **amplitude**.

angle of rotation or moment in time at which the measurement was taken. Of course, nothing is accomplished by calculating what might be called the **mean instantaneous amplitude** of a sine wave, because for every positive instantaneous amplitude there is a corresponding and exactly equal negative instantaneous amplitude. Therefore the *mean instantaneous amplitude of sine waves normally will be zero* (unless what is called a "dc bias" exists).

Maximum Amplitude (A)

The **maximum** amplitude (**A**), which is sometimes called the "peak amplitude," is *the instantaneous amplitude that corresponds to 90°* (or 270°). Thus wave **A** in Figure 2–11 has a maximal or peak amplitude of 2 Pa and wave **B** has a maximal amplitude of 4 Pa.

Peak-Peak Amplitude

The **peak-peak** amplitude is *the absolute (not algebraic) difference between the maximum amplitude at 90° and 270°*. Thus,

Equation 2.1   Peak-to-Peak = 2P.

For the two sine waves in Figure 2–11, the peak-to-peak values are 4 Pa for Wave **A** and 8 Pa for Wave **B**.

Root-Mean-Square Amplitude (rms)

The **Root-Mean-Square (rms)** amplitude is probably the most common metric that will be encountered for expressing the amplitude of sine waves, but it often seems difficult to achieve an intuitive grasp of what **rms** means. We can achieve an *approximate* understanding of **rms amplitude** by defining it as the *standard deviation of all the instantaneous amplitudes in a sine wave*.

Recall that if we calculate the mean or average of instantaneous amplitudes or pressures, the result is zero (unless there is a dc bias). However, the standard deviation is the square root of the mean of the squared deviations of the instantaneous pressures about their mean of zero. When we square the deviations, we remove the algebraic sign (all values become positive) and the problem is solved.

In Figure 2–12 we show one sinusoidal waveform, and with considerable statistical hazard, we will sample only six of the infinite number of instantaneous amplitudes: +0.50, +1.00, and +0.50 during the positive half of the cycle, and −0.50, −1.00, and −0.50 during the negative half of the cycle. Table 2–1 summarizes the steps that are taken to calculate the standard deviation of any set of numbers (**X**). In this case, the set of numbers is the six instantaneous amplitudes.

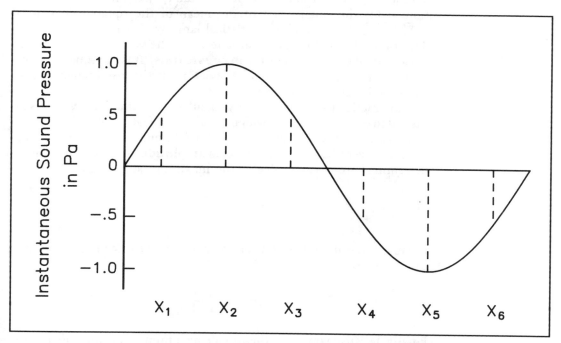

Figure 2–12. Sampling of instantaneous amplitudes to illustrate the concept of **root-mean-square (rms)** amplitude.

Table 2-1. Procedures for calculating the standard deviation

X	$X - \bar{X}$	$(X - \bar{X})^2$
0.50	0.50	0.25
1.00	1.00	1.00
0.50	0.50	0.25
−0.50	−0.50	0.25
−1.00	−1.00	1.00
−0.50	−0.50	0.25
$\Sigma X = 0.00$		$\Sigma(X - \bar{X})^2 = 3.00$
$\Sigma X/N = 0.00$		

$$\sigma^2 = \Sigma(X - \bar{X})^2/N = 0.50$$

$$\sigma = \sqrt{\Sigma(X - \bar{X})^2/N} = 0.707$$

In the calculation, we see that the sum (ΣX) and the mean $(\Sigma X/N)$ of the instantaneous amplitudes are 0.00 (left column). In the second column, the mean of 0.00 is subtracted from each instantaneous amplitude in the first column. Thus, the numbers in the second column are *deviations of the instantaneous amplitudes from the mean*. In the right column each deviation is squared. At the bottom of the right column we see that the sum of the squared deviations $(\Sigma[X - \bar{X}]^2)$ is 3.00.

The next computation shows that the mean of the squared deviations $(\Sigma[X - \bar{X}]^2/N)$ is 0.50. In statistics, that value is called the variance (σ^2) of the distribution of the six numbers (X). The final computation yields the square root of the mean of the squared deviations $(\sqrt{\Sigma[X - \bar{X}]^2/N}$), which in statistical language is called the standard deviation (σ). For this particular sine wave, the value is 0.707. This is one origin of the name **root mean square (rms)**. It is the square *root (r)* of the *mean (m)* of the *squared (s)* deviations of the instantaneous pressures, and, hence, it is the **rms pressure**.

In practice we do not actually calculate the standard deviations of instantaneous amplitudes, which would be a feat of considerable accomplishment because there are an infinite number of them. In fact, with the use of Equation 2.2, the **rms amplitude** *of a sine wave* can be determined from knowledge of the maximum amplitude (A):

Equation 2.2
$$rms = \frac{A}{\sqrt{2}}$$

Because the square root of 2 is a constant equal to 1.414, Equation 2.2 can be rewritten as:

Equation 2.3
$$rms = \frac{A}{(1.414)}$$

Finally, because you can either divide by a number *or multiply by the reciprocal of that number*, Equation 2.3 can be changed to read:

$$\text{rms} = A\left(\frac{1}{1.414}\right)$$

$$= A\,(.707),$$

Equation 2.4

because 0.707 is the reciprocal of 1.414.

Thus to calculate the **rms** amplitude *of a sine wave*, either divide the maximal amplitude by 1.414 (Equation 2.3) or multiply the maximum amplitude by 0.707 (Equation 2.4).[3] What is the unit of measure? The unit of measure of **instantaneous sound pressure** is the pascal. Similarly, the unit of measure of **rms sound pressure** is the pascal. Thus, the **rms pressures** of the two sine waves in Figure 2–11 are 1.414 Pa for wave **A** and 2.828 Pa for wave **B**.

Mean Square Amplitude

Mean Square sound pressure relates to **rms** sound pressure as the variance (σ^2) in statistics relates to the standard deviation (σ). Thus, the variance equals the standard deviation squared and mean square sound pressure equals the rms pressure squared.

$$\text{Because rms} = \frac{A}{\sqrt{2},}$$

$$\text{and because mean square} = \text{rms}^2,$$

$$\text{mean square} = \frac{A^2}{2.}$$

Equation 2.5

Mean square amplitude has some utility for those who are concerned with measurements in mechanical dynamics, but it is not likely to be encountered as a useful metric for acoustics in the speech and hearing literature. It was presented here only to complete the picture of statistical–acoustical equivalents.

Full Wave Rectified Average Amplitude (FW$_{avg}$)

Before we consider the equation for the **full wave rectified average** (**FW$_{avg}$**), it might be useful to discuss briefly what is meant by **rectification**. When you connect some electronic device such as a cassette tape deck into an electrical wall outlet, the recorder receives a sinusoidally alternating electrical current that looks just like (i.e., has the same shape of waveform) the acoustical sine waves we have described. It is called an *alternating* electrical current because during half of its cycle the current is flowing in one direction (+), and during the other half the current is flowing in the opposite direction (−). The frequency of that electrical current is exactly 60 Hz (in the United States), which means it has a period of 0.0167 sec (T = 1/f).

The waveform at the top of Figure 2–13 shows the sinusoidal electrical current that is directed to the cassette player. However, a problem arises because the player cannot function with the alternating current that the power company provides. It must have a direct current, which

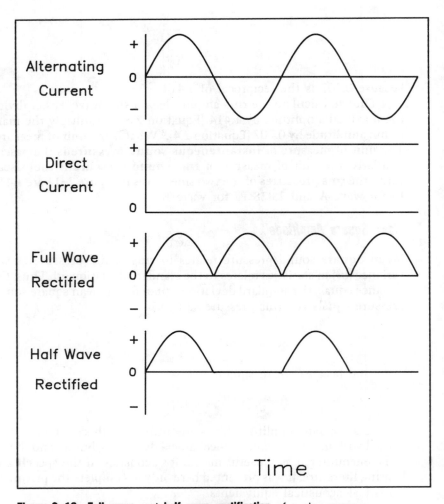

Figure 2–13. Full wave and **half wave rectification** of a sine wave.

is current that flows in only one direction such as you get from a battery. Thus, the alternating electrical current shown at the top of Figure 2–13 must be converted into direct current such as is shown by the second curve in Figure 2–13.

We need not explain all of the steps that are required to accomplish that conversion, but the first step is important for us. In the third curve of the figure, the negative half of each cycle has been "flipped" to become positive. That process is called **full wave rectification**. We learned previously that it makes no sense to calculate the arithmetic mean of the instantaneous amplitudes of the sinusoid because we would obtain precisely the same answer, zero, for all sinusoids regardless of differences in their maximum sound pressure unless a dc bias exists. That circumstance no longer exists with the full wave rectified sinusoid shown in the figure; all of the instantaneous amplitudes are now positive. Suppose, therefore, that we calculate *the arithmetic* *average of all of the instantaneous amplitudes in the rectified wave.* That is defined as the **full wave rectified average (FW$_{avg}$)**.

Fortunately, we do not have to perform such a computation. Instead we can use Equation 2.6:

$$FW_{avg} = 2\frac{A}{\pi}$$

$$= 2\frac{A}{3.1416} \quad \text{(substituting the value of } \pi)$$

$$= A(.636) \quad \text{(dividing 2 by 3.1416).} \qquad \textbf{Equation 2.6}$$

Thus, we see that the **FW$_{avg}$** is almost two-thirds as large as the maximal sound pressure, whereas the **rms** is approximately 70% as large as the maximal pressure.

Half Wave Rectified Average Amplitude (HW$_{avg}$)

The last metric that we will consider is called the **half wave rectified average (HW$_{avg}$)**. In **half wave rectification**, the negative half of each cycle is eliminated rather than flipped to become positive. The bottom curve of Figure 2–13 shows the result. It should be obvious that the average of the instantaneous amplitudes that remain will be exactly half of what was obtained when we calculated the full wave rectified average. Thus,

$$HW_{avg} = \frac{A}{\pi} \qquad \text{(rather than } 2A/\pi)$$

$$= \frac{A}{3.1416}$$

$$= A(.318) \quad \text{(taking the reciprocal of 3.1416).} \qquad \textbf{Equation 2.7}$$

The **FW$_{avg}$** is almost two-thirds as large as the maximal sound pressure, and because **HW$_{avg}$ = 0.5 FW$_{avg}$,** the **HW$_{avg}$** is almost one-third as large as the maximal sound pressure.

Comparisons Among Metrics. The waveform at the top of Figure 2–14 represents a sinusoidal wave that has a maximum amplitude of 4 Pa. Thus, the instantaneous amplitudes vary sinusoidally from a minimum value of −4 Pa through 0 Pa to a maximum value of +4 Pa. The lower portion of the figure shows the **rms** (Equation 2.4), **mean square** (Equation 2.5), **FW$_{avg}$** (Equation 2.6), and **HW$_{avg}$** (Equation 2.7).

It is important to note that whereas the instantaneous amplitudes vary sinusoidally over time, the other metrics are described by straight lines that remain horizontal to the baseline. They do not vary. Suppose we direct the sinusoid to some kind of measuring instrument that has an indicating meter or needle like you might have seen on the VU meter of some tape recorders. If the measuring instrument had been

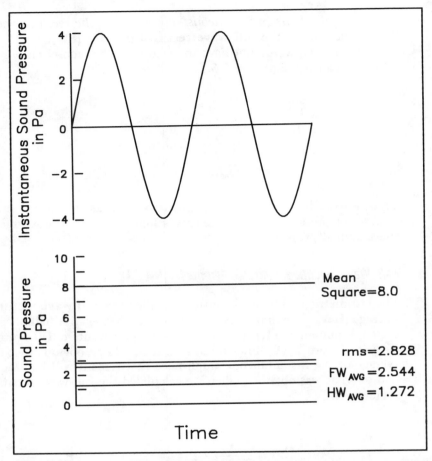

Figure 2–14. Comparison of **mean square, root-mean-square, full-wave rectified average,** and **half-wave rectified average** measures of amplitude of a sine wave.

designed to respond to the instantaneous pressure, it would move back and forth about some average value at a rate corresponding to the frequency of the sinusoid. However, if the instrument had been designed to respond to any of the other measures of amplitude, the needle would remain perfectly stationary — those values remain constant over time because each is time-averaged.

Frequency (f) and Period (T)

The second dimension of the sinusoidal wave is the **frequency** and its reciprocal the **period**. As we learned earlier, frequency is defined as *the rate, in hertz, at which the sinusoid repeats itself.* The period is defined as *the amount of time, in seconds, that is required to complete one cycle.*

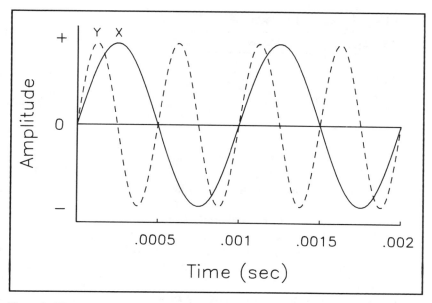

Figure 2-15. Sinusoidal distribution of sound pressure for two sound waves of identical amplitude that differ in **frequency**.

Consider the two sinusoids that are shown in Figure 2-15. Wave **X** has a period of .001 sec, which means that the frequency is 1000 Hz (see Equation 1.12). Wave **Y**, on the other hand, has a period of .0005 sec, and thus its frequency is 2000 Hz. The inverse relationship between frequency and period should be apparent. As frequency is doubled (from 1000 Hz to 2000 Hz), period is halved from .001 sec to .0005 sec.

You might observe that we have to resort to rather cumbersome numbers when the frequency is very large or the period is very small. Suppose, for example, that the frequency were 2,345,129 Hz. If that seems cumbersome to write, think about its period (0.0000004264 sec). Fortunately, we can at least partially avoid such cumbersome expressions by using multiples of **hertz** for frequency and submultiples of **second** for period. The various alternatives that are commonly used to describe both frequency and period are shown in Table 2-2.

We can see from the table that 1 kilohertz (1 kHz) = 1000 Hz, that 1 Megahertz (1 MHz) = 1,000,000 Hz, that 1 MHz also = 1000 kHz, and so on. For period, a msec is 0.001 (one thousandth) sec, a μsec is 0.000001 (one millionth) sec, and so on.

Those multipliers are encountered frequently. Consider your AM radio dial. The AM tuner is designed to receive radio signals with frequencies that range from 550 kHz to 1600 kHz. Thus, if you set your dial to 1560, that means the tuner is adjusted to receive a signal with a frequency of 1560 kHz. (If you happen to be driving [very] near to where the Walhonding and Tuscarawas rivers join to form the Muskingum river, you will be tuned to station WTNS in Coshocton, OH.) However, suppose that you set your FM tuner to 91.2. That does not

Table 2–2. Standard units of measure for frequency and period.

Frequency		Multiplier	Period		Multiplier
Hertz	(Hz)	1	sec	(sec)	1
Kilohertz	(kHz)	1,000	millisec	(msec)	.001
Megahertz	(MHz)	1,000,000	microsec	(μsec)	.000001
Gigahertz	(GHz)	1,000,000,000	nanosec	(nsec)	.000000001

mean 91.2 Hz, but rather it means 91.2 MHz, which is equivalent to 91,200,000 Hz. The FM tuner covers the range from 88 MHz to 108 MHz, and it is more convenient to label the dial in megahertz rather than hertz.

The tuner on your television set receives frequencies that are both below and above the range of frequencies for FM radio stations. VHF (very-high-frequency) tuners range from 54 MHz to 88 MHz (below the FM frequencies) for channels 2 through 6, but from 174 MHz to 216 MHz (above the FM frequencies) for channels 7 through 13. UHF (ultra-high-frequency) tuners lie in a much higher frequency range that extends from 470 MHz to 890 MHz.

In Equations 1.11 and 1.12, we learned that frequency and period are reciprocally related. Thus, to determine period from knowledge of frequency, you simply calculate the reciprocal of frequency ($1/f$) and, correspondingly, to determine frequency from knowledge of period, you calculate the reciprocal of period ($1/T$). If frequency is expressed in hertz and you take the reciprocal, *period will be expressed in seconds*. However, if frequency is expressed in kilohertz, when you calculate the reciprocal, the result for period will be in milliseconds, not seconds. Similarly the reciprocal of frequency in megahertz will be period in microseconds.

Suppose that the frequency of a sinusoid is 2 kHz, but you want to express the corresponding period in *seconds rather than milliseconds*. You must proceed in either of two ways. You can convert 2 kHz to hertz by multiplying by 1000 (see Table 2–2), and the reciprocal of 2000 Hz is .0005 sec. Alternatively, you can calculate the reciprocal of 2 kHz, which is 0.5 msec, and then convert 0.5 msec to seconds by multiplying by 0.001 (see Table 2–2). The answer, of course, is the same — 0.0005 sec.

Determinants of Frequency

We learned earlier that the frequency at which a source of sound vibrates is governed by *properties of the source of sound*. Specifically, the frequency of vibration of some simple harmonic oscillator such as a spring–mass system depends on the **mass** and **stiffness** of the system.

The frequency with which that system oscillates can be called the **natural frequency** of the system. The **natural frequency** is inversely proportional to the square root of the **mass** (frequency decreases as mass increases) and directly proportional to the square root of the stiffness (frequency increases as stiffness increases). For different sources of sound, different properties must be considered. We know, for example, that vibratory frequency of a pendulum depends almost entirely on its length (Equation 1.13). What about the string or wire on a guitar, violin, or piano? In that case, the frequency of vibration depends on the **length, cross-sectional mass,** and **tension** of the string, and the relation of each of those three factors to the *frequency of a vibrating string* is shown in Equation 2.8:

$$f = \frac{1}{2L} \sqrt{\frac{t}{m}},$$

Equation 2.8

where L = length, **t** = tension, and **m** = cross-sectional mass.

We can see that the frequency of vibration of a string increases (1) as length decreases (inversely proportional to twice the length), (2) as tension increases (directly proportional to the square root of tension), or (3) as mass decreases (inversely proportional to the square root of mass). This makes sense if you think about the wires on a piano. Tones of lower frequency are produced by longer and more massive wires (inverse relations). To increase the frequency of vibration of any of the wires, you increase the tension — the same process that you go through when you "tune" any stringed instrument such as a guitar.

The equation for the frequency of a vibrating string is particularly important for those who are interested in voice production, because the frequency of vibration of the vocal folds depends mainly on the length, cross-sectional mass, and tension of the folds. The nature of the proportionalities (direct or inverse) for vocal fold vibration is the same as we just learned for a string.

Other sources of sound depend upon different characteristics. The frequency of a drum's membrane, for example, is directly related to the *tension* of the membrane, but inversely related to its *radius, thickness, and density.* The equations for calculating frequency of vibration of sources such as stretched membranes, bars, and the like, however, are beyond the scope of this book.

Angular Velocity (ω)

There are occasions in which it is useful to describe frequency by reference to what is called **angular velocity**. Before we attempt to define angular velocity, let us consider some alternative ways that *could* be used to express frequency, *although they have not been adopted*. We learned earlier that back and forth vibration is analogous to a point on a turning wheel moving about the circumference of a circle. Consider the circle shown at the left of Figure 2-16. If the reference point **X** moves completely around the circumference of a circle, it has completed 360° of rotation. If the 360° rotation is accomplished in 1 sec, we ordinarily say that the frequency is 1 Hz, and if the rotation is accomplished in 1 msec, we say that the frequency is 1000 Hz or 1 kHz.

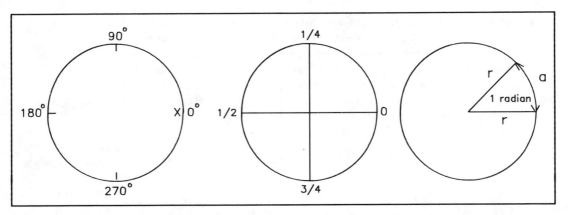

Figure 2–16. An explanation of **angular velocity** in which point **X** moves around the circumference of a circle. At the left, the frequency of rotation of point **X** is represented in "degrees per sec" because the circle is divided into 360 equal parts. At the middle, frequency of rotation is represented in "quarter cycles per sec" because the same circle is divided into only 4 equal parts, rather than 360. At the right, frequency of rotation is represented in "2π radians per sec" because the same circle is divided into 6.2832 equal parts, where 6.2832 equals 2π. See text for an explanation of a radian.

Suppose, instead, that the unit of measure for frequency were *degrees of rotation per second* rather than hertz. If that were the case, we would say that the frequency is "360° per sec" in the first case and "360,000° per sec" in the second. Frequency has *not* been described in that way, but it would be perfectly valid. Of course, it would often result in frequency being described by rather large numbers.

We could try a different approach such as that illustrated in the middle circle in the figure. We might reason that because one cycle consists of *four quarter cycles* (each of which corresponds to 90°), 360° per sec could be expressed as *4 quarter cycles per sec* (dividing 360 by 90), and 360,000° per sec could be expressed as "*4000 quarter cycles per sec.*" With either of these approaches, the full circle of 360° is simply divided into some arbitrary number of segments—360 equal segments to arrive at "degrees per second," and four equal segments to arrive at "quarter cycles per second."

It turns out, of course, that no one has described frequency by dividing the circle into either 360 equal parts, or four equal parts. Instead, *the circle is divided into 6.2832 parts of equal size.* Why 6.2832 parts? One cycle equals 360°, and 360° corresponds to 2π radians, which equals 6.2832 radians (2 x 3.1416). For the circle shown at the right of Figure 2–16, we show one of the 6.2832 possible segments, and it has been drawn to equal 1 radian.

You might read in a geometry textbook that a radian is equal to the angle subtended by an arc whose length is equal to the radius. Stated differently, *an angle equals a radian when the intersection of the two sides of the angle with the circumference yields an arc whose length is exactly equal to the length of the radius.* For the angle shown in the figure, the two sides of the angle are both of equal length and both are the radius (**r**). An arc (**a**) is formed by the intersection of those two radii with the circumference, and the length of the arc **a** equals the length of the radius **r**.

Any circle has 360°, and for any circle there are exactly 2π radians. Because π equals 3.1416, any circle therefore has 6.2832 (2 x 3.1416) radians, and 1 radian corresponds to 57.3° (360° divided by 2π). Another way to conceptualize what is meant by radians is to imagine that we "snip" a circle and then "unroll" it. *Regardless of the size of the circle that we unroll*, the length of the line that we are left with will be *exactly* (to four decimal places) 6.2832 times the length of the radius of the circle, or 3.1416 times the length of the diameter of the circle.

How can radians be used to express frequency? When we used degrees to express frequency, we said that one cycle = 360°, and therefore 1 Hz (cps) corresponds to 360° per sec. In the same vein, because one cycle = 2π radians, 360° per sec corresponds to 2π radians per sec. *When frequency is expressed in radians per sec, the unit of measure is called the **angular velocity** (ω).*

Equation 2.9 shows the relation between angular velocity and frequency:

$$\omega = 2\pi f,$$

Equation 2.9

which means that to determine the angular velocity in radians per second, you simply multiply the frequency in hertz by 2π. Thus, if f = 1 Hz, ω = 6.28 rps (radians per sec), if f = 100 Hz, ω = 628 rps, and if f = 1 kHz, ω = 6,280 rps. In practice, angular velocity is not often used in this way. However, it will be useful to keep angular velocity in mind when we describe the third dimension of the sine wave — **phase**.

Phase

Consider the wheel that is shown in Figure 2–17. This time we have four reference points (A, B, C, & D) rather than one. In terms of the Ferris wheel analogy, four people are seated at 90° intervals, and each is aiming a flashlight at the same wall. The wheel is turning in a counterclockwise direction and the sinusoidal projections from the four sources are shown at the right of the figure. Note, also, that the degrees of rotation that have been used to label the abscissa refer to the course of travel of person **A**, where 0° is the starting point, 90° is 1/4 of the way around the circle, and so on.

The four curves cannot be superimposed upon one another, of course, because the passengers are seated at different locations around the circumference of the wheel. In fact, we could specify their relative positions by reference to degrees of separation. Thus, **B** *leads* **A** (**B** ahead of **A**) by 90°, **C** leads **B** by 90° and **C** leads **A** by 180°, and so on. Just as the position of the passengers could be described in degrees, so could the differences among the four sinusoidal projections. Curve **B** *leads* **A** by 90°, or we could say that curve **A** *lags* curve **B** by 90°; either is perfectly acceptable.

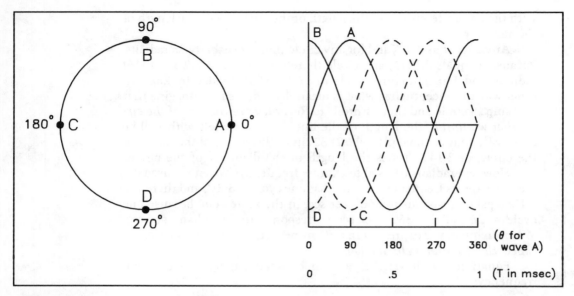

Figure 2–17. An explanation of **starting phase**. At the left, four reference points (A, B, C, and D) are located at different angles, 0°, 90°, 180°, and 270°. When the wheel commences to turn, each point rotates around the circumference with the same amplitude and frequency as the other points. Projections of the sinusoidal motions of the four different points are shown at the right. The only difference among the four functions is the angle of rotation at T_0, which is the **starting phase**.

It is important to remember that all four sinusoids in Figure 2–17 *have exactly the same frequency and exactly the same amplitude*, and that must be the case in this example because there is only one wheel with a fixed circumference (determinant of amplitude), and the rate at which the wheel turns (determinant of frequency) will result in all four reference points rotating with the same frequency.

Starting Phase

Even though the four curves in the figure have the same amplitudes and frequencies, they obviously are different and the difference is in what we can call the **starting phase**. Wave **B** starts at 90°, whereas wave **A** starts at 0°, wave **C** starts at 180°, and wave **D** starts at 270°. By **starting phase** we refer to the *displacement, in degrees, from 0° at the instant the vibration, or rotation, begins*. The four curves in the figure all have different starting phases.

Phase Angle: Instantaneous Phase

We can also speak of **phase angle**, and in this case similarities or differences in frequency are irrelevant. With starting phase, we referred to what can be called **time zero**, a reference time where displacement commenced. The **phase angle**, which also is called the **instantaneous**

phase, is the *angle of rotation at any specified moment in time.* Thus, at t = 0.5 msec in Figure 2–17 the **phase angles** are 180° for **A**, 270° for **B**, 360° for **C**, and 90° for **D**. **D** has a starting phase of 270° and therefore leads **A** by 270°, and that separation will always remain because **D** and **A** rotate with the same frequency. This contrasts with what we saw in Figure 2–15 that displayed two sine waves with different frequencies.

When the frequencies are different, the two waves will move in and out of phase rather than maintain a constant phase separation, even though the starting phases of the two waves happened to be the same. We will capitalize on this concept in Chapter 8 when the phenomenon of **beats** is described.

Phase angles also can be described in radians rather than degrees. Recall that a circle has 360° and 2π radians. The relation between these two for describing phase angle is shown in Figure 2–18. If 360° corresponds to 2π radians, then 0° = 0 radians, 90° = π/2 (1/4 of 2π), 180° = π (1/2 of 2π), and 270° = 3π/2 (3/4 of 2π).

Another Application of Radians

Those who elect to study **psychoacoustics**, a branch of science that is concerned with *psychological correlates* of the physical dimensions of sound waves, will almost certainly encounter instances in which phase angle is described in radians.

Imagine the following experiment. A sinusoid is presented to a listener who is wearing a pair of earphones. The signal will be delivered simultaneously to both ears. Thus, the frequency and the amplitude of the signal will be the same in both ears.

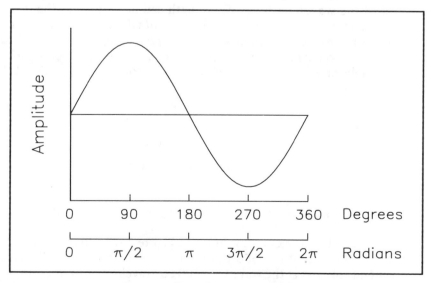

Figure 2–18. The relation between **instantaneous phase** expressed in **degrees** and in **radians**.

Suppose, that in one portion of the experiment the *starting phase* of the signal is exactly the same in the left ear as in the right ear. The two signals are said to be *in phase* because there is no difference in phase angle. That condition could be called S_0, which means that the *difference* in phase angle of the signals (S) between the two ears is 0 radians.

In a second portion of the experiment, suppose that the starting phase of the signal in the left ear is 0°, but the starting phase of the signal in the right ear is 180°. Curves **A** and **C** in Figure 2–17 are examples of this condition. The two signals are obviously out of phase by exactly 180°. Because 180° corresponds to π radians, that circumstance can be called S_π (see Figure 2–18).

Wavelength (λ)

The final dimension of the sinusoidal wave is called the **wavelength**. In the course of our discussion of sound to this point, we have described two quantities that are measured by reference to *time*. One quantity is **frequency**, which was described as the rate at which the sinusoid repeats itself and is measured in cycles per second or hertz. Frequency is determined by characteristics of the sound source.

The second quantity is **speed of sound**, which is the rate at which a disturbance is propagated through the medium and is measured in feet per second (**fps**), meters per second (**MKS**), or centimeters per second (**cgs**). Propagation speed is determined by the elasticity and density of the transmitting medium.

The fourth and final dimension of the sine wave shows the relation between the two quantities, frequency and propagation speed; it is called the **wavelength** (λ). Wavelength can be defined as the *distance traveled by a sine wave during one period of vibration*, or as the *distance between two identical points (identical phase angles) on two adjacent cycles*. Wavelength is directly proportional to the speed of sound and inversely proportional to frequency, as is shown by Equation 2.10:

Equation 2.10

$$\lambda = \frac{s}{f,}$$

where λ is wavelength in meters,

f is frequency in hertz,

and

s is the speed of sound in meters per second.

Consider the examples shown in Figure 2–19 where two sinusoids (f = 1100 Hz and f = 550 Hz) travel in two different media, air and water. Look first at the wave f = 1100 Hz traveling in air. Its period (**1/f**) is 0.9 msec. After 1 sec has elapsed, the wave will have traveled 340 m (assuming the speed of sound is 340 m/sec). Therefore, during just one

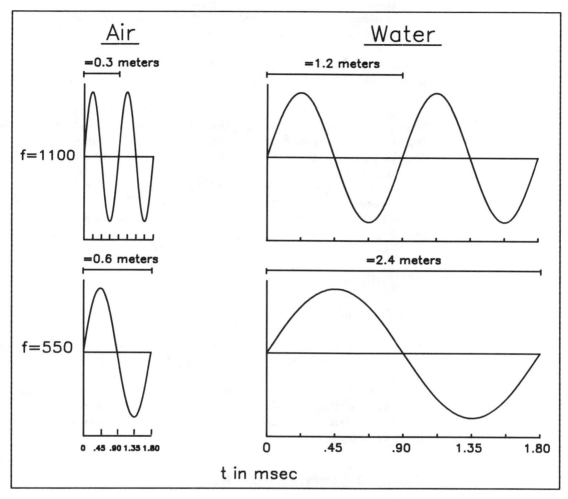

Figure 2-19. An illustration of the dependence of **wavelength** on both frequency and speed of sound wave propagation. Comparison of the two functions within a column (left for air; right for water) shows how wavelength varies with frequency when speed of propagation is held constant. Comparison of the two functions within a row (top for 1100 Hz; bottom for 550 Hz) shows how wavelength varies with speed of propagation when frequency is held constant.

period it will have traveled only 1/1,100 of that distance, which is 0.3 m. That is the distance traveled during one period, which is a definition of wavelength, and that is the answer we would obtain with Equation 2.10: $\lambda = 340/1,100 = 0.3$m.

Compare that outcome with what we would obtain if f = 550 Hz in air. The speed of sound is still 340 m/sec, which means that the sinusoid will still travel 340 m in 1 sec. However, the period now is 1.8 msec. During that 1.8 msec (one period), the wave will have traveled 0.6 m.

What happens when the same sine waves are propagated through water? For convenience, we will treat the speed of sound in water as if it were four times the speed in air (1,360 m/sec), which is a reasonable approximation. When f = 1100 Hz, the wave will travel 1,360 m in 1 sec, the period is still 0.9 msec, and the distance traveled during 1 period will be four times as great (1.2 meters). If f = 550 Hz, the wavelength will be increased from 0.6 m in air to 2.4 m in water. Thus, we see that wavelength is directly proportional to the speed of sound and inversely proportional to its frequency.

The period of most sound waves that are likely to be encountered is typically very small. For example, the period of the vocal fold wave during vowel production by an average adult male is only about 10 msec and the period for the average adult female is just a little over 4 msec. However, the wavelengths of those sounds in air are relatively large — about 1.5 m (5 ft) for the female and about 3 m (10 ft) for the male. In other words, one complete cycle of vibration will span a distance of about 1.5 m for the vowel produced by the female and 3.0 m for the vowel produced by the male.

■ DAMPING

When the vibratory motions of, for example, a simple spring–mass system were presented in Chapter 1, and when sine waves were described early in this chapter, each cycle of (sinusoidal) motion was represented as being identical in every respect to every other cycle. That representation is appropriate when the sine wave is conceptualized from a strict mathematical perspective *and when there is no opposition to motion*. However, oscillating systems do encounter opposition to motion in the form of **friction**, or **frictional resistance**, and **friction** serves to limit **velocity**.

Review of Simple Harmonic Motion

When amplitude of vibration diminishes over time, the oscillations, or vibrations, are said to be **damped**. To further our understanding of damping, it might be helpful to review and expand on some of the characteristics of vibratory motion described previously.

A spring–mass system, or other simple harmonic oscillator, vibrates sinusoidally. In Figure 2–20 we see that the amplitude of **displacement** (dashed line) of the system varies sinusoidally over time. In accordance with Hooke's law, the restoring force of **elasticity** also varies sinusoidally over time. The magnitude of the restoring force of elasticity is directly proportional to the magnitude of displacement. Elasticity is *in phase* with displacement and, hence, the sinusoidally varying elastic force is shown by the same dashed line that is used to describe displacement.

Velocity (solid line) also changes sinusoidally over time, and as you recall, velocity *leads* displacement by 90°. Also recall that whereas velocity leads displacement by 90°, velocity *lags* **acceleration** (dotted line) by 90°, and acceleration is 180° out of phase with displacement. As the

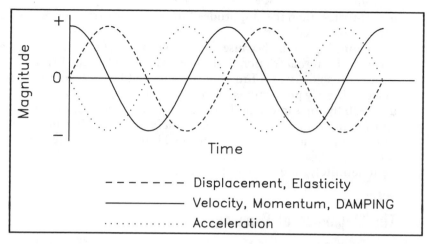

Figure 2–20. The relations among sinusoidal waveforms for **displacement, elasticity, velocity, momentum, damping (frictional resistance)**, and **acceleration**.

mass of the system moves from maximum displacement toward equilibrium, acceleration increases because of the restoring force of elasticity, the velocity of motion increases, and the system gains **momentum**.

Because **momentum** is given by the product of **mass** and **velocity** ($M = mc$; Equation 1.9), momentum is directly proportional to velocity of motion. Momentum also varies sinusoidally over time, and momentum is *in phase* with velocity. Thus, momentum is shown by the same solid line that is used to represent velocity. Because momentum is in phase with velocity, elasticity is in phase with displacement, and velocity leads displacement by 90°, we can see that momentum also *leads* the restoring force of elasticity by 90°. Therefore, momentum is greatest when velocity is greatest, and velocity is greatest when displacement is zero (i.e., when the vibrating mass is passing through the equilibrium point), and the force of elasticity is zero when displacement is zero.

Effects of Friction on Vibratory Motion

Once energy is imparted to an object, vibratory motion would continue indefinitely with no decrement in amplitude over time if there is no opposition to motion. However, because **frictional resistance** serves to limit velocity, vibratory motion is prevented from continuing indefinitely.

The amplitude of vibration of the mass diminishes over time, and the vibrations are therefore **damped**. The same is true of the child's swing in the park and all other forms of vibratory motion. One push is sufficient to cause the swing and child to move to and fro, but because of friction, the amplitude of each successive excursion (displacement) is slightly less than the amplitude of the previous excursion, and **damping** has occurred.

Damping occurs because of the **resistance** of the air medium and because of internal friction within an oscillating system. Damping also varies sinusoidally as a function of time, and because frictional resistance is directly proportional to velocity, damping is represented in Figure 2–20 by the same solid line that is used to represent both velocity and momentum. Thus, as velocity increases, damping increases because the kinetic energy is transformed into thermal energy (heat). Because of the loss of energy due to damping, free vibrations do not continue indefinitely, and the amplitude of vibration diminishes over time.

The Magnitude of Damping

How long will the vibrations of a damped system continue? We learned earlier that the magnitude of the *initial* displacement of the mass depends upon the magnitude of force applied. Therefore, it should make sense that the duration of vibratory motion depends on the *amount of damping present* relative to the *magnitude of the force applied*. Thus, the duration of vibrations is directly proportional to the force applied and inversely proportional to damping.

Vibratory systems are not all characterized by the same amount of damping. In systems that are **low damped**, the vibrations last for a relatively long time. A tuning fork is a good example of a low-damped system. Energy is imparted to the fork by striking it, and once struck, it might continue to vibrate freely for several seconds, depending, of course, on the force with which it was struck. In contrast, in systems that are **high damped**, the vibrations are very brief and there is a steep decrement in the amplitude of vibration over time.

Figure 2–21 displays examples of the vibrations of a "lossless" system (panel A), a theoretical concept in which no damping exists, and also of low-damped (panel B) and high-damped (panel C) systems. We can see that in a low-damped system, the amplitude diminishes fairly gradually over time. In a high-damped system, the vibrations last for only a brief period of time and the decrement in amplitude is steep.

The Damping Factor

Regardless of whether we are considering low-damped or high-damped systems, the *ratio of the amplitudes (A) of any two consecutive cycles of vibration is a constant*. Thus, for example, in the low-damped system, $A_1/A_2 = A_2/A_3 = A_3/A_4$, and so forth. We will learn in Chapter 3 that *constant ratios* can be expressed logarithmically. For that reason, the *magnitude of damping* (the **damping factor**), which we will symbolize as d_f, is given by what is called the natural log ($\log_e$ or ln) of the ratio of the amplitudes of any two consecutive cycles:

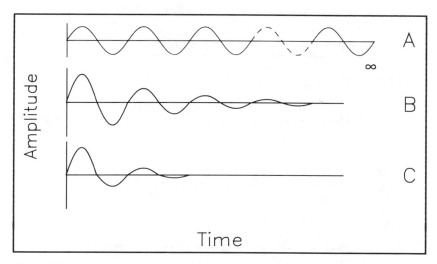

Figure 2–21. Illustrations of **damping** that occurs because of resistance to motion.

$$d_f = \ln\left(\frac{A_1}{A_2}\right).$$

Equation 2.11

Figure 2–22 shows examples of vibration resulting from five systems with different damping factors d_f. For convenience of computation, $A_1 = 1$ (in arbitrary units). The values of A_2 decrease progressively from 0.5 units to 0.0625 units for the first four examples in panels A through D, and a constant ratio of 2:1 is preserved between the amplitudes of any two consecutive cycles. As the amplitude decreases, the damping factor increases from 0.693 (a relatively low-damped system) to 2.77 (a relatively high-damped system).

After completing the review of logarithms and antilogarithms in Chapter 3, the interested reader might return to this discussion of damping. It should then be apparent that because we have seen that a constant ratio of 2:1 is preserved between the amplitudes of any two consecutive cycles, the damping factor increases linearly in equal (if you carry the calculation to sufficient decimal places) log units of 0.69315 because a constant ratio of 2:1 is preserved and the natural log of 2 is 0.69315.

In a theoretically lossless system, $d_f = 0$, because the ratio of any two amplitudes would equal one, and the log of 1 (regardless of the base) equals 0. The lowest curve in panel E of Figure 2–22 shows what is called **critical damping**. In this case, the system is displaced and then returns to equilibrium, but not beyond.

Examples of Damped Systems

We are all familiar with practical examples of damped systems in our daily lives. For example, shock absorbers on cars are usually designed to

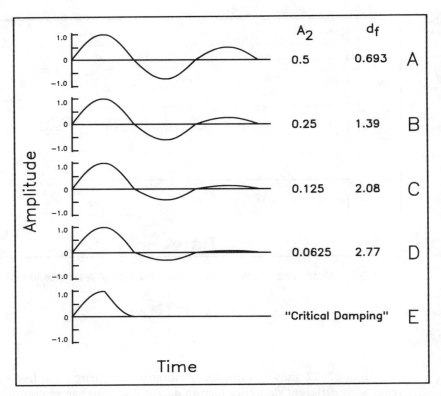

Figure 2–22. Examples of waveforms with different damping factors that range from 0.693 to 2.77 to what is called **critical damping**.

give critical damping (or nearly so) so that the car will not bounce up and down excessively. Of course, as the shock absorbers wear out, they become underdamped and the car will tend to bounce up and down several times when it hits a bump.

Another example is the level indicator, or needle, on a VU meter of a tape recorder. It too is typically designed to be close to critically damped. If underdamped, the needle would swing back and forth on either side of the "correct value" before finally settling down. On the other hand, if the needle is overdamped, too much time would be required for the needle to reach the correct value, and the rapid changes in the level of signals such as speech or music could not be detected.

■ **ACOUSTIC IMPEDANCE**

The tuning fork, pendulum, and simple spring–mass system introduced in Chapter 1 all engage in simple harmonic motion. Moreover, they all engage in what is called **free vibration**, and each system vibrates at its own **natural frequency**.

By **free vibrations** we mean that once energy is imparted to a body that has a low **damping factor**, it vibrates *freely* for some considerable period of time, and no additional outside force is required to urge the continued vibrations. Thus, once an external force is applied to a system and vibration is initiated, the only force that is operating is the restoring force of **elasticity** (except for the pendulum, where the restoring force is gravity).

What will be the frequency of vibration? The **natural frequency** of a simple harmonic oscillator is dependent upon the **mass** and the **stiffness** of the system. Specifically, the natural frequency of a system is *directly proportional to the square root of its stiffness and inversely proportional to the square root of its mass*. Thus, if the **natural frequency** of a system were 200 Hz and its stiffness were increased by a factor of 4:1, the **natural frequency** would *increase* by a factor of 2:1 (square root of 4) to a frequency of 400 Hz. If, instead, the mass of that same system were increased by a factor of 4:1, the natural frequency would **decrease** by a factor of 2:1 to a frequency of 100 Hz.

We know, of course, that **free vibrations** will not continue indefinitely. The oscillations will be damped because of **resistance**. There is no such thing as perpetual motion because forces exist that oppose or **impede** all motion.

Resistance (R)

All motion is opposed by **resistance (R)**, and resistance contributes to, but is not synonymous with, what is called **acoustic impedance**. We may think of acoustic impedance as the *total opposition to motion*. In other words, there are forces in addition to resistance that help determine the total opposition to motion, which is the **impedance**.

We have learned previously that because **friction** opposes or resists motion, it serves to limit the velocity of motion. Energy is transformed from **kinetic energy** to **thermal energy** (heat). Importantly, **resistance**, which is measured in units called **ohms**, *is independent of frequency*. Thus, a given magnitude of resistance provides a specified opposition to motion of a system, regardless of the frequency with which that system oscillates. There are, however, additional forces that oppose motion of an elastic system *in a frequency selective way*. Those forces are called **reactance forces** or, simply, **reactances**.

Reactance (X)

When a force is applied to a simple harmonic oscillator, some of the energy associated with the applied force is converted to thermal energy because of resistance. However, some of the energy that is applied to a system is *stored in the elastic system as potential energy* (**PE**). The component of a system that is responsible for storage of energy is called **reactance**.

Reactance opposes motion, but in a way that is very different from the opposition to motion attributable to **resistance**. In the case of resistance, *energy is dissipated.* In the case of reactance, *energy is stored.* Thus, we can say that the **impedance** of a system has two components: an *energy-dissipating component* called **resistance** and an *energy-storage component* called **reactance.**

Resistance, the energy-dissipating component of impedance, *is independent of frequency.* Reactance, the energy-storage component of impedance, *is frequency dependent.* We shall see, subsequently, that the total opposition to motion, the **acoustic impedance**, is the complex sum of frequency-independent resistance and frequency-dependent reactance.

The opposition to motion in frequency-selective ways, the reactance, depends upon the **mass** and **compliance** of the system. Although a system's **mass** and **compliance** both serve to oppose or impede motion, they do so in opposite ways. To explain this, it will be helpful to return to Figure 2–20 and review the phasic relations among displacement, velocity, acceleration, and so forth. The following phasic relations are important for understanding impedance.

1. **Resistance,** which is independent of frequency, is *in phase with velocity;*
2. **Compliance** (elasticity), which is frequency dependent, *lags resistance by 90°;*
3. **Mass,** which is proportional to acceleration and also frequency dependent, *leads resistance by 90°;* and it follows that:
4. **Mass** *is 180° out of phase with compliance.*

Reactance has two components. One is called the **mass reactance** (**X$_m$**) and the other is called the **compliant reactance** (**X$_c$**). Some writers refer to compliant reactance as **elastic reactance.** The two components of reactance, mass reactance and compliant reactance, always act in opposition to one another. When one is storing energy, the other is giving it up.

Mass Reactance (X$_m$)

The magnitude of **mass reactance** (**X$_m$**), which is measured in **ohms**, is given by:

Equation 2.12

$$X_m = 2\pi fm,$$

where **f** is frequency; **m** is the effective mass,

and

2π is a constant.

Recall that $2\pi f$ defines the angular velocity (ω). Therefore it is equally appropriate to say that **mass reactance** is given by the product of angular velocity and mass. **Mass reactance** (**X$_m$**) *is directly proportional to frequency* and is essentially negligible at very low frequencies.

However, for each octave increase in frequency $(f_2 = 2f_1)$, mass reactance *increases* by a factor of 2:1. Hence, mass reactance contributes to the frequency-dependent nature of impedance.

Compliant Reactance (X_c)

The magnitude of **compliant reactance** (X_c), which also is measured in **ohms**, is given by:

$$X_c = \frac{1}{2\pi fc,}$$

Equation 2.13

where **c** is the compliance.

Compliant reactance also can be defined as the reciprocal of the product of compliance and angular velocity, and as we can see in Equation 2.13, *compliant reactance is inversely proportional to frequency.* Thus, compliant reactance also contributes to the frequency-dependent nature of impedance.

Whereas mass reactance is negligible at low frequencies, **compliant reactance** is quite large at low frequencies. For each octave increase in frequency, the **compliant reactance** *decreases* by a factor of 2:1.

When $X_m = X_c$, the two opposing reactances cancel one another (because they are 180° out of phase), and the only opposition to motion is resistance. When that circumstance exists with a free vibrating, simple harmonic oscillating system, the frequency at which the two opposing forces cancel one another defines the **natural frequency** with which the system will vibrate.

Impedance (Z)

Resistance causes energy to be dissipated, whereas **mass reactance** and **compliant reactance** cause energy to be stored. Although all three factors serve to oppose motion and the transfer of energy, we cannot add their respective magnitudes algebraically to determine the total opposition (**impedance**) because the three components are not in phase: X_m (**mass reactance**) leads R (**resistance**) by 90°; X_c (**compliant reactance**) lags R by 90°; and X_m **leads** X_c by 180°.

Because the three components of impedance are not in phase with one another, they must be treated as vector-like quantities called **phasor quantities**, or just **phasors**, but the mathematics are the same as for vector solution. Consider the phase diagrams in Figure 2–23. In panel A, we show only **mass reactance** (X_m) and **resistance** (R). Mass reactance leads resistance by 90°, and the two quantities are drawn at right angles to one another. The resultant **impedance** (Z) **vector**, which is shown by the dashed line, is determined by the use of Pythagoras' theorem, just as we learned to do with the velocity (Equation 1.2) in Chapter 1:

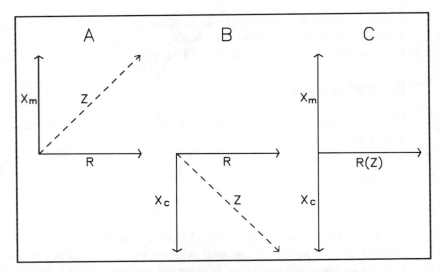

Figure 2–23. Phase diagrams that show the **impedance vectors** resulting from **mass reactance** and **resistance** in panel A, **compliant reactance** and **resistance** in panel B, and **mass reactance, compliant reactance,** and **resistance** in panel C.

Equation 2.14
$$Z = \sqrt{R^2 + X_m^2},$$

where **R** is the resistance,

and

X_m is the mass reactance.

In panel B, we show only **compliant reactance** (X_c) and **resistance** (**R**), but of course in this case, compliant reactance lags resistance by 90°. Again, the impedance (**Z**) vector is shown by the dashed line, and the resultant impedance is given by:

Equation 2.15
$$Z = \sqrt{R^2 + X_c^2},$$

where X_c is the compliant reactance.

In panel C, all three components of **impedance** (**R, X_m,** and X_c) are included with the appropriate phasic relations. The impedance vector is now given by:

Equation 2.16
$$Z = \sqrt{R^2 + (X_m - X_c)^2}.$$

Thus, **acoustic impedance (Z)**, which is expressed in **ohms**, may be defined as *the square root of the sum of the square of the resistance* (**R**) *and the square of the reactance* (**X**). In the case of the specific example that is shown in panel C in Figure 2–23, $X_m = X_c$, the two components of reactance cancel, and **Z = R**. As we learned previously, the frequency at which $X_m = X_c$ defines the **natural frequency** of the sys-

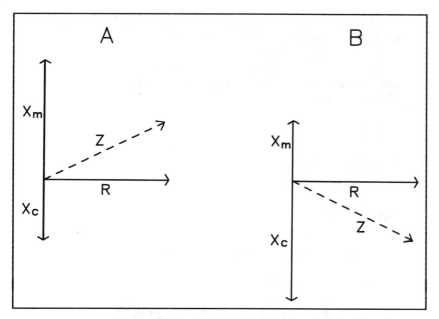

Figure 2–24. Phase diagrams that show the **impedance vectors** that result from all three components of impedance. In panel A, **mass reactance** is dominant, and in panel B, **compliant reactance** is dominant.

tem. In Chapter 6, we will learn to say that when $X_m = X_c$ (the two reactance components equal one another), *the system is "in resonance."*

Panel A of Figure 2–24 shows a phase diagram in which $X_m > X_c$. In this case, the contribution of mass reactance to impedance is greater than the contribution of compliant reactance. The opposite relation $X_c > X_m$ is shown in panel B of the figure.[4] You should also note that in those two instances, **impedance** is not determined exclusively by **resistance**. The **reactance** components also contribute to the total opposition to motion, the **impedance**. When $X_m = X_c$, **impedance** (**Z**) is at its minimum.

■ SUMMARY

We have seen that simple harmonic oscillators engage in sinusoidal motion. Once a force is applied to such an oscillator, it engages in free vibration. The waveform has four dimensions of interest: amplitude, frequency (and period), phase, and wavelength. Finally, we have learned that free vibrations of a system do not last indefinitely because of opposition to motion from friction. The amplitudes decay over time, and those vibrations are called damped vibrations. The total opposition to motion or energy transfer is called impedance, and impedance has two components, resistance and reactance (mass reactance and compliant reactance).

Chapter 4 will concern the use of **decibels** to express the "magnitude" of a sound wave. To understand the decibel requires knowledge of logs and antilogs. Readers who feel comfortable with those concepts might wish to move directly to Chapter 4. For those who would profit from a review, Chapter 3 contains a detailed description of logs and antilogs.

■ PRACTICE PROBLEMS

Set 1

1. If rms $= A/\sqrt{2}$, A must then $=$?

2. If $A =$ rms(1.414), then rms must $=$?

3. Given rms, write the equation for peak-to-peak.

4. Solve for rms sound pressure for each of the following values of peak sound pressure.

    a. 1.0   b. 1.5   c. 0.6   d. 3.8

5. Solve for peak-to-peak sound pressure for each of the following values of rms sound pressure.

    a. .707   b. 1.0   c. 3.5

6. Solve for rms sound pressure that corresponds to each of the following peak-to-peak values.

    a. 1.0   b. 1.414   c. 10   d. 2.0   e. 18   f. x

7. Given a sinusoid with a maximum amplitude of 5 volts (where voltage is an electrical analog to acoustic pressure), solve for:

    a. rms $=$ b. P $-$ P $=$ c. mean square $=$
    d. FW$_{avg}$ $=$ e. HW$_{avg}$ $=$ f. A $=$

8. For each tenfold increase in maximum amplitude, rms increases by a factor of:

9. For each twofold increase in maximum amplitude, the full-wave rectified average increases by a factor of:

10. If rms increases by a factor of two,

    a. mean square increases by a factor of:
    b. the full-wave rectified average increases by a factor of:

11. If rms voltage were increased from 10 volts to 100 volts, mean square voltage would increase by a factor of:

12. Under what condition will rms equal mean square?

13. If $FW_{avg} = 2A/\pi$, then $HW_{avg} = $:

14. If $HW_{avg} = 1.3$, $FW_{avg} = $:

15. If rms = 1.5V, mean square = :

16. If rms increases by a factor of N, mean square increases by a factor of:

Set 2

1. If the period of a sinusoid is 150 msec, f = :

2. If 1.5 cycles are completed within 5 msec, f = :

3. Calculate f, in Hz, for each period:

    a. .002 sec   b. 3 msec   c. 1,000 μsec

4. Calculate T, in msec, for each frequency.

    a. 400 Hz   b. 800 Hz   c. 100 Hz   d. 500 Hz   e. 8000 Hz

5. Calculate f, in kHz, for each of the following.

    a. 100 Hz   b. .002 sec   c. 1 MHz   d. 5 msec

6. Draw a sinusoidal pressure function (instantaneous pressure) where f = 1000 Hz and rms sound pressure = 1.414 Pa. Label both coordinates.

7. Draw a function that shows the distribution of rms sound pressure as a function of time for a sinusoid with a frequency of 500 Hz and a maximum sound pressure of 0.707 Pa.

■ ANSWERS TO PRACTICE PROBLEMS

Set 1

1. rms $(\sqrt{2}\,)$; or rms(1.414); or rms/0.707

2. A/1.414; or A(.707)

3. 2 $(rms\sqrt{2}\,)$; or 2(rms × 1.414); or 2(rms/0.707)

4. a. 0.707   b. 1.06   c. 0.42   d. 2.69

5. a. 2   b. 2.828   c. 9.9

6. a. 0.35   b. 0.50   c. 3.5   d. 0.707   e. 6.36   f. .5x (.707)

7. a. 3.53   [Given by 5 × 0.707]
   b. 10   [Given by 5 × 2]
   c. 12.5   [Given by $A^2/2$]
   d. 3.18   [Given by $2A/\pi$; or A(.636)]
   e. 1.59   [Given by A/π; or A(.318)]
   f. 5   [Given]

8. 10

9. 2

10. a. 4   b. 2

11. 100

12. rms = 1   [Because mean square = rms^2, and 1^2 = 1.]

13. A/π

14. 2.6

15. 2.25V

16. N^2

Set 2

1. 6.67 Hz

2. 300 Hz   [Note that 1.5 cycles is to 5 msec as 1 cycle is to X msec. This is generally noted in the form 1.5/5 : 1/X. This equation then is solved by cross-multiplication: 1.5X = 5/1; X = 3.33 msec. Therefore, if T = 3.33 msec, f = 1/3.33 = .3 kHz = 300 Hz]

3. a. 500   b. 333   c. 1000

4. a. 2.5   b. 1.25   c. 10   d. 2   e. 0.125

5. a. 0.1   b. 0.5   c. 1000   d. 0.2

6.

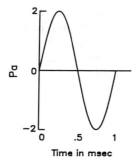

Time in msec

7.

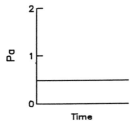

Time

■ NOTES

1. Those who are familiar with calculus will understand that the particle velocity curve in Figure 2–10 is shifted relative to the particle displacement curve because velocity is the first derivative of displacement.
2. The relations between acceleration and displacement or velocity exist because acceleration is the first derivative of velocity and the second derivative of displacement.
3. These equations provide an approximate, but perfectly acceptable, *estimate* of the **rms** sound pressure of sine waves. Precise calculations of the **rms** pressure require knowledge of calculus, which is beyond the scope of this book. For the interested reader, however, the defining equation for **rms** is

$$\text{rms} = \sqrt{\frac{1}{T}\int_0^T x(t)^2 dt} \quad,$$

where **x(t)** is the time-domain waveform, **T** is the period, and the integral sign $(\int)$ indicates summation of an infinite number of instantaneous amplitudes during one period (one cycle) of the wave. For our purposes and for all practical purposes that most readers will encounter, Equation 2.4 will suffice for calculating the **rms sound pressure** for sine waves.
4. Impedance is, of course, a vector-like quantity called a phasor. Solution of Equation 2.16 reveals the *length* of the impedance vectors

in Figure 2–24. However, the impedance vector in each panel of the figure also must reflect the appropriate phase angle, θ. The phase angle of impedance is given by $\theta = \mathbf{arctan\ [(X_m - X_c)/R]}$, which is the same as $\theta = \mathbf{tan^{-1}\ (X/R)}$. $\mathbf{Tan^{-1}}$ is the same as **arctan**, and $\mathbf{tan^{-1}}$ is likely to be the label that you will find on your pocket calculator.

Logarithms and Antilogarithms

In Chapter 2 we learned that the magnitude, or amplitude, of a sine wave can be expressed by reference to its sound pressure in newtons per square meter or pascals. However, most of the time the magnitude of the sine wave is described by what is known as the decibel (dB). It is apparent from reading popular literature such as newspapers and magazine articles and, unfortunately, even from reading some professional papers, that the decibel is sometimes used incorrectly and apparently is often misunderstood. We will consider the decibel (actually the decibels) in detail in Chapter 4, but because decibel notation requires a facility with logarithms (logs) and antilogarithms (antilogs), those concepts will be reviewed here.

■ THE CONCEPT OF LOGARITHMS AND ANTILOGARITHMS

Some readers might not know the answers to the two antilog problems below:

$$\text{antilog}_2 \ 2 = \underline{\hspace{2cm}} \ ?$$

or

$$\text{antilog}_{10} \ 2 = \underline{\hspace{2cm}} \ ?$$

However, almost everyone will know the answers to the next two problems, which might appear to be easier to understand and solve:

$$2^2 = \underline{\hspace{2cm}} \ ?$$
$$10^2 = \underline{\hspace{2cm}} \ ?$$

Actually, the two sets of problems are equal in difficulty because the second set is identical to the first. If you know that $2^2 = 4$ and that $10^2 = 100$, the *concept* of antilogs will be easily understood. The reason for that assurance lies in the following statement of equivalence:

$$\text{antilog}_2 \ 2 = \ 2^2 = 4$$

and

$$\text{antilog}_{10} \ 2 = \ 10^2 = 100.$$

In other words, asking, "$\text{antilog}_{10} \ 2 = \ ?$" is identical to asking, "What is 10 raised to the second power, or, more simply, what is 10 squared?" The concept of *any* antilog problem is no more difficult than that, and all that remains is to learn some simple steps that make it possible to solve problems that are computationally, but not conceptually, more difficult. For example, it will not be immediately obvious that:

$$\text{antilog}_{10} \ 1.7 = 50.12,$$

but the fact remains that asking, "$\text{antilog}_{10} \ 1.7 = \ ?$" is identical to asking, "what is 10 raised to the 1.7 power?"

We shall see subsequently that the *concept* of logarithms is as easy to grasp as the concept of antilogs. However, before proceeding to some computational details, it will be helpful to review "scales of measurement" briefly.

■ SCALES OF MEASUREMENT

The word "measurement" describes a process whereby *numerals* are assigned to objects according to specific rules. The word "numerals" was emphasized, because, as we shall see, it is important to distinguish between numerals and numbers. A **numeral** is a symbol such as 8, 25, III, A, and so forth. In contrast, a **number** is a symbol that bears some fixed relationship to other symbols. For example, the numbers 12 and 13 will always sum to the number 25, whereas the numerals 12 and 13 are nothing but names or designators — they cannot be added or manipulated in other mathematical ways. The importance of distinguishing between numerals and numbers should become more clear as we review the various scales of measurements that are available to us.

We can speak of four different scales of measurement: **nominal, ordinal, interval,** and **ratio** (Stevens, 1951).[1] Before any measurement is undertaken, we should be careful to determine which type of scale applies.

Nominal Scale

With the **nominal** scale, we can sort things into different categories by observing that one object is the *same* as or *different* from another. That is the only requirement. For example, we could sort according to two categories of male/female, adult/child, fruit/vegetable, basic/derived quantities, 1s/0s, and so forth, or according to three categories of beef/pork/poultry, or whatever. Within each category, then, we simply count the number of objects that belong: 6 male/14 female, 13 adults/7 children, and so on. This is not a very powerful scale because, basically, the only arithmetic operation that can be performed legitimately on the entries in the categories is to count them.

Ordinal Scale

With the **ordinal** scale, we still can say that two or more things are different, but we also can say that one object has *more or less* of (or the same as) some quantity than another object. Thus, with the familiar letter grades that often are used to describe performance or achievement, we are accustomed to saying that:

$$A > B > C > D > F.$$

In such a scale, we have an implicit ordering of the letters, but *the letters are not numbers and they cannot legitimately be added or subtracted.* We know that A exceeds B, but we do not know by how much A exceeds B. Of equal importance, we have no guarantee that A exceeds B by the same amount that B exceeds C. We often assign *numerals* to represent those letter grades, and from that we generate another ordinal scale,

$$4 > 3 > 2 > 1 > 0.$$

However, you still cannot perform many arithmetic operations on those numerals even though Offices of Admission and Records do calculate grade point averages (perhaps only athletic departments realize that the g.p.a. is invalid anyway). When the numerals above are used on an ordinal scale, you do know that $4 > 3$ and that $3 > 2$, but you do *not* know the amounts by which 4 exceeds 3 or 3 exceeds 2. Furthermore, you do *not* know that 4 exceeds 3 by the same amount that 3 exceeds 2 anymore than you did for the As, Bs, and Cs that the numerals replaced. That is why addition and subtraction of the numerals in the ordinal scale can lead to misleading results.

Interval Scale

The **interval** scale, which also is called a **linear** scale, represents a large leap in mathematical power. Order is still preserved as it was with the ordinal scale, but now *the size of the interval is some constant value.*

The interval is called the **base**. If the numerals 4, 3, 2, 1, and 0 appear on an interval scale, they can be called *numbers* rather than numerals. In this case, then, because the base (the size of the interval between adjacent numbers) is a known constant, we know that 4 exceeds 3 by *exactly* the same amount (1) that 3 exceeds 2 (1).

The interval, or linear, scale consists of successive units that are generated by adding (or subtracting) some specified **base** (size of interval) to each successive number along the scale. Consider the examples for different bases that are shown in Table 3-1. In the first series where the base = 1, we add the base of 1 to each successive number to generate a series 1, 2 (1 + 1), 3 (2 + 1), 4 (3 + 1), and so on. Note also that there is no restriction on the starting number in the series. The only difference between the first and second series is that the first series starts with 1 and the second series starts with 0; the base is the same. The third series is formed in an identical way, except that now a base of 2 is added to each successive number in the series: 0, 2 (0 + 2), 4 (2 + 2), 6 (4 + 2), and so on. In the fourth series, another interval scale has been constructed, but in this case a base of 2 is *subtracted* from each successive number: 10, 8 (10 − 2), 6 (8 − 2), 4 (6 − 2), and so forth. In the final series in the table, a base of 10 is added to form the successive numbers.

With each of the five examples in the table, the interval between any two successive units is exactly equal to the interval between any other two successive units, *and that interval is equal to the* **base**. Thus,

Table 3-1. Examples of interval scales

Base	Scale	Interval Size
1	1, 2, 3, 4, 5, 6, ... , n	1
1	0, 1, 2, 3, 4, 5, ... , n	1
2	0, 2, 4, 6, 8, 10, ... , n	2
2	10, 8, 6, 4, 2, 0, ... , n	2
10	10, 20, 30, 40, 50, ... , n	10

with an interval scale, we can say that one object is different from another (as with the nominal scale), we can say that one object has more or less of some quantity than another (as with the ordinal scale), and we can say that one object or event is *a certain number of units more or less than another.*

Ratio Scale

The final scale is called a **ratio scale**. We shall see in a moment that it also can be called an **exponential**, or **logarithmic**, scale. The ratio scale has the additional requirement that we have an absolute zero point. The principal characteristic of the ratio scale is that we can say that *one unit on the scale is so many times greater (or less) than another.*

One easy way to understand the necessity of an absolute zero for a ratio scale is to consider the fundamental physical quantity of **time**. Calendar time has no absolute zero. The year 1992 A.D., therefore, is not twice as late in time as the year 996 A.D. because we do not know when time began. On the other hand, periods of time can be expressed in terms of ratios. Thus, a person who requires only 5 minutes to run a mile can be said to run twice as fast as a person who requires 10 minutes to finish the same distance.

The ratio scale consists of successive units that are generated by multiplying (or dividing) each successive number along the scale by the **base**. Consider the five examples in Table 3-2. In those examples, a base of 1, 2, 1.5, 10, or 0.1 is multiplied by each successive unit along the scale. Thus, in the first series we obtain 1, 1 (1 $\times$ 1), 1 (1 $\times$ 1), and so forth; in the second series we obtain 1, 2 (1 $\times$ 2), 4 (2 $\times$ 2), 8 (4 $\times$ 2), 16 (8 $\times$ 2), and so on; and in the fourth series we obtain 1, 10 (1 $\times$ 10), 100 (10 $\times$ 10), 1,000 (100 $\times$ 10), 10,000 (1,000 $\times$ 10), and so forth.

In the scales that result with the five different bases in Table 3-2, we see that successive units always are different by some *constant ratio* (1:1, 2:1, 1.5:1, 10:1, and 0.1:1), and *the constant ratio is always equal to the base.* Thus, when the base = 2: 64/32 = 2; 16/8 = 2; and so on. Similarly, when the base = 10: 10,000/1,000 = 10; 1,000/100 = 10; 100/10 = 10; and 10/1 = 10. The same must be true for the more unusual base of 1.5, and in fact we find that 5.0625/3.375 = 1.5; 3.375/2.25 = 1.5; and 2.25/1.5 = 1.5. In all cases, the ratio between two adjacent numbers in the series is equal to the base.

The **ratio scale** also can be called an **exponential scale** because any such scale of numbers can be represented as a certain **base** that is

Table 3–2. Examples of ratio scales

Base	Scale
1	1, 1, 1, 1, 1, ..., 1
2	1, 2, 4, 8, 16, 32, 64, ..., n
1.5	1, 1.5, 2.25, 3.375, 5.0625, ..., n
10	1, 10, 100, 1,000, 10,000, ..., n
0.1	1, .1, .01, .001, .0001, ..., n

raised to successively higher and higher **powers,** or **exponents**. For example, if the base = 2, we can describe the series by either of two ways:

$$1, \quad 2, \quad 4, \quad 8, \quad 16, \quad 32, \quad 64$$

$$(or)$$

$$2^0, \quad 2^1, \quad 2^2, \quad 2^3, \quad 2^4, \quad 2^5, \quad 2^6.$$

The general expression that defines the exponential series shown above is:

$$X^n = \#,$$

which means that the base (X) is used *n* times in multiplication. Thus, in the example above where the base was 2, we used the base some specified number of times (0, 1, 2, 3, 4, 5, or 6) in multiplication, and we generated a scale that consisted of 1, 2, 4, 8, 16, 32, and 64. If the base of 2 is used either 3, 4, or 5 times in multiplication, we obtain the outcome shown in Table 3–3. Thus, 2^3 means that the base of 2 is used 3 (the power) times in multiplication ($2 \times 2 \times 2$) to yield 8; 2^4 means the base of 2 is used 4 times in multiplication to yield 16; and 2^5 means $2 \times 2 \times 2 \times 2 \times 2 = 32$.

Table 3–4 shows two exponential (ratio) series that are generated with different base numbers: base = 2 and base = 10. Two generalizations can be made from the examples in Table 3–4. First, *any base that is raised to the zero power* (X^0) *equals 1*. From the first rule we learn that: $2^0 = 1$; $10^0 = 1$; $3.1416^0 = 1$; and so forth. Second, *any base that is raised to the first power* (X^1) *equals the base*. From the second rule we learn that: $2^1 = 2$; $10^1 = 10$; $3.1416^1 = 3.1416$; and so forth.

■ MORE ON EXPONENTS

We have seen that exponents (or powers) specify how many times a base (X) is used in multiplication or division. When the operation is *multiplication,* the expression is:

Table 3–3. Base = 2 raised to powers of 3, 4, and 5

X^n	Operation	Result
2^3	$2 \times 2 \times 2$	8
2^4	$2 \times 2 \times 2 \times 2$	16
2^5	$2 \times 2 \times 2 \times 2 \times 2$	32

Table 3–4. Exponential series for base = 2 and base = 10

Base = 2		Base = 10	
X^n	Result	X^n	Result
2^0	1	10^0	1
2^1	2	10^1	10
2^2	4	10^2	100
2^3	8	10^3	1,000
2^4	16	10^4	10,000
2^5	32	10^5	100,000

$$X^n = \#.$$

Equation 3.1

For example,

$$3^4 = 3 \times 3 \times 3 \times 3 = 81.$$

The exponent (4) indicates that the base (3) is used 4 times in multiplication. When the operation is *division,* the expression is written as:

$$X^{-n},$$

Equation 3.2

where $X^{-n} = 1/X^n$.

Thus, $3^{-4} = 1/3^4 = 1/(3 \times 3 \times 3 \times 3) = 1/81$ or, less precisely, $= 0.01234567$.

The two expressions shown as Equations 3.1 and 3.2 will be encountered frequently in decibel notation. There are other defining equations for exponents, although only one of them will appear often:

$$X^0 = 1.$$

Equation 3.3

The importance of remembering the rule given by Equation 3.3 cannot be emphasized too strongly. *Any base (X) raised to the zero power will always equal 1.* Thus,

$$X^0 = 1,$$
$$1^0 = 1,$$
$$2^0 = 1,$$
$$10^0 = 1, \text{ and}$$
$$[(2.36)/(a+bx)]^0 = 1.$$

Laws of Exponents

There are three laws that govern the use of exponents, and they will be of tremendous value in helping to solve decibel problems simply.

Law 1 of Exponents

LAW 1

$$X^m \times X^n = X^{m+n}.$$

According to Law 1, if you wish to determine the product of some *common base* (X) that is raised to two different powers (m and n), you simply raise the base (X) to the sum of the two powers (m + n). For example,

$$2^3 \times 2^2 = 2^{3+2} = 2^5 = 32.$$

It might not seem very useful to use Law 1 to solve such a simple problem, because we certainly know that $2^3 = 8$ and $2^2 = 4$, so it indeed is simpler to just multiply 8×4 to get 32. But, consider the next example.

$$2^{1.5} \times 2^{1.5} = ?$$

It might not be immediately obvious how we proceed to determine the value of $2^{1.5}$, and it also might not be intuitively obvious what is meant by *using the base of 2 one and a half times in multiplication*. However, the solution is easy if we employ Law 1.

$$2^{1.5} \times 2^{1.5} = 2^{1.5+1.5} = 2^3 = 8.$$

It is important to remember that in order to use Law 1 in solution of exponent problems, *the value of the base* (X) *must be the same in both terms of the product*. Thus, Law 1 does not apply for a problem such as $X^m \times Y^n$ (e.g., $2^3 \times 10^4$).

Law 2 of Exponents

The second law is undoubtedly the most useful of the three laws in solution of decibel problems:

$$\frac{X^m}{X^n} = X^{m-n}.$$

According to Law 2, the ratio of some base (X) raised to two different powers is equal to the base (X) raised to the difference between the two powers (m−n). For example:

$$\frac{2^4}{2^2} = 2^{(4-2)} = 2^2 = 4.$$

That problem also is not difficult to solve without use of Law 2 because we know that $2^4 = 16$, and $2^2 = 4$, and $16/4 = 4$. Nevertheless, the example does illustrate that the law works. The next example would be more difficult to solve without Law 2:

$$\frac{2^{17.5}}{2^{15.5}} = 2^{(17.5-15.5)} = 2^2 = 4.$$

As can be seen from Law 2, as long as the same base appears in both the numerator and the denominator of the ratio, you simply subtract the exponents and then raise the base to the difference.

As was mentioned previously, Law 2 will be encountered frequently in decibel problems, and in virtually all instances the base will equal 10. Consider, therefore, four additional examples of Law 2 with the base = 10.

$$\frac{10^{-9}}{10^{-12}} = 10^{(-9)-(-12)} = 10^3.$$

Example 1

Note that in this example you are subtracting one negative number from another negative number. To accomplish this, remember that *minus a minus is a plus*. Thus, the difference between −9 and −12 is +3 because it becomes a −9 and a +12 (minus a minus is a plus). The solution could have been carried one step further to show that $10^3 = 1,000$, but an additional computational step generally is not necessary. It should be perfectly acceptable to show the answer simply as 10^3.

$$\frac{10^{-12}}{10^{-9}} = 10^{(-12)-(-9)} = 10^{-3}.$$

Example 2

Minus a minus is a plus, but in this case that translates to a −12 and a +9, which is a −3.

$$\frac{10^{-9}}{10^{-16}} = 10^{(-9)-(-16)} = 10^7.$$

Example 3

You should see that Example 3 is identical in form to Example 1.

$$\frac{10^{-9}}{10^{-9}} = 10^{(-9)-(-9)} = 10^0 = 1.$$

Example 4

The answer of 1 is consistent with Equation 3.3, which defined $X^0 = 1$ (any base raised to the zero power equals one). You should see from Example 4 that this makes sense, because any number (e.g., 10^{-9}) divided by itself (i.e., 10^{-9}) must equal one.

Law 3 of Exponents

The third law of exponents will not be used extensively in decibel problems, but it might be encountered occasionally.

LAW 3

$$(X^m)^n = X^{mn}.$$

For example,

$$(2^2)^3 = 2^{(2\times3)} = 2^6 = 64.$$

■ LOGS AND ANTILOGS

Antilogs

In Table 3–4 we showed two exponential series that were generated with different base numbers, 2 and 10. Those two series are shown again in Table 3–5, but this time the table is organized differently. We can ask either of two questions and then perform either of two arithmetic operations, depending on how the entries in Table 3–5 are arranged. As the table is presently arranged, we are asking the question:

$$X^n = ?$$

For those examples, therefore, we are asking, "what is the value of 2 raised to the 0 power, 2 raised to the 1st power, 2 raised to the 2nd power, and so on?" Stated differently, we are asking, "what is the value of the base (X) raised to the nth power?" That question also is called *determining the **antilog** of the number*. Thus, the question can be written in either of two forms, and they are equivalent.

Table 3–5. Two exponential series of numbers for base = 2 and base = 10

Base = 2		Base = 10	
X^n	Answer	X^n	Answer
$2^0 = ?$	1	$10^0 = ?$	1
$2^1 = ?$	2	$10^1 = ?$	10
$2^2 = ?$	4	$10^2 = ?$	100
$2^3 = ?$	8	$10^3 = ?$	1,000
$2^4 = ?$	16	$10^4 = ?$	10,000

$$X^n = ?$$

is exactly the same as

$$antilog_X n = ?$$

In other words,

$$X^n = antilog_X n.$$

Stated differently, "what is the antilog to the base X of n?" is the same as "what is the value of X raised to the nth power?" In the examples below, the same questions are posed both ways.

$$2^3 = 8 \text{ and } antilog_2 3 = 8.$$ **Example 1**

$$10^3 = 1,000 \text{ and } antilog_{10} 3 = 1,000.$$ **Example 2**

Thus, with a base of 2, we could ask, "2 raised to the third power equals what number?" (Answer = 8), or we could ask, "what is the antilog to the base 2 of 3?" (Answer = 8).

Logs

In Table 3–6 you will see the same two series of numbers that appeared in Table 3–5, but now they are arranged differently so that we can ask a different question. With this new arrangement of the table, *the exponent is not given,* and we are asking "to what power must some specified base be raised to equal some particular number?" In other words, we are asking:

$$X^? = \#.$$

Consider the following two examples.

To what power must the base of 2 be raised to equal 8? (Answer = 3.) **Example 1**

Table 3–6. Two exponential series for base = 2 and base = 10

Base = 2		Base = 10	
X^n	Answer	X^n	Answer
$2^? = 1$	0	$10^? = 1$	0
$2^? = 2$	1	$10^? = 10$	1
$2^? = 4$	2	$10^? = 100$	2
$2^? = 8$	3	$10^? = 1,000$	3
$2^? = 16$	4	$10^? = 10,000$	4

Example 2   To what power must the base of 10 be raised to equal 10,000?
(Answer = 4.)

When you solve problems of that kind, you are *taking the log of a number,* and the following two expressions are identical to each other in every respect.

$$X^? = \#$$

is exactly the same as

$$\log_X \# = ?$$

Thus, the question, "to what power must the base X be raised to equal the number in question?" is equivalent to asking, "what is the log to the base X of the number?" In the examples below, the same questions are posed both ways.

Example 1 $2^? = 16$ (Answer = 4) *and* $\log_2 16 = ?$ (Answer = 4.)

Example 2 $10^? = 1,000$ (Answer = 3) *and* $\log_{10} 1,000 = ?$ (Answer = 3.)

Bases for Logs and Antilogs

When you attempt to solve either **log** or **antilog** problems, it should be apparent that *the base must always be specified.* Thus, log 1,000 = ? is a meaningless question that cannot be solved. How would one possibly know whether you are asking for the power to which 2 must be raised to equal 1,000 or for the power to which 10 must be raised to equal 1,000, or whatever? *Any number can serve as the base,* but in practice there are three bases that are most common: "2," "10" (which is called the **common log** or **Briggsian log**), and "e" (2.718, which is called the **natural log** or **Naperian log**).

Summary

It is important to note that when you "take the log of a number" (e.g., $\log_{10} 100 = 2$), *you are solving for an exponent.* An exponent is a log, a log is an exponent, and they will forever be one and the same. That is why the title to this chapter is "Logarithms and Antilogarithms" rather than "Exponents, Logarithms, and Antilogarithms."

By now you might be able to solve the simple examples of log and antilog problems fairly quickly by inspection. Thus, you undoubtedly know that $\log_{10} 1,000 = 3$ and that $\log_{10} 100 = 2$. You might, for example, have simply counted the number of zeroes and accepted that as your answer. That turns out to be perfectly acceptable for those particular problems. It might be less obvious, though, that:

$$\log_{10} 121 = 2.08279.$$

Conceptually, the problem $\log_{10} 121 = ?$ is no different from the problem $\log_{10} 100 = ?$. You are asked to answer the questions, "to what power must the base of 10 be raised to equal 121 in one case and to equal 100 in the other?" The concept is the same, but counting zeroes will not always provide you with the correct solution. All that remains, then, is to identify a series of computational steps that will permit us to determine the log of any (positive) number.

■ PROCEDURES FOR SOLVING LOG AND ANTILOG PROBLEMS

Components of a Logarithm

A logarithm consists of one or more **integers** (whole numbers) and an endless string of decimal values. Thus,

$$\log_{10} 100 = 2.00000000 - - - -$$

and

$$\log_{10} 121 = 2.08278537 - - - -.$$

When we take the log of 100, the solution gives us an integer or whole number of 2, and the endless string (usually limited to four, and sometimes only two) of decimals that is composed entirely of zeroes. When we take the log of 121, the integer also is 2, but in this case the first four values in the string of decimals are 0.0828. Recall, of course, that in the first example we have learned that 10 (the base) must be raised to a power of 2.0000 to equal 100, and in the second example that the base of 10 must be raised to a power of 2.0828 to equal 121.

Because a log is an exponent, we can rephrase both problems to conform to the language that we used previously with exponents. The base of 10 must be used 2.0000 times in multiplication to equal 100, and it must be used 2.0828 times (just a little more than 2.0000 times) in multiplication (a seemingly strange concept) to equal 121.

The **integer** is called the **characteristic** of a log. The decimal values are called the **mantissa** of a log. Thus, in the two examples above, the **characteristic** (integer) was 2 in both cases, but the **mantissa** (decimal values) was 0.0000 when we took the log of 100 and 0.0828 when we took the log of 121.

To find the log of some (positive) number, the pocket calculator is an indispensable aid. The steps to be followed might vary with different brands, but the calculator's manual should specify the steps. Most generally, to find the log of some number such as, for example, 121, you enter the number 121 and depress the key labeled [**LOG**]. The display, depending upon how many decimals your calculator will show, should read "2.08278537," where the integer 2 is the **characteristic** and 0.08278537 is the **mantissa**.

Some might find it useful to solve a few log problems by using a table of logarithms so that you have an opportunity to become more familiar with the concept of logarithms. Therefore, we shall specify the few easy steps by which the log, both the characteristic and the mantissa, can be found for any positive number. Before taking the log of a number, it is convenient to first transform the number from what can be called **conventional notation** to **scientific notation**.

Scientific Notation

In the course of discussing frequency and period in Chapter 2, we encountered examples of both very large and very small numbers such as 890 MHz (890,000,000 Hz) and its reciprocal (0.001123596 μsec or 0.00000001123596 sec). In Chapter 4, when the concept of sound intensity is introduced, we will encounter numbers such as 0.0000000000000001 watt/cm^2.

It should be obvious that there are at least two problems with this kind of notation, which we will call "conventional notation." The expression is cumbersome, and it would be quite easy to drop or add a zero or so without noticing it. Those two problems should be minimized by using, instead, what is called **scientific notation**. We will learn that for the example of sound intensity cited above, the number would be written as 1×10^{-16} in scientific notation rather than 0.0000000000000001 in conventional notation.

Let us begin more simply. We know that 100 could be written as 10^2 because $100 = 10 \times 10$. Similarly, 1,000 could be written as 10^3 because $1,000 = 10 \times 10 \times 10$. That being the case, then it should make sense that 2,000 could be written as $2 \times 10 \times 10 \times 10$ or, more simply, as 2×10^3.

When a number such as 2,000 is expressed as 2×10^3, we are using **scientific notation**. With scientific notation, a number is written *as the product* of some "simple number" (e.g., 2) and the base of 10 raised to some power. Hence $2,000 = 2 \times 10^3$, $5,000 = 5 \times 10^3$, and $6,000 = 6 \times 10^3$. What about the number 5,500, which of course is halfway between 5,000 and 6,000? We will see in a moment that it would be written as 5.5×10^3.

The "simple number," which is the first term in the product, is called the **coefficient**, and in scientific notation, the coefficient is always multiplied by the base 10 raised to some power. The coefficient can be any number that is greater than or equal to 1.00, but less than 10 (e.g., 9.99). You could add as many additional decimal places as might be required to preserve the desired degree of precision, but two decimal places will be sufficient for most of the applications that we will encounter.

Conversion from Conventional Notation to Scientific Notation

Table 3–7 contains several examples in which the same number is written conventionally and in equivalent scientific notation. In the first

Table 3–7. Comparison of conventional and scientific notation

Conventional Notation	Scientific Notation
10	1.00×10^1
100	1.00×10^2
1,000	1.00×10^3
121	1.21×10^2
800	8.00×10^2
0.1	1.00×10^{-1}
0.0121	1.21×10^{-2}

five examples in the table, the conventional numbers are converted into scientific notation by counting the number of places that the decimal point must be moved to the *left (successive division by 10)* to yield an integer between 1 and 9. That specifies the *value of the exponent* in scientific notation.

To transform 10, the decimal point must be moved one place to the left (divided by 10 once) to arrive at an integer between 1 and 9, and the exponent in scientific notation is 1. For 100, the decimal is moved two places to the left (divided by 10 twice) to get the integer, and the exponent is therefore 2. The same is true for the number 121; when the decimal is moved two places to the left, we have a coefficient of 1.21, and thus the exponent is 2.

In the last two examples in the table, the decimal point must be moved to the *right (successive multiplication by ten)* to yield an integer between 1 and 9. That process also provides the value of the exponent, *but in these cases the exponent is negative.* For example, with 0.0121, the decimal point must be moved two places to the right to yield an integer between 1 and 9 (coefficient = 1.21), and therefore the exponent is −2. A few more examples are shown below.

$$.002 = 2.00 \times 10^{-3}.$$ **Example 1**

$$.0002 = 2.00 \times 10^{-4}.$$ **Example 2**

$$2002 = 2.00 \times 10^3 .$$ **Example 3**

More precisely, 2002 equals 2.002×10^3, but for convenience we are limiting ourselves to two decimal values in the coefficient.

$$222 = 2.22 \times 10^2.$$ **Example 4**

Solution for Logs

When a number is expressed initially in conventional notation, only three steps are required to take the log of that (positive) number. In stating the steps, we will use the example of $\log_{10} 121 = ?$

Step One: Express the conventional number in scientific notation.

$$121 = 1.21 \times 10^2.$$

Obviously, this step is omitted if the number is expressed in scientific notation form in the problem, that is, $\log_{10} 1.21 \times 10^2$.

Step Two: The exponent in the scientific notation expression is the **characteristic** of the log. Thus,

$$\log_{10} 121 = \log_{10} 1.21 \times 10^2 = 2.????.$$

We now know the characteristic of the log (the integer), but we also need to know the mantissa (the decimal values).

Step Three: If the base is 10, as it will be most of the time, use a Common Log Table to find the **mantissa**. Use the three-numbered *multiplier* in the scientific notation expression to find the appropriate row and column in the log table; for this purpose, we ignore the decimal point and view the multiplier simply as three numbers. The first two numbers specify the correct *row* in the table; the third number specifies the correct *column*. The *cell entry* corresponding to that row and column is the **mantissa** of the logarithm. For our example, we locate row 12 and column 1, and the cell entry (the **mantissa** of the logarithm) is .0828. The answer, then, after completing all three steps is:

$$\log_{10} 121 = \log_{10} 1.21 \times 10^2 = 2.0828.$$

By way of brief review, when we say that the log to the base 10 of 121 is 2.0828, that means that we must raise the base of 10 to the 2.0828 power (use the base 2.0828 times in multiplication) to equal 121. We should be able to perform a quick mental check to see if that answer is reasonable. We know without use of a log table that the log of 100 is 2 and that the log of 1,000 is 3. Therefore, the log of 121 (which is larger than 100 and smaller than 1,000) must be a number between 2 and 3, and 2.0828 falls within that range.

That kind of check to determine if an answer is reasonable is generally a good idea. It will not necessarily reveal if the answer that you obtained is precisely correct, but it will tell you if it is approximately correct or at least if it is wildly wrong. For example, suppose you calculated (incorrectly) that the $\log_{10} 163 = 3.2122$. You then think for a moment and realize that the log of 100 is 2 and that the log of 1,000 is 3. Because the number 163 lies between 100 and 1,000, the $\log_{10} 163$ must be 2.????, not 3.????.

Following are additional examples that you might wish to work for yourself before reading the answer.

$$\log_{10} 648 = \log_{10} 6.48 \times 10^2 = 2.8116.$$

$$\log_{10} 707 = \log_{10} 7.07 \times 10^2 = 2.8494.$$

$$\log_{10} 1,000 = \log_{10} 1.00 \times 10^3 = 3.0000.$$
$$\log_{10} 1 \quad = \log_{10} 1.00 \times 10^0 = 0.0000.$$

If $X^0 = 1$ (Equation 3.3), and if an exponent is a log, then it must be the case that the log, to any base, of $1 = 0$.

$$\log_{10} 2 \quad = \log_{10} 2.00 \times 10^0 \quad = 0.3010.$$
$$\log_{10} 0.0002 = \log_{10} 2.00 \times 10^{-4} = \bar{4}.3010.$$

Solution of the first five problems above should be accomplished easily if the three suggested steps are followed: (1) convert the number to scientific notation; (2) the exponent in scientific notation is the characteristic of the log; and (3) the multiplier in scientific notation is used to find the mantissa in the log table.

However, the last example, in which we solved for $\log_{10} 0.0002$, deserves additional explanation. Notice, that a negative sign is placed *above the 4* rather than in front of it. That is because *the **characteristic** can be either positive or negative,* but *the **mantissa** can only be positive.* Thus, $\bar{4}.3010$ does not equal -4.3010. When we say "-4.3010," we imply that the number is 4.3010 units *less than zero.* However, with "$\bar{4}.3010$," we have a negative characteristic of 4, but a positive mantissa of .3010. With a very loose analogy, that is like having roughly 30 cents in your pocket (an asset — a positive value) and owing a friend $4.00 (a liability — a negative value). In that case, your net is a deficit of $3.70.

You approach the log problem in the same conceptual manner. Thus, $\bar{4}.3010 = -4.0000 + 0.3010 = -3.6990$. In other words, $\bar{4}.3010$ is really 3.6990 units below zero, not 4.3010 units below zero. Fortunately, when you solve the problem $\log_{10} 0.0002$ with a calculator that has a log function, the answer will automatically show as -3.6990.

Logs with Bases Other than 10

There might be a few occasions in which you will need to solve a log problem that has a base other than 10, and you might not be able to locate a published log table to help you. However, there is an equation that will enable you to solve such problems using a base of 10. Suppose you want to solve the problem $\log_2 8$. Because we have practiced these simple kinds of problems, you probably can see immediately that the answer is 3, which means that the base of 2 must be raised to the third power ($2 \times 2 \times 2$) to equal 8. Now try to get the answer in a different way by use of Equation 3.4.

$$\log_Y X = \frac{\log_{10} X}{\log_{10} Y.} \qquad \text{**Equation 3.4**}$$

Substitute the values from our problem into Equation 3.4.

$$\log_2 8 = \frac{\log_{10} 8}{\log_{10} 2} = \frac{0.9031}{0.3010} = 3.0000.$$

The equation tells us that to find the $\log_2 8$, we first find the $\log_{10} 8$ (0.9031) and divide that answer by the $\log_{10} 2$ (0.3010). The answer is 3.0 (if you ignore the fourth decimal place), which is the answer that we knew by inspection.

Solutions for Antilogs

If your calculator has a log function, it almost certainly also has an anti-log function. The key normally is not labeled as "antilog," but rather as 10^X. So, to take the antilog of 2.0828, we enter that number, activate the antilog function, and the number 121 should appear in the display.

Solution of antilog problems without a calculator is just as easy as solution of log problems. We simply use the same three steps that were described for solving log problems, but in reverse order. Consider the following example:

$$\text{antilog}_{10} \ 2.0828 = ?,$$

which means

$$10^{2.0828} = ?$$

Regardless of the way in which the problem is posed, we are seeking the answer to the question "what is 10 raised to the 2.0828 power?", which as you should recall, means "what is the value of 10 used 2.0828 times in multiplication?"

Step One: The exponent, 2.0828, is a logarithm and it consists of a characteristic (2.) and a mantissa (0.0828). The **mantissa** is 0.0828 and you first locate the cell entry of that value in the log table. The row (12) and column (1) that correspond to the cell entry of 0.0828 yields the *multiplier,* or coefficient, in scientific notation. Because the coefficient always includes an integer *between 1 and 9* followed by some number of decimal values, row 12 and column 1 tell you that the multiplier is 1.21; that is the only place within those three digits that the decimal can be located to produce an integer between 1 and 9.

Step Two: If an exponent in scientific notation is the **characteristic** of a log, then the characteristic of a log must be the exponent in the scientific notation expression. Thus, the characteristic of 2 tells us to raise the base 10 to the 2nd power (10^2). The answer, in scientific notation, is 1.21×10^2.

Step Three: If you wish to complete the process by expressing the answer in conventional notation, you simply multiply (or divide) the answer obtained in Step Two by ten by moving the decimal point to the right (for positive exponents) the number of places specified by the exponent or to the left for negative exponents. For most of the problems that will be encountered in this book, the third step will not be executed, and the answer will remain in scientific notation.

$$1.21 \times 10^2 = 121.$$

(Because the exponent is 2, the decimal point is moved two places to the right.)

To provide an example for the three steps in determining both logs and antilogs, the number 121 was used. From those solutions we can see that:

$$\log_{10} 121 = 2.0828$$

and

$$\text{antilog}_{10} 2.0828 = 121.$$

Laws of Logarithms

Earlier we presented three laws of exponents that permit us to accomplish certain computations more easily. There are four laws of logarithms (not all independent), and they will permit us to solve many decibel problems easily. Each of the four laws applies to logarithms with any base, but only a base of 10 will be used in the examples.

Law 1 of Logarithms

$$\log ab = \log a + \log b. \qquad \text{LOG LAW 1}$$

The first law tells us that the log of any product is equal to the sum of the logs of the factors. Thus,

$$\log_{10} 3 \times 2 = \log_{10} 3 + \log_{10} 2$$
$$= 0.4771 + 0.3010$$
$$= 0.7781.$$

The answer of 0.7781 can be verified by calculating the $\log_{10} 6$. As with some of the earlier examples, we have not saved much time by using Law 1 to solve such a simple problem because it would have been just as simple to multiply 3 by 2 and take the log of 6. However, use of Law 1 will simplify the solution of more difficult problems.

Actually, we have already applied Law 1 in solution of more difficult log problems without having identified it as such. Look back to

Step One in solution of log problems. When the number 121 was converted into scientific notation, we formed the product 1.21×10^2. We can think of that as the log of the product **ab**, in which **a** (the coefficient) = 1.21 and **b** = 10^2. We then found the log of 10^2, which is 2.????, and that became the **characteristic**. Next, we found the log of 1.21 in the log table, which was 0.0828, and that became the **mantissa**. The log of 1.21×10^2, then, is the sum of the characteristic (2.0000) added to the mantissa (0.0828), which equals 2.0828.

That kind of reasoning is particularly helpful when we express the log of a number less than one as having a negative characteristic and a positive mantissa. The log is the algebraic sum of the negative characteristic and the positive mantissa, which is an application of Law 1 of logarithms. Below are three more examples of the application of Law 1.

$$\log_{10} 10 \times 10 = \log_{10} 10 + \log_{10} 10 = 1 + 1 = 2.$$

$$\log_{10} 20 \times 20 = \log_{10} 20 + \log_{10} 20 = 1.3010 + 1.3010 = 2.6020.$$

$$\log_{10} 648 \quad = \log_{10} 6.48 \times 10^2 \text{ (log of a product)}$$

$$= \log_{10} 10^2 + \log_{10} 6.48$$

$$= 2.0000 + 0.8116$$

$$= 2.8116.$$

Law 2 of Logarithms

LOG LAW 2
$$\log \frac{a}{b} = \log a - \log b.$$

The second law of logarithms states that the log of some ratio is equal to the difference between the logs of the factors. Thus,

$$\log_{10} \frac{3}{2} = \log_{10} 3 - \log_{10} 2 = 0.4771 - 0.3010 = 0.1761.$$

The answer, 0.1761, can be verified by calculating the log of 1.5, which corresponds to the ratio of 3/2. It should be apparent that the major advantage to Law 2 is that it allows us to subtract logs rather than perform potentially cumbersome division. It is not imposing to divide 3 by 2, but use of the law will certainly simplify solutions to the two problems below.

Example 1
$$\log_{10} \frac{1.8}{1.2} = (\log_{10} 1.8) - (\log_{10} 1.2) = 0.2553 - 0.0792 = 0.1761.$$

Example 2
$$\log_{10} \frac{(1 \times 10^0)}{(2 \times 10^{-4})} = (\log_{10} 1 \times 10^0) - (\log_{10} 2 \times 10^{-4})$$

$$= 0.0000 - (\bar{4}.3010)$$

$$= 0.0000 - (-3.6990)$$

$$= 3.6990.$$

Law 3 of Logarithms

$$\log a^b = b \log a \qquad \text{LOG LAW 3}$$

The third law of logarithms states that the log of the number **a** raised to the **b**th power is equal to **b** times the log of **a**. This law will be particularly helpful in Chapter 4 when we explain the difference in the equations for decibels intensity and decibels pressure.

The first example below is a simple problem that will allow you to find the answer with and without use of Law 3. In the second example, you should see how use of the law simplifies computation greatly.

$$\log_{10} 2^2 = 2 \log_{10} 2 = 0.6020. \qquad \textbf{Example 1}$$

The answer of 0.6020 should be easy to verify by calculating the log of 4 (2^2).

$$\log_{10} 2^{1.65} = 1.65 \times \log_{10} 2 = 0.4967. \qquad \textbf{Example 2}$$

Law 4 of Logarithms

$$\log \frac{1}{a} = -\log a. \qquad \text{LOG LAW 4}$$

The fourth and final law states that the log of a reciprocal is equal to minus the log of the number. Thus,

$$\log_{10} \frac{1}{2} = -\log_{10} 2 = -0.3010.$$

You should be able to see that Law 4 is not an independent law, but rather is a special application of Law 2. Law 2 stated that,

$$\log \frac{a}{b} = \log a - \log b.$$

When we take the log of 1/2, that fits the form of the second law. But, of course, the log of 1 in the numerator is always 0.0000. Therefore, the answer will always be a negative number because you will be subtracting some positive number in the denominator from zero in the numerator. Hence, Law 4 is written simply as **−log a**.

Logs Without Log Tables

You can get an approximate answer to many log problems without use of a log table, and to do so it is necessary to memorize the logs of only four numbers: 1, 2, 3, and 7. This will be particularly useful because it will enable you to check to see if the answer you obtained by following all of the steps and using a log table is *approximately* correct. Consider the numbers between 1 and 10, and because we are only interested in getting an approximate answer, we will only use one or two decimal places in the computations.

1. The log of 1 is 0.0.	**Memorize**
2. The log of 2 is 0.3.	**Memorize**
3. The log of 3 is 0.48.	**Memorize**
4. The log of 4 is ?	Law 1 stated that log ab = log a + log b. Because $4 = 2 \times 2$, the log of 4 must equal the log of 2 + the log of 2, which has already has been memorized, and $0.3 + 0.3 = 0.6$.
5. The log of 5 is ?	Law 2 stated that log a/b = log a − log b. Because $5 = 10/2$, the log of 5 must equal the log of 10 − the log of 2 = 1.0 − 0.3 = 0.70.
6. The log of 6 is ?	Because $6 = 3 \times 2$, the log of 6 must equal the log of 3 + the log of 2 = 0.48 + 0.30 = 0.78.
7. The log of 7 is 0.85.	**Memorize**
8. The log of 8 is ?	Because $8 = 4 \times 2$, the log of 8 must equal the log of 4 + the log of 2 = 0.60 + 0.30 = 0.90. Alternatively, you might see that 8 equals 2^3 (i.e., $2 \times 2 \times 2$). Therefore the log of 8 = 0.30 + 0.30 + 0.30 = 0.90.
9. The log of 9 is ?	log of 3 + log of 3 = 0.96.
10. The log of 10 is ?	With only a little practice you should see that the answer is 1.

It should be helpful to try to use that system to solve the following problems without log tables.

$\log_{10} 20 = $?	$20 = 10 \times 2$. Therefore, the answer is 1.3.
$\log_{10} 30 = $?	$30 = 10 \times 3$. Therefore, the answer is 1.48.
$\log_{10} 100 = $?	$100 = 10 \times 10$. Therefore, the answer is 2.0.
$\log_{10} 300 = $?	Can you see easily that the answer is 2.48?

A Final Comment About Logarithms

You might have noticed that when you take the log of a series of numbers from a ratio scale, the logs are *linearly* spaced. That concept is illustrated below by comparing the two columns of numbers. The first column shows numbers that progressively increase by powers of 10 (1, 10, 100, . . ., 1,000,000). The second column shows that the logs of those numbers are linearly spaced (0, 1, 2, . . ., 6).

Column I	Column II
1	0
10	1
100	2
1,000	3
10,000	4
100,000	5
1,000,000	6

Because logs are linearly spaced, you can convert linear graph paper into logarithmic units by calculating the logs of the numbers you wish to display. That operation enables you to display a large range of numbers in an economical space. Suppose each dot below represents a tick mark on your graph paper, and you wish to display information that ranges from 1 to 1,000,000 units of measurement. Only 60 lines on the graph paper will be required if the resolution that you desire is restricted to one decimal place.

```
I.........I.........I.........I.........I.........I.........I
0         1         2         3         4         5         6
1         10        100       1,000     10,000    100,000  1,000,000
```

In Chapter 4 we will introduce the concept of the decibel, and in all decibel computations we will make considerable use of logs and antilogs. The base for all computations involving decibels will be 10.

■ PRACTICE PROBLEMS

Set 1

1. Express the following values in scientific notation.

   a. 6875   b. .0064   c. 109.6

2. What is the base of 8^2?

3. Solve each of the following.

a. 7^3 b. 0.2^4 c. $10^{2.2} \times 10^{1.8}$

d. $2^5 \times 2^{-2}$ e. $2^2 + 2^2$ f. $(5 \times 10^3) \times (2 \times 10^2)$

g. $(xyz)^0$ h. 5.764^1 i. $(1.6/5.2)^0$

j. $(10^2)^3$ k. $(3^2)^2$ l. $(2^{2.5})^2$

m. $(4^2)^{1/2}$ n. $3^{4/2}$ o. 2^{-2}

p. 10^{-3}

Set 2

1. Solve the following.

a. $\log_3 27$ b. $\log_4 16$ c. $\log_4 16^2$ d. $\log_4 16^{-2}$

e. $\log_{10} 10$ f. $\log_2 2$ g. $\log_{67} 67$ h. $\log_e e$

i. $\log_{10} 10^2$ j. $\log_{10} 100$ k. $\log_2 4$ l. $\log_3 9$

m. $\log_{12} 144$ n. $\log_e e^2$ o. $\log_{4.4} 4.4^{16}$ p. $\log_{10} 1/10$

q. $\log_{10} 3+4+1+2$

2. Assume a base of 10 for the following.

a. $\log 54$ b. $\log 3.6$ c. $\log 0.4$

d. antilog 0.3010   e. antilog 1.5315   f. antilog 6.7202

■ ANSWERS TO PRACTICE PROBLEMS

Set 1

1. a. 6.875×10^3 b. 6.4×10^{-3} c. 1.096×10^2

2. 8

3. a. 343 or 3.43×10^2 $(7 \times 7 \times 7)$

b. .0016 or 1.6×10^{-3} $(.2 \times .2 \times .2 \times .2)$

c. 10,000 or 10^4 $(10^{2.2+1.8} = 10^4)$

3. d. 8 or 8×10^0 $(2^{5+(-2)} = 2^3)$

    e. 8 or 8×10^0 (You are adding, not multiplying; Law 1 does not apply.)

    f. 10^6 $(10 \times 10^{3+2})$

    g. 1   (Any base raised to the 0 power = 1)

    h. 5.764   (Any base raised to the 1st power = base)

    i. 1   (Same rule as for Problem 3-g; therefore, you need not divide 1.6 by 5.2)

    j. 10^6 $(10^{2 \times 3})$

    k. 81 or 8.1×10^1 (3^4)

    l. 32 or 3.2×10^1 (2^5)

    m. 4 $(4^{2 \times 0.5} = 4^1 = 4)$

    n. 9 (3^2)

    o. 1/4 or 25×10^{-1} $(2^{-2} = 1/2^2 = 1/4)$

    p. .001 $(1/10^3)$

    q. 1 $(3+4+1+2 = 10; \log_{10} 10 = 1)$

Set 2

1. a. 3   b. 2   c. 4   d. −4

    e. 1   f. 1   g. 1   h. 1

    i. 2   j. 2   k. 2   l. 2

    m. 2   n. 2   o. 16   p. −1

    q. 1

2. a. 1.7324   b. 0.5563   c. $\bar{1}.6021$

    d. 2   e. 34   f. 5,250,000 or 5.25×10^6

■ NOTES

1. The discussion of the four scales of measurement is largely a condensed version of the extensive treatment of the topic by S. S. Stevens (1951). Readers who wish to explore this important topic in greater detail are advised to read his chapter in the *Handbook of Experimental Psychology.*

Sound Intensity and Sound Pressure: The Decibel

We learned in Chapter 1 that sound is a form of wave motion in which a pattern of pressure — or a change in density — is propagated through an elastic medium. **Energy** is transferred through the medium and the transfer of energy occurs at some particular rate. *The rate at which sound energy is transferred through the medium* is called the **acoustic power**.

More generally, **power** is defined as the rate at which work is accomplished, or as the rate at which energy is transformed or transferred:

**Power = work/unit time = energy transformed
or transferred/unit time.**

For example, **power** refers to the amount of work accomplished by an engine per second, or the amount of electrical energy that is transformed into heat energy per second by an electrical heater.

It is important to realize that **power** and **energy** are not equivalent. Consider the case of a person who is engaged in a physical activity such as shoveling snow. The person might be able to shovel for an hour at a rate of two shovelfuls per minute before the amount of energy stored in the muscles is used up and exhaustion results. However, if the person is anxious to complete the job more quickly and picks up the pace to four shovelfuls each minute, exhaustion will occur earlier. Thus, our ability to complete such tasks is limited not only by our **energy**, the capacity to do work, but also by the rate at which the energy is expended, the **power**.

The unit of measure of power, including acoustic power, is the **watt (W)**, which was named in honor of James Watt, the developer of the steam engine. If we expend energy at a rate of 1 joule per sec (**MKS** system) or 10,000,000 ergs per sec (**cgs** system), we have expended *one watt of power*. Therefore,

$$1 \text{ watt} = 1 \text{ joule/sec} = 10{,}000{,}000 \text{ ergs/sec} \ (10^7 \text{ ergs/sec}).$$

■ ABSOLUTE AND RELATIVE MEASURES OF ACOUSTIC POWER

Absolute Measure of Power

If we say that a particular sound wave has an acoustic power of some number of watts, we are referring to the **absolute acoustic power**. In the case of sound waves, we should not expect to encounter large amounts such as 60, 100, or 200 watts, and we certainly will find no acoustic rival to the megawatt electrical power station. Instead, we commonly deal with very small magnitudes of acoustical power such as, for example, 10^{-8} watt or 2.13×10^{-9} watt. Even though the value of acoustic power is small, the absolute measure of acoustic power in watts refers to *the rate at which energy is consumed*.

Relative Measure of Power

We frequently speak of **relative acoustic power** rather than absolute power. In this case, *the absolute power in one sound wave is compared with the absolute power in another (reference) sound wave,* and the two absolute sound powers are used to form a ratio. Thus, we might say, for example, that the acoustic power of wave A is 10 times greater than the acoustic power of wave B.

$$A = 10B.$$

We do not know the absolute power in watts of either wave A or wave B, but we do know the relation between the two. If the absolute power of B is 10^{-6} watt, the power of A must be 10^{-5} watt if we are to preserve the ratio of A $=$ 10B. With the example above, if A $=$ 10B, then

$$B = \frac{A}{10}$$

Thus, if the absolute power of wave A were 6.21×10^{-3} watt, then the power of wave B must be 6.21×10^{-4}.

$$B = \frac{(6.21 \times 10^{-3})}{(1 \times 10^{1})} = 6.21 \times 10^{-4}.$$

That is the only solution in which the 1:10 ratio would be preserved.

Summary

In summary, with relative power we are expressing the **level** of power in a sound wave by forming a ratio of two absolute powers: the ratio of the absolute acoustic power of the sound wave in question (W_x) to the absolute acoustic power of some reference sound wave (W_r).

$$\text{Level} = \frac{W_x}{W_r.}$$

Equation 4.1

Importance of Specifying the Reference Power

Because level of power is simply the ratio of *any* two absolute powers, *the measure of level is generally meaningless unless the value of the reference power is specified.* If we determine that the level of a particular sound wave is 1,000, we know only that its power is 1,000 times greater than the power of some unspecified reference sound wave. It could be that the power of W_x is 10^{-1} relative to (re:) W_r of 10^{-4}. But, of course, a level of 1,000 would apply equally to $W_x = 10^{-13}/W_r = 10^{-16}$. In either case, the ratio of 1,000 is preserved.

A more explicit statement, therefore, would be: "the level of acoustic power is 1,000 re: 10^{-4} watt." When the reference (W_r) is specified, there should be no ambiguity. *If the reference is not known, the concept of level has little meaning.*

■ SOUND INTENSITY

Imagine that we have what is called an "idealized point source of sound" that operates in a "free, unbounded medium." By an "idealized point source," we mean a very small sphere that is capable of pulsating in and out in a manner similar to the pulsation of the balloon in Figure 2–9. By "free and unbounded medium" we mean that there are no reflecting surfaces or energy-absorbing materials in the medium to affect sound transmission in any way. In such a case, sound energy is transferred uniformly through the medium in all directions.

In essence, the *energy is transferred outward from the point source as an ever-expanding sphere.* To measure the acoustic power in such a wave at some distance from the point source, we would have to integrate over the entire surface of the sphere. However, we generally are more interested in the *amount of power that acts upon or that is dissipated upon, or passes through, some much smaller area.* The area is the square meter (**m²**) in the **MKS** metric system or the square centimeter (**cm²**) in the **cgs** metric system. Thus, instead of referring to the *energy per second* (the **acoustic power**), we speak of the *energy per second per square meter,* and that is called the **intensity** of the sound wave.

Intensity is the *amount of energy transmitted per second over an area of one square meter.*

1. If the unit of measure of **acoustic power** is the **watt** (energy per second); and
2. if **intensity** is the amount of energy per second per square meter, then it follows that
3. the unit of measure for **intensity** must be the **watt per square meter (watt/m²)**.

Absolute and Relative Measures of Sound Intensity

Sound power was expressed in both absolute and relative terms, and the same is true of sound intensity. If we say that a sound has an intensity of 10^{-8} watt/m², we are referring to the **absolute intensity** of the sound wave. Alternatively, we can speak of the **relative intensity**, or the level of intensity (not to be confused with "intensity level," because the label "intensity level" implies a specific reference intensity that will be introduced later), by reference to the same kind of ratio that was used for power.

$$\text{Level} = \frac{I_x}{I_r}.$$

Equation 4.2

Importance of Specifying the Reference Intensity

It is just as important to specify the reference for level of sound intensity as it is to specify the reference for level of sound power. Consider the examples in Table 4–1 in which each of six absolute sound intensities in **watt/m²** is referenced to two different reference intensities: $I_r = 10^{-10}$ watt/m² and $I_r = 10^{-12}$ watt/m².

For each absolute intensity (I_x), the ratio (I_x/I_r) depends on the reference intensity. Thus, for example, the level of intensity in the first example is 10^2 when referenced to 10^{-10} watt/m², but 10^4 when referenced to 10^{-12} watt/m². In a similar vein, it is not acceptable to say that some sound has a level of intensity of 10^{-1} because, for the examples in Table 4–1, that would apply equally to 10^{-13} re: 10^{-12} and to 10^{-11} re: 10^{-10}.

■ THE DECIBEL

When we speak of the level of power or the level of intensity in a sound wave, we often are faced with a rather cumbersome number. For example, a conservative estimate of the range of intensities to which the human auditory system can respond is about $10^{12}:1$, and the range of acoustic powers of interest in noise measurements is even greater: about $10^{18}:1$. Thus, we are faced with a wide range of intensities, and that presents us with awkward numerical notations.

The awkwardness can be minimized, though, by some elementary transformations of the numbers. Look again at Table 4–1. Entries in the second and the third columns are the ratios of the absolute intensities (I_x) to each of the two reference intensities (I_r). Each of those entries is the base 10 raised to some power.

Table 4–1. Ratios I_x/I_r for two different reference intensities

Absolute Intensity in watt/m² I_x	Relative Intensity, I_x/I_r in watt/m²	
	$I_r = 10^{-10}$	$I_r = 10^{-12}$
10^{-8}	10^2	10^4
10^{-9}	10^1	10^3
10^{-10}	10^0	10^2
10^{-11}	10^{-1}	10^1
10^{-12}	10^{-2}	10^0
10^{-13}	10^{-3}	10^{-1}

It should be obvious that the base is redundant from one example to another in the table; it is always 10. Thus, we could just as well eliminate the base and only list the exponents. We also know that an *exponent is a log* (Chapter 3). In other words: $\log_{10} 10^2 = 2$; $\log_{10} 10^0 = 0$; $\log_{10} 10^{-3} = -3$; and so on. The numbers are simplified, therefore, by *calculating the logarithm to the base ten of the ratio of two intensities.*

$$\log_{10} \frac{I_x}{I_r}.$$

The Bel

For the first example in Table 4-1 where the absolute intensity (I_x) equaled 10^{-8} watt/m², we calculated that its level re: 10^{-10} watt/m² was 10^2. Now we see that one further transformation, the log of the ratio, yields a value of 2. This unit of measurement of relative intensity is called the **bel** in honor of Alexander Graham Bell, an inventor who patented the first telephone. Thus,

Equation 4.3
$$N \text{ (bels)} = \log_{10} \frac{I_x}{I_r},$$

where I_x is the absolute intensity of the wave in question in watt/m²,

I_r is the absolute intensity of a *reference* sound wave in watt/m²,

and

the **bel** is a unit of level of intensity.

Thus, the relative intensities of the six sounds in Table 4-1 can be described as 2, 1, 0, −1, −2, and −3 Bels re: 10^{-10} watt/m², and as 4, 3, 2, 1, 0, and −1 bels re: 10^{-12} watt/m².

Summary

Before proceeding further, it might be helpful to provide a brief review of the transformations that have been accomplished for specifying the intensity of a sound wave. Consider the first example in Table 4-1.

1. The absolute intensity is 10^{-8} watt/m².
2. The relative intensity, referenced to 10^{-12} watt/m², is 10,000, which can be expressed more simply as 10^4.
3. The base 10 is redundant because the level of intensity will always be described as the base 10 raised to some power. The expression can be simplified further, therefore, by calculating the log of the ratio. Because an exponent is a log, the log of 10 raised to some power (exponent) is the exponent. The level in this example, therefore, is 4 (**bels**).

4. Thus, a sound wave with an absolute intensity (I_x) of 10^{-8} watt/ m^2 has a relative intensity of 4 Bels re: 10^{-12} watt/m^2. Because relative intensity varies with the reference that is chosen for comparison, that same sound has a relative intensity of 2 Bels re: 10^{-10} watt/m^2.

From the Bel to the Decibel

The **bel** as a measure of relative intensity is less cumbersome than the ratio of intensities because the wide-range linear scale of intensities has been compressed by transformation to a logarithmic scale. Thus, instead of expressing the relative intensity for various sounds as 0.0001, 0.01, 1,000, 100,000, or 1,000,000,000,000, we could say simply that the relative intensities are -4, -2, 3, 5, and 12 bels respectively.

Although the bel might be less cumbersome than a ratio (a level of 10^{12} is expressed simply as 12 bels), the scale has been compressed so much that fractional values often are required to reflect an appropriate accuracy of measurement. For example, a sound intensity of 2×10^{-12} watt/m^2 has a relative intensity of 4.3 bels re: 10^{-16} watt/m^2.

$$\text{Bels} = \log \frac{(2 \times 10^{-12})}{(1 \times 10^{-16})}$$

$$= \log 2 \times 10^4$$

$$= 4.3.$$

Excessive use of decimals can be minimized if we use **decibels (dB)** rather than bels in the same way that we sometimes use inches rather than feet and centimeters or millimeters rather than meters. A length of 5.5 ft can be expressed as 66 in. because each foot contains 12 in.

The prefix, deci, means 1/10. Therefore, *a decibel* **(dB)** *is 0.1 of a bel*. Because 1 dB = 0.1 bel and, conversely, 1 bel = 10 dB, Equation 4.3 for bels can be rewritten for decibels as:

$$N \text{ (dB)} = 10 \log_{10} \frac{I_x}{I_r.} \qquad \text{Equation 4.4}$$

Thus, with the preceding example, we can say that the relative intensity is 43 dB rather than 4.3 bels. What, then, is a decibel? To say that "a decibel is one-tenth of a bel" is a true statement, but such a definition is not sufficient unless the mathematical definition of the bel is understood. Instead, the decibel is defined most appropriately by reference to Equation 4.4: *the decibel is ten times the log of an intensity ratio or a power ratio.*[1]

A comment about grammar is in order. The singular forms are **bel, decibel,** and **dB,** but the plural forms are **bels, decibels,** and **dB** (not dBs). Only d'birds can rightfully be linked with "dBs."

Intensity Level (dB IL)

The decibel, as with intensity ratios and the bel, is ambiguous unless the reference intensity is specified. How, then, can utter confusion be avoided? First, *no confusion should exist if the reference intensity is specified.* A statement that the relative intensity of a sound is 86 dB re: 10^{-12} watt/m^2 is explicit: we know the relative intensity (86 dB), we know the reference intensity (10^{-12}) to which some absolute intensity has been compared, and we can calculate (with the use of antilogs) that the absolute intensity of the sound is 3.99×10^{-4} watt/m^2.

Second, the possibility of confusion has been lessened by adoption of a *conventional reference intensity of 10^{-12} watt/m^2* (**MKS** system).[2] Any intensity can be used as the reference for expressing relative intensity, but *when the reference is 10^{-12} watt/m^2, the result is called **intensity level (dB IL)*** rather than just "level of intensity." Strictly speaking, the label **intensity level** and its abbreviation **dB IL** should only be used when the reference is 10^{-12} watt/m^2. However, there is still sufficient departure from the convention to warrant one final admonition: *the reference intensity should always be specified when the term **decibel** is used.*

The relation between absolute intensity (I_x) in watt/m^2 and dB IL re: 10^{-12} watt/m^2 is shown in the following illustration.

dB IL	I_x
70	= 10^{-5}
$\mid$	
60	= 10^{-6}
$\mid$	
50	= 10^{-7}
$\mid$	
40	= 10^{-8}
$\mid$	
30	= 10^{-9}
$\mid$	
20	= 10^{-10}
$\mid$	
10	= 10^{-11}
$\mid$	
0	= **10^{-12}**
$\mid$	
-10	= 10^{-13}
$\mid$	
-20	= 10^{-14}

When $I_x = 10^{-12}$, dB IL = 0 because $I_x = I_r$, the reference intensity. As you move up the scale, I_x increases *multiplicatively* by powers of 10 to the quantities 10^{-11}, 10^{-10}, and so on, to a maximum intensity of 10^{-5} in the illustration. For each tenfold increase in sound intensity, dB IL increases *additively* by 10 dB to a maximum of 70 dB IL when $I_x = 10^{-5}$

watt/m^2. Similarly, if you move down the scale, I_x decreases progressively by powers of 10, and for each power of 10 decrease in sound intensity, dB IL decreases by 10 dB to a minimum of -20 dB IL at a sound intensity of 10^{-14} watt/m^2.

Sample Problems

Two steps should be followed to solve decibel problems for relative intensity (any reference) or **intensity level (dB IL)** (reference = 10^{-12} watt/m^2):

1. *Select the proper equation.* If the problem concerns the **intensity** of a sound wave, use Equation 4.4. Later in this chapter we will focus instead on the **pressure** of a sound wave, and that will necessitate a slight modification of Equation 4.4.

2. *Form a ratio and solve the problem.*

Problem 1: An increase in intensity by a factor of two (2:1) corresponds to how many decibels?

1. Because we are dealing with **intensity**, use Equation 4.4. The ratio is 2:1, which means that some absolute intensity whose value is unknown is twice as large as some unknown reference intensity. It might be that the intensity of one sound wave (A) is twice as great as the intensity of another sound wave (B). Alternatively, it might be that the intensity of one sound wave (A) at one point in time (t_1) has been doubled at another point in time (t_2). In either case, *the ratio is 2:1.*

2. dB = 10 log 2/1
       = 10 × 0.3010
       = 3.01   (which normally is rounded to 3 dB)

3. Because the problem could have involved any absolute intensity and any reference intensity that preserved the ratio of 2:1, we see that *as any sound intensity is doubled (the ratio of absolute to reference = 2:1), the level is increased by 3 dB.* Correspondingly, if intensity were halved (ratio = 1:2), the level is decreased by 3 dB because:
       dB = 10 log 1/2
          = −10 log 2   (**Log Law 4**)
          = −3.

Problem 2: An increase in intensity by a factor of ten corresponds to how many decibels?

1. dB = 10 log 10/1
       = 10 × 1
       = 10.

2. Thus, as intensity increases *multiplicatively* by 10, relative intensity increases *additively* by 10 dB. Similarly, if intensity were decreased by a factor of 10, intensity would decrease by 10 dB.

$$dB = 10 \log 1/10$$
$$= -10 \log 10$$
$$= -10.$$

Problem 3: What is the intensity level re: 10^{-12} watt/m^2 of a sound whose absolute intensity is 10^{-6} watt/m^2?

1. Follow the same steps that were used with the first two problems, but note that the ratio is now different. The intensity was not simply increased (or decreased) from some unknown value by a stated ratio such as 2:1 or 10:1, but rather a specific absolute intensity was compared with a specified reference intensity.

$$dB = 10 \log 10^{-6}/10^{-12}$$
$$= 10 \log 10^{6}$$
$$= 10 \times 6$$
$$= 60.$$

Problem 4: What is the intensity level re: 10^{-12} watt/m^2 of a sound whose intensity is 2×10^{-6} watt/m^2?

1. There are two approaches that can be taken. First, you can solve the problem in the same way that was used for Problem 3.

$$dB = 10 \log (2 \times 10^{-6})/(1 \times 10^{-12})$$
$$= 10 \log 2 \times 10^{6}$$
$$= 63.$$

2. However, a quicker solution is available. We learned in Problem 3 that a sound whose absolute intensity is 10^{-6} has an intensity level of 60 dB. The sound in Problem 4 has an intensity of 2×10^{-6}, which is twice as great as an intensity of 1×10^{-6}. We also know from Problem 1 that any time you increase the intensity by 2:1, relative intensity increases by 3 dB. Therefore, if the intensity level of $1 \times 10^{-6} = 60$ dB, the intensity level of 2×10^{-6} must $= 63$ dB. It will almost always be a useful shortcut to inspect a problem to see if it involves powers of 2 (3 dB) or powers of 10 (10 dB). For example, see if such shortcuts can be used to solve Problem 5.

Problem 5: What is the intensity level re: 10^{-12} watt/m^2 of a sound whose intensity is 4×10^{-5} watt/m^2?

1. We know from Problem 4 that 2×10^{-6} corresponds to 63 dB. In addition, we should see that 10^{-5} is 10 times greater than 10^{-6} (10 dB), and 4 is 2 times greater than 2 (3 dB). Therefore,

we should expect the answer to be 13 dB (10 + 3) greater than for Problem 4, which is 76 dB.

2. If we solve the problem step-by-step without taking answers to previous problems into account, we must get the same result.

$$\text{dB} = 10 \log (4 \times 10^{-5})/(10^{-12})$$
$$= 10 \log 4 \times 10^{7}$$
$$= 10 \times 7.6$$
$$= 76.$$

Problem 6: 3 dB corresponds to what intensity ratio?

1. This is an antilog problem, and the solution requires following the steps suggested in Chapter 3.

2. 3 dB = 10 log X
   0.3 = log X   (Divide both sides by 10.)
   X = 2 × 10⁰.   (Zero is the characteristic of the log and also the exponent in scientific notation; 0.3 is the mantissa of the log and, with the aid of pocket calculator or a log table, we determine that the multiplier in scientific notation is 2.)

Problem 7: 13 dB corresponds to what intensity ratio?

1. Try to solve the problem initially without paper and pencil. You know that 3 dB corresponds to a ratio of 2:1 and that 10 dB corresponds to a ratio of 10:1. Because 13 dB consists of 3 + 10, the ratio must consist of 2 × 10 = 20:1.

2. Check the answer above by solving the problem step-by-step.
   13 dB = 10 log X
   1.3 = log X
   X = 2 × 10¹   (which is 20:1).

Problem 8: 14 dB corresponds to what intensity ratio?

1. There might not be an obvious combination of 3 dB (2:1) and 10 dB (10:1) that adds to 14 dB, which means that a shortcut that involves powers of 2 and/or powers of 10 does not *seem* to be available. However, you can use your knowledge of powers of 2 and powers of 10 to at least "bracket your answer." We know that 13 dB corresponds to a ratio of 20:1. We should also know that 16 dB would correspond to a ratio of 40:1 because another 3 dB represents another doubling. Therefore, the answer must lie between 20:1 and 40:1.

2. 14 dB = 10 log X
   1.4 = log X
   X = 2.51 × 10¹   (and 25.1 lies between 20 and 40).

3. Actually, *a shortcut is available,* even if it is not obvious at first glance. We know that 20 dB corresponds to a ratio of 100:1.

Therefore, 17 dB, which is 3 dB less, must correspond to a halving of sound intensity, or a ratio of 50:1. Finally, 14 dB represents another halving of sound intensity, which corresponds to a ratio of 25:1.

Problem 9: An intensity level of 65 dB re: 10^{-12} watt/m^2 corresponds to what intensity?

1. Combinations of 10 dB and 3 dB will not add to 65 (unless you use a long string such as $10 + 10 + 10 + 10 + 10 + 3 + 3 + 3 + 3 + 3 = 65$). In this case it might be less cumbersome to solve the problem step-by-step. However, we can determine a range within which the answer must lie by use of powers of 10 and 2, and that will enable us to determine if the answer we calculate is reasonable. We should know that 63 dB consists of $10 + 10 + 10 + 10 + 10 + 10 + 3$. Each 10 dB involves a tenfold increase in intensity relative to the reference, which therefore corresponds to 10^{-6} (the reference increased by a factor of 10^6). Similarly, each 3 dB involves a twofold increase in intensity relative to the reference. Thus 63 dB would correspond to an intensity of 2×10^{-6}, and that is a lower boundary of the bracket. To get an upper boundary add another 3 dB. 66 dB would represent another doubling of intensity, which would be 4×10^{-6}. Because 65 dB lies between 63 and 66, we should expect that the intensity corresponding to 65 dB would lie between 2×10^{-6} and 4×10^{-6}.

2. $$65 \text{ dB} = 10 \log I_x/10^{-12}$$
$$6.5 = \log I_x/10^{-12}$$
$$3.16 \times 10^6 = I_x/10^{-12}$$
$$I_x = 3.16 \times 10^6 \times 10^{-12}$$
$$= 3.16 \times 10^{-6}.$$

■ SOUND PRESSURE

We often wish to refer to the **pressure** associated with a sound wave rather than its acoustic power or intensity. We saw previously (Equation 1.5) that **pressure** is the *amount of force per unit area*. The unit of measure in the **MKS** system is the **Nt/m^2** (newton per square meter) or **Pa** (pascal), and we learned in Chapter 2 that 1 Nt/m^2 = 1 Pa. It has now become more common to use the **μNt/m^2** (microNt/m^2) or the **μPa** (microPa) as the unit of measure, and we will use **μPa** in all future computations involving sound pressure.[3]

If we say that a particular sound has a pressure of 200 μPa (2×10^2 μPa), we are referring to the **absolute pressure** of the wave. As with intensity, we also can speak of **relative pressure** in decibels by calculating the log of a pressure ratio. However, Equation 4.4 *cannot be used for decibels of sound pressure.* That equation for decibels of intensity must, therefore, be modified in an appropriate manner. In order that we might understand the reasons for the transformation of Equation 4.4, it will be helpful first to reconsider the concepts of sound intensity and sound pressure in relation to **impedance**.

Impedance

We learned in Chapter 2 that the **impedance** of any vibratory system, including a volume of air through which sound is transmitted, is determined by the **resistance, mass reactance,** and **compliant reactance** of the system. Moreover, we learned in Chapter 1 that the speed of sound in a medium such as air also is determined by properties of the medium, namely, the **elasticity** and the **density**. We might reason, therefore, that **impedance** also would be dependent on the speed of sound in a medium.

The **acoustic impedance** for a plane progressive wave is given by the product of the ambient **density** (ρ_o) in kg/m^3 and the **speed of sound (s)**.[4] Thus,

$$Z_c = \rho_o s.$$
    Equation 4.5

The subscript **(c)** is used in the equation because the impedance of the medium with plane progressive waves is called the **characteristic impedance**.

We previously defined intensity as *energy per second per square meter.* Intensity also can be defined as the *ratio of the square of rms pressure to the characteristic impedance:*

$$I = \frac{P_{rms}^2}{\rho_o s,}$$
    Equation 4.6

where **I** is intensity,

P_{rms} is root mean square pressure,

and

the product $\rho_o s$ is the characteristic impedance.

Decibels for Sound Pressure

We can see from Equation 4.6 that intensity is proportional to the square of rms pressure, and conversely, **rms pressure** is proportional to the square root of sound intensity.

$$P \propto \sqrt{I,}$$

$$I \propto P^2, \text{ and}$$

$$I = \frac{P^2}{Z_c,}$$

where **P** refers to rms sound pressure,

I refers to sound intensity,

and

Z_c is the characteristic impedance.

Thus, if intensity increases by 16:1, pressure increases by only 4:1 (square root of 16); if intensity increases by 10:1, pressure increases by only 3.16 (square root of 10); or if sound intensity is doubled, pressure increases by only 1.414 (square root of 2). It is important to keep in mind that:

1. As sound intensity increases by some factor, rms pressure increases only by the *square root* of the factor.
2. As rms pressure increases by some factor, sound intensity increases by the *square* of that factor.

Equation 4.4 *cannot* be used for decibels of pressure because rms pressure is proportional to the square root of intensity, not to intensity. However, Equation 4.4 can be modified to be appropriate for measures of pressure from our knowledge of the relation between sound intensity and rms pressure.

$$dB = 10 \log_{10} \frac{I_x}{I_r} \qquad \textbf{(Equation 4.4)}$$

Because

$$I = \frac{P^2}{Z_c}$$

$$dB = 10 \log \frac{(P_x^2/Z_c)}{(P_r^2/Z_c)} \qquad \text{(by substitution)}$$

$$= 10 \log \frac{(P_x^2)}{(P_r^2)} \qquad \text{(canceling } Z_c)$$

$$= 10 \log \left(\frac{P_x}{P_r}\right)^2$$

$$= 10 \times 2 \log \frac{P_x}{P_r} \qquad \textbf{(Log Law 3: } \log a^b = b \log a)$$

Equation 4.7 $$dB = 20 \log_{10} \frac{P_x}{P_r}.$$

Equation 4.4 should be used to solve problems that involve sound intensity, and Equation 4.7 should be used to solve problems that involve sound pressure. Thus, the decibel now can be defined as *10 times the log of a power or intensity ratio and as 20 times the log of a pressure ratio*. The only difference between the two equations is that a multiplier of 10 is used for intensity problems and a multiplier of 20 is used for pressure problems.

Sound Pressure Level (dB SPL)

Equation 4.7 applies for all instances in which we wish to represent a pressure ratio by decibels, and it is imperative that the reference pressure be specified. We have learned that the standard reference intensity for **dB IL** is 10^{-12} watt/m^2. The standard reference for **sound pressure** in the **MKS** system is 20 µPa (2×10^1 µPa), which is the pressure created in air by a sound wave whose intensity is 10^{-12} watt/m^2 under what are called "standard conditions."

"Standard conditions" generally mean a temperature of 20^0 Centigrade and a barometric pressure of 760 mm of mercury. When the reference is 20 µPa, we refer to decibels **sound pressure level (dB SPL)**[5]. This does not mean that 20 µPa is always the reference for sound pressure level. On the contrary, sound pressure level could be (and on occasion has been) referenced to 1 dyne/cm^2 (**cgs**) or to other values. However, the moral by now should be obvious: *all uses of decibel notation require that the reference be specified.*

In Chapter 1 we emphasized that when an air medium is energized by a vibrating source of sound, *the individual air particles are displaced over a very small distance.* We are now in a position to specify the magnitude of that "small displacement" more precisely to provide some perspective. If the sound wave is a 1000 Hz sinusoid with a sound pressure of 20 µPa (0 dB SPL), the displacement of the air particles is approximately 7.68×10^{-8} m, which is about 1/300 of the diameter of a hydrogen molecule (2.34×10^{-6} m).

Think for a moment about the vastly different magnitudes that we encounter in the study of sound. For the 1000 Hz sine wave, air particles are displaced a nearly infinitesimal distance (7.68×10^{-8} m), whereas the wavelength of that sound wave is about 0.34 m. If we substitute a 100 Hz sine wave at the same sound pressure level, air particle displacement will be unchanged, but now the wavelength will equal about 3.4 m.

The Relation Between Absolute Pressure and Decibels

The relation between absolute pressure (P_x) in µPa and dB SPL re: 20 µPa is illustrated on the next page. When $P_x = 2 \times 10^1$, dB SPL = 0 because $P_x = P_r$. As you move up the scale, P_x increases *multiplicatively* by powers of 10 to the magnitudes 2×10^2, 2×10^3, and so on, to a maximum pressure of 2×10^6 in the illustration. For each tenfold increase in sound pressure, dB SPL increases *additively* by 20 dB to a maximum of 100 dB SPL when $P_x = 2 \times 10^6$ µPa. Similarly, if you move down the scale, P_x decreases progressively by powers of 10, and for each power of 10 decrease in sound pressure, dB SPL decreases by 20 dB to a minimum of -40 dB SPL in the illustration at a sound pressure of 2×10^{-1} µPa.

dB SPL	P_X
100	$= 2 \times 10^6$
80	$= 2 \times 10^5$
60	$= 2 \times 10^4$
40	$= 2 \times 10^3$
20	$= 2 \times 10^2$
0	$\mathbf{= 2 \times 10^1}$
−20	$= 2 \times 10^0$
−40	$= 2 \times 10^{-1}$

Sample Problems

The same two steps that were used to calculate decibels for intensity should be used to calculate decibels for pressure: (1) Select the proper equation, and (2) form a ratio and solve the problem.

Problem 1: An increase in sound pressure by a factor of two (2:1) corresponds to how many decibels?

   1. dB = 20 log 2/1
        = 20 × 0.3010
        = 6.02   (which normally is rounded to 6 dB).

   2. We learned previously that as sound intensity increases by a factor of 2:1, the level is increased by 3 dB. However, from this problem we see that as sound pressure increases by a factor of 2:1, the *pressure level* is increased by *6 dB*. That difference, of course, occurs because with intensity we multiply the log of 2 (0.3) by 10 and with pressure we multiply the log of 2 (0.3) by 20. Correspondingly, if pressure is *halved* (ratio = 1:2), the pressure level is *decreased* by 6 dB.

Problem 2: An increase in pressure by a factor of ten corresponds to how many decibels?

   1. dB = 20 log 10/1
        = 20 × 1
        = 20.

   2. As pressure increases *multiplicatively* by 10, relative pressure increases *additively* by 20 dB. If the pressure is decreased by a factor of 10 (1:10), the level is decreased by 20 dB.

Problem 3: What is the sound pressure level re: 2×10^1 µPa of a sound whose absolute pressure is 2×10^4 µPa?

$$dB = 20 \log (2 \times 10^4)/(2 \times 10^1)$$
$$= 20 \log 10^3$$
$$= 60.$$

Problem 4: What is the sound pressure level re: 2×10^1 µPa of a sound whose absolute pressure is 4×10^4 µPa?

1. First you should note that the pressure in this problem (4×10^4) is exactly twice as great as the pressure in Problem 3 (2×10^4). Because a doubling of pressure corresponds to 6 dB, you should expect that the answer would be 6 dB greater than the answer for Problem 3 ($60 + 6 = 66$).

2. $dB = 20 \log (4 \times 10^4)/(2 \times 10^1)$
   $= 20 \log 2 \times 10^3$
   $= 66.$

3. By now, it should not be necessary to use a calculator or log table for this kind of problem, and you might not even need scratch paper. You know that the log of 10^3 is 3 (a log is an exponent), and you should remember that the log of 2 is 0.3. Law 1 of logarithms stated that the log of a product is equal to the sum of the logs of the factors, so the log of 2×10^3 must equal $3 + 0.3$, which multiplied by 20 yields 66.

Problem 5: 26 dB corresponds to what pressure ratio?

1. Before using paper and pencil, see if you can determine the answer by recalling powers of 2 and 10.

2. $\quad$ $26 \text{ dB} = 20 \log X$
   $\quad\quad\quad 1.3 = \log X$
   $2 \times 10^1 = X$
   $\quad\quad\quad\quad = 20.$

3. With powers of 2 and 10 in mind, you might have noticed that 26 dB was composed of 20 dB (10:1) and 6 dB (2:1). Because 26 dB consists of $20 + 6$, the ratio must be $10 \times 2 = 20:1$.

Problem 6: A sound pressure level of 65 dB re: 2×10^1 µPa corresponds to what sound pressure?

$$65 \text{ dB} = 20 \log P_x/(2 \times 10^1)$$
$$3.25 = \log P_x/(2 \times 10^1)$$
$$1.78 \times 10^3 = P_x/(2 \times 10^1)$$
$$P_x = 1.78 \times 2 \times 10^3 \times 10^1$$
$$P_x = 3.56 \times 10^4.$$

■ THE RELATION BETWEEN dB IL AND dB SPL

In Table 4-2 we see that an *intensity ratio* of 10:1, for example, corresponds to 10 dB, whereas a *pressure ratio* of 10:1 corresponds to 20 dB. Would you conclude, therefore, that 60 dB IL = 120 dB SPL? *You should not!*

It is true that an intensity ratio of 10:1 corresponds to 10 dB and a pressure ratio of 10:1 corresponds to 20 dB. However, if the intensity of a particular sound were increased by a factor of 10:1, the pressure of the same sound wave would be increased only *by the square root of 10:1* (3.1623), and the decibel equivalent would still be 10 (20 log 3.1623 = 10 dB).

Recall that *pressure is proportional to the square root of intensity*, and conversely, *intensity is proportional to the square of pressure*. Other examples of this same relation can be seen in the table. An intensity ratio of 100:1 corresponds to 20 dB and a pressure ratio of 100:1 corresponds to 40 dB. However, if the intensity of a particular wave were increased by 100:1, the pressure would be increased by only 10:1 and, in either case, the decibel equivalent would be 20 dB.

Thus, we see that 60 dB IL does *not* equal 120 dB SPL. Recall from the derivation of Equation 4.7 that the multiplier of 10 in decibels for intensity was changed to a multiplier of 20 in decibels for pressure. As long as equivalent references are used in the two equations, dB IL = dB SPL, and as we learned previously, 2×10^1 µPa is the pressure equivalent to an intensity of 10^{-12} watt/m^2.

The equivalence of dB IL and dB SPL is illustrated in Figure 4-1, which shows what might be called isodecibel contours. At the left of the figure, intensity in watt/m^2 increases from 10^{-13} at the bottom to 10^{-4} at the top. At the right of the figure, *corresponding* pressure values in µPa increase from 6.32×10^0 to a maximum of 2×10^5.

Thus, we see that as intensity is increased or decreased by a power of 10, pressure changes only by the square root of 10. Each contour is a line that connects a given intensity at the left with a corresponding pressure at the right. The parameter of the figure, then, is decibels, *either dB IL or dB SPL*. They are equivalent.

Table 4-2. Relation between decibels for intensity and decibels for pressure

Intensity		Pressure	
Ratio I_x/I_r	dB $10 \log_{10} I_x/I_r$	Ratio P_x/P_r	dB $20 \log_{10} P_x/P_r$
1	0	1.0000	0
10	10	3.1623	10
100	20	10.0000	20
1,000	30	31.6228	30
10,000	40	100.0000	40
100,000	50	316.2278	50
1,000,000	60	1,000.0000	60

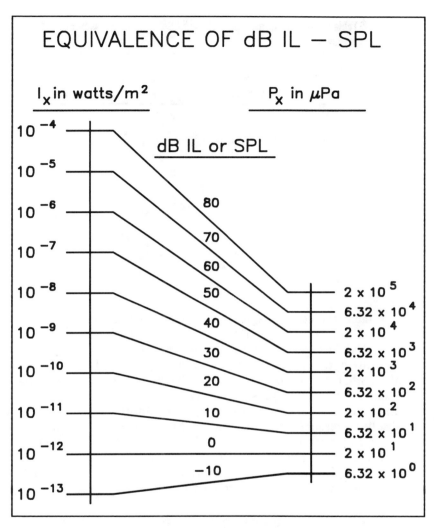

Figure 4-1. Equivalence of dB IL and dB SPL. The reference intensity for dB IL is 10^{-12} watt/m². The pressure created in air by a sound wave that has an intensity of 10^{-12} watt/m² is 20 μPa. Thus, the reference pressure for dB SPL is equivalent to the reference intensity for dB IL, and dB IL *always* equals dB SPL.

■UNITS OF MEASURE FOR PRESSURE

In Chapter 1 we indicated that force is measured in **newtons (MKS)** or **dynes (cgs)** and therefore that pressure (the amount of force per unit area) is measured in **newtons/m² (MKS)** or **dynes/cm² (cgs)**. The popularity of these and other units of measure for pressure have changed over the past several years, and it is necessary to compare and understand the relations among the various systems if we are to read and understand all of the scientific literature, not just the literature written in the past few years.

Table 4–3. Comparisons of various units of **measure for pressure**

dB SPL	dynes/cm² or microbar	Nt/m² or Pa	μNt/m² or μPa
100	2×10^1	2×10^0	2×10^6
94	10^1	10^0	10^6
80	2×10^0	2×10^{-1}	2×10^5
74	10^0	10^{-1}	10^5
60	2×10^{-1}	2×10^{-2}	2×10^4
54	10^{-1}	10^{-2}	10^4
40	2×10^{-2}	2×10^{-3}	2×10^3
34	10^{-2}	10^{-3}	10^3
20	2×10^{-3}	2×10^{-4}	2×10^2
14	10^{-3}	10^{-4}	10^2
0	$\mathbf{2 \times 10^{-4}}$	$\mathbf{2 \times 10^{-5}}$	$\mathbf{2 \times 10^1}$
−6	10^{-4}	10^{-5}	10^1

Table 4–3 compares, in approximate order of their appearance in the literature, the dyne/cm² (*and its equivalent, the **microbar***) with the **Nt/m²** (and its equivalent, the **pascal [Pa]**) and with the μNt/m² (and its equivalent, the **μPa**). The first column of Table 4–3 lists various values of dB SPL ranging from 100 to −6. The second column shows the corresponding *absolute* pressure in **dynes/cm²** or **microbar**. Those two units are equal to each other. The third column shows the equivalent absolute pressures in **Nt/m²** and **pascals (Pa)**, which are equal to each other, and the fourth column lists the corresponding absolute pressures in **μNt/m²** and **μPa**, which also are equivalent to one another.

We can make several observations from the entries in Table 4–3, some of which have been stressed previously.

1. The **reference pressures** for dB SPL appear in the row for 0 dB SPL, and *the three entries are all equivalent.* Thus, 2×10^{-4} dyne/cm² (or microbar) = 2×10^{-5} Nt/m² (or Pa) = 2×10^1 μNt/m² (or μPa). In a similar vein, all entries of absolute pressure *in any single row are equivalent.* Thus, for the row corresponding to 74 dB SPL, 10^0 dyne/cm² (or microbar) = 10^{-1} Nt/m² (or Pa) = 10^5 μNt/m² (or μPa).

2. Regardless of which unit of measure of sound pressure is selected, any twofold change in pressure corresponds to 6 dB: +6 dB if pressure increases and −6 dB if pressure decreases. For example, 2×10^{-2} Pa = 60 dB SPL; a pressure of 10^{-2} is only half as great as a pressure of 2×10^{-2}, and it corresponds to 54 dB SPL, which is 6 dB less. Similarly, 10^1 μPa = −6 dB SPL, and 2×10^1 μPa, which is twice as great, corresponds to 0 dB SPL, which is 6 dB more.

3. Any tenfold change in sound pressure corresponds to 20 dB: +20 dB if pressure increases and −20 dB if pressure decreases.

Thus, 10^{-3} microbar = 14 dB SPL and 10^{-2} microbar (change in pressure by 10:1) corresponds to 34 dB SPL (+20 dB).

4. What does 0 dB SPL mean? *It does not mean absence of sound.* It simply means that the pressure in question, P_x, is exactly equal to the reference pressure, P_r. When $P_x = P_r$, the ratio is 1, the log of 1 = 0, and 20 times 0 will always equal 0 dB. Of course, the same is true for dB IL or any other decibel. A decibel is always 10 or 20 times the log of a ratio, and 0 dB always mean that $P_x = P_r$ or that $I_x = I_r$.

5. What do negative decibels mean? It does not matter whether we are dealing with decibels for pressure or decibels for intensity. Negative decibels mean that the value of the reference pressure (P_r) or reference intensity (I_r) exceeds the value of the pressure (P_x) or intensity (I_x) in question, that is, $P_r > P_x$ or $I_r > I_x$. That situation can be seen in the last row of Table 4-3 for all of the units of measure.

■ CONVERSION FROM ONE REFERENCE TO ANOTHER

The values of absolute pressure listed in Table 4-3 opposite 0 dB SPL are the **standard reference pressures** for decibels sound pressure level. However, there are occasions in which a different reference might be adopted for some reason. In that circumstance, it might be important to compare decibels corresponding to one reference pressure with decibels referenced to a different pressure to determine whether or not they are equivalent.

You are likely to encounter older, but still important, literature in which decibels **sound pressure level** are expressed re: 1 dyne/cm^2 instead of 2×10^{-4} dyne/cm^2 in the **cgs** metric system. Suppose, for example, one author contends that level of some particular noise is 74 dB SPL re: 2×10^{-4} dyne/cm^2. A second investigator describes the level of the same noise as 0 dB re: 1 dyne/cm^2. Are the results equivalent? We shall see that the answer is "yes," and only a few calculations are necessary to demonstrate the equivalence.

You might encounter a "conversion rule" that says: to convert from a reference pressure of 2×10^{-4} dyne/cm^2 to a reference of 1 dyne/cm^2, subtract 74 dB, or, conversely, to convert from 1 dyne/cm^2 to 2×10^{-4} dyne/cm^2, add 74 dB. That is in fact a correct rule — if you can remember when to add and when to subtract — but it only applies to those two values. What we need, then, is a system that will permit us to convert between any two reference pressures expressed in the same metric system. Two alternative approaches can be used.

One choice, albeit more cumbersome, is to calculate P_x (an antilog problem) from knowledge of the original reference pressure and then recalculate decibels (a log problem) using the new reference pressure.

1. 74 dB SPL re: 2×10^{-4} dyne/cm^2 = how many dB SPL re: 1 dyne/cm^2? Calculate the pressure, P_x, corresponding to 74 dB re: 2×10^{-4}.

$$74 = 20 \log (P_x)/(2 \times 10^{-4})$$
$$3.7 = \log (P_x)/(2 \times 10^{-4})$$
$$5 \times 10^3 = (P_x)/(2 \times 10^{-4})$$
$$P_x = 10 \times 10^{-1}$$
$$= 1 \times 10^0.$$

2. From that calculation we know that the sound had an absolute pressure $(P_x) = 1$ dyne/cm^2 (1×10^0). The next step, then, is to recalculate dB SPL using Equation 4.7, but with the new reference pressure, 1 dyne/cm^2, in the denominator.

$$dB = 20 \log (1 \times 10^0)/(1 \times 10^0)$$
$$= 0 \text{ dB SPL.}$$

Consider a second example. 20 dB SPL re: 1 dyne/cm^2 = ? dB SPL re: 2 dynes/cm^2?

1.
$$20 = 20 \log (P_x)/(1 \times 10^0)$$
$$1 = \log (P_x)/(1 \times 10^0)$$
$$10^1 = (P_x)/(1 \times 10^0)$$
$$P_x = 10^1 \times 1 \times 10^0$$
$$= 1 \times 10^1.$$

2.
$$dB = 20 \log (1 \times 10^1)/(2 \times 10^0)$$
$$= 20 \log .5 \times 10^1$$
$$= 20 \log 5 \times 10^0$$
$$= 20 \times 0.7$$
$$= 14.$$

The approach just described required two steps: (1) solve an antilog problem to determine the value of P_x; and (2) solve a log problem to express P_x in decibels re: the new reference. An easier alternative is to use Equation 4.8, where only one step is necessary.

Equation 4.8

$$dB_{Pr(2)} = dB_{Pr(1)} - 20 \log_{10} \frac{P_{r(2)}}{P_{r(1)},}$$

where $P_{r(1)}$ = the original reference

and

$P_{r(2)}$ = the new reference.

Equation 4.8 tells us that decibels re: a second (new) reference are given by subtracting 20 log of the ratio of the two references from decibels re: the first (original) reference. To illustrate that the two approaches yield identical results, we shall solve the first of the two problems listed above: 74 dB SPL re: 2×10^{-4} dyne/cm^2 = ? dB re: 1 dyne/cm^2.

$$dB = 74 - 20 \log (1 \times 10^0)/(2 \times 10^{-4})$$
$$= 74 - 20 \log .5 \times 10^4$$
$$= 0.$$

■ COMBINING SOUND INTENSITIES FROM INDEPENDENT SOURCES

If the intensity of some sound is 10^{-5} watt/m^2, we can calculate with Equation 4.4 that the intensity level is 70 dB IL re: 10^{-12} watt/m^2. Suppose, then, that two independent sound sources are operating simultaneously and that each produces a sound with an intensity of 10^{-5} watt/m^2. We know that each source has an intensity level of 70 dB, but what is the *total intensity level* from the two sources combined? It is *not* 140 dB. Work through the problem and see why 140 dB is not a reasonable answer. To have an intensity level of 140 dB would require an absolute intensity of 10^2 watt/m^2.

$$140 = 10 \log I_x/10^{-12}$$

$$14 = \log I_x/10^{-12}$$
$$I_x = 10^{14} \times 10^{-12}$$
$$= 10^2.$$

It should be apparent that it is clearly *impossible* to have a total intensity of 10^2 watt/m^2. Each independent source produces a finite amount of energy. If the intensity (**energy/sec/m²**) from each source is an identical 10^{-5} watt/m^2, then the total intensity from the combined sources can only be twice as great, 2×10^{-5} watt/m^2, not 10^2 watt/m^2. If the total **intensity** from the two sources combined is 2×10^{-5} watt/m^2, what is the **intensity level** from the two combined?

$$dB = 10 \log 2 \times 10^{-5}/10^{-12}$$
$$= 73.$$

If the **intensity level** is 73 dB, what is the **sound pressure level** from the combined sources? If the reference pressure is 2×10^1 µPa, *dB SPL also equals 73*. First, a brief calculation should demonstrate the equivalence. The **intensity** from the combined sources was twice as great as for either source alone. A doubling of intensity corresponds to +3 dB, and we saw that the total of 73 dB was 3 dB greater than the intensity level from only one of the sources. However, if the intensity were increased by a factor of 2:1, what would have happened to the pressure? It would have increased by the square root of 2 ($P \propto \sqrt{I}$), or 1.414. From Equation 4.7 we see that sound pressure level also would have increased by 3 dB from 70 dB SPL.

$$dB = 20 \log 1.414$$
$$= 3.$$

Second, we learned previously (see Figure 4–1) that dB IL always equals dB SPL *when equivalent reference intensities and pressures are used.* Thus, 70 dB IL (the level for either source alone) equals 70 dB SPL, and if the intensity level increases by only 3 dB, the same must be true for the sound pressure level, which produces a total level of 73 dB SPL.

Unfortunately, the equivalence of dB IL and dB SPL is not always understood. Several years ago a person took a national examination that is required for certification by the American Speech-Language-Hearing Association and encountered the following kind of problem: If two sound sources each produce an identical sound pressure level, by how much will the total sound pressure level of the two combined sources exceed the level for either source alone?

By now, you should know that the answer is 3 dB because it is the energies, powers, or intensities that should be added, which requires us to use the "10-log" equation (Equation 4.4). The person wrote a letter-to-the-editor of the journal *Asha* to complain that the examination was unfair because the alternative answers included 3 dB, but not 6 dB, and the writer was certain that 6 dB was the correct choice.

That letter produced some lively (and correct) responses from Mitchell Kramer, who then was a doctoral student at Northwestern University, and from Professors Larry Feth and W. Dixon Ward that were published in *Asha* (March, 1977). Some comments from those three individuals should serve to emphasize the main point that has been stressed in this section:

Both sound pressure and power change with a change in energy of an acoustic signal, with power changing as the square of pressure. But, a 3 dB change in pressure is equal, identical, and the very same as a 3 dB change in power or intensity. Of course, a doubling of pressure results in a 6 dB increase (of both pressure and intensity or power) but unless two signals are (1) the same frequency, and (2) added in phase, the intensities add, and a 3 dB increase results. This is equivalent to doubling the sound power, or increasing pressure by a factor of 1.41. But a dB is still a dB. (Kramer, p. 225)

What students often carry away from the lecture on combining sound sources is the rule of thumb: "Double the intensity means a 3 dB increase; double the sound pressure results in a 6 dB increase." That rule by itself is correct. The errors arise in not understanding how sound pressure waveforms are added and in thinking that there is a difference between intensity level (IL) and sound pressure level (SPL) . . . . It must be kept in mind that sound pressure level (SPL) and intensity level (IL) are always synonymous and further are always numerically equal . . . . When two independent sound sources are combined, one must always add their intensities. Two sound pressure waveforms can only be added if their relative phase is known, and it seldom is. (Feth, pp. 225–226)

What I suspect happened is that the problem went something like this: "If we put two machines side by side, each of which develops an SPL of 80 dB, what will be the SPL when they are both running?" The question is designed to lead the unwary down the primrose path by using SPL instead of IL, so that he or she is hoodwinked into thinking: "Oh yes, doubling the pressure is a 6-dB increase" — which is correct, but, alas, irrelevant, because the pressure simply does not get doubled in this situation. The correct answer is indeed 83 dB SPL — and, assuming that it is still taking place here on earth, also 83 dB IL. In air at standard temperature and pressure, the zeroes on the SPL and IL scales have been chosen to represent the same acoustic conditions, so X dB SPL is also X dB IL . . . . To double the pressure (still under optimum conditions) would require four equal machines. (Ward, p. 226)

It is important to remember that when the total intensity level or sound pressure level from uncorrelated (independent) sound sources is desired, it is *the **energies**, or **powers**, or **intensities** that should be summed, not the pressures.* As Feth stated in his letter cited above, we cannot add the pressures unless the relative phases are known, and they seldom are.

There are two approaches that can be taken to solving problems such as these.

Equal Source Intensities

We will consider first the easier situation in which all of the contributing sources are characterized by an identical intensity level or sound pressure level. In that case,

$$dB_N = dB_i + 10 \log_{10} N, \qquad \text{**Equation 4.9**}$$

where i = dB SPL (or dB IL) from one of the equal sources

and

N = the number of sources combined.

We do not have to determine the **intensity** of any of the sources or of the total. We simply want to know the total **intensity level** in dB.

Two snowmobiles each produce 94 dB IL. What is the total level from   **Example 1**
the two combined?

$$dB_N = 94 + 10 \log 2$$
$$= 97.$$

Each source produces some finite amount of intensity that we do not need to calculate. Because there are two such sources, *the two sources combined must produce twice the intensity as either one alone.* Anytime we increase intensity by a factor of 2:1, decibels increase by 3: 94 + 3 = 97. Why does Equation 4.9 "apparently" not contain a ratio? Actually it does. We are asking what happened to the intensity level when we increased from one source to two sources. Thus, the reference is 1 and need not be shown in the denominator.

Example 2   What is the total **sound pressure level** for eight sound sources, each of which produces 92 dB when operating alone?

Even though the level in the problem is expressed in SPL rather than IL, it is the intensities that must be added, not the pressures. Thus, we proceed just as we did with Example 1.

$$dB_N = 92 + 10 \log 8$$
$$= 92 + 9$$
$$= 101.$$

By now you should be able to work this kind of problem mentally by thinking of powers of 2. 8 is 2^3, which means that 8 is the result of the base 2 being used 3 times in multiplication. Each doubling corresponds to 3 dB. Thus, eight sources would produce a sound whose intensity is 9 dB (3 + 3 + 3) greater than just one of the sources alone.

Unequal Source Intensities

When the contributing sources are not all characterized by equal intensity, Equation 4.9 will not apply, but the problem can still be solved by following three steps: (1) calculate the **intensity** of each source, (2) add the intensities, and the sum of the intensities becomes the numerator of the ratio, and (3) calculate decibels with Equation 4.4 with a reference of 10^{-12} watt/m^2. The result will be either dB IL or dB SPL because the two are equivalent.

Example 1   What is the total SPL that results from combining one source that produces 90 dB SPL with a second source that produces 80 dB SPL?

1. $90 = 10 \log I_x/10^{-12}$,   Therefore, $I_{x(1)} = 10^{-3}$,
     and
     $80 = 10 \log I_x/10^{-12}$,   Therefore, $I_{x(2)} = 10^{-4}$,
2. $10^{-3} + 10^{-4} = 1.1 \times 10^{-3}$,
3. $dB = 10 \log 1.1 \times 10^{-3}/10^{-12}$
     $= 10 \log 1.1 \times 10^9$
     $= 90.4.$

There are two important observations to make. First, when the levels of two sources differ by 10 dB, the total level is only 0.4 dB greater than the level of the source with the higher intensity. That is true of any two levels that differ by 10 dB: 90 and 80 (90.4), 80 and 70 (80.4), 0 and −10 (0.4), and so on. Second, one must be careful with addition of the intensities in Step 2 because the exponents are different.

$$I_{x(1)} = 1 \times 10^{-3}$$
$$+ \; I_{x(2)} = 1 \times 10^{-4}$$
$$= \; ?$$

Before the two intensities can be added, the exponent for one must be converted to be the same as the other exponent. We will illustrate the process by converting $I_{x(2)}$ to have an exponent of -3 rather than -4. To convert from -4 to -3 we *multiply* by 10. To preserve equivalence, therefore, we must *divide* the other term in the product, the coefficient, by 10: Thus,

$$1 \times 10^{-4} = .1 \times 10^{-3}.$$

Now when we add the two intensities, we obtain:

$$1 \times 10^{-3}$$
$$+ \; .1 \times 10^{-3}$$
$$= 1.1 \times 10^{-3}.$$

If the validity of that series of steps is not obvious, the two intensities are added below in conventional notation rather than scientific notation,

$$1 \times 10^{-3} = .001$$
$$+ \; 1 \times 10^{-4} = .0001$$
$$= .0011$$

and .0011 in conventional notation equals 1.1×10^{-3} in scientific notation.

A fan is operating at an unknown level in a noisy environment. You wish to determine the sound pressure level of the fan, but it cannot be removed from its location and the surrounding noise cannot be turned off.   **Example 2**

1. Measure the sound pressure level of the combined noise produced by the fan and the surrounding equipment. This measurement would be accomplished with the aid of a sound level meter, which will not be discussed in this book. Suppose this total level is 90 dB SPL.

2. Turn off the fan and measure the level produced by the surrounding equipment. Suppose that this new measurement is 86 dB SPL.

3. From those two measurements we know that the surrounding equipment and the fan together produce a noise of 90 dB SPL

and that the surrounding equipment alone produces a noise of 86 dB SPL. The fan, therefore, must be responsible for the difference of 4 dB, but *do not conclude that its level is 4 dB SPL.* Before we solve the problem, try to approximate the answer by mentally using powers of 2. Recall the earlier problem involving the two snowmobiles. We learned that combining two sound sources that have the same intensity produced a 3 dB increase from the level produced by either machine alone. In the present problem, the surrounding noise is 86 dB. Therefore, if the noise from the fan also were 86 dB, the two combined would produce a noise of 89 dB, which is just 1 dB less than the 90 we measured. Therefore, we should expect the true noise level of the fan to be just a little more than 86.

a. (Intensity of fan plus surrounding noise)
$90 = 10 \log I_x/10^{-12}.$ Therefore, $I_{x(2)} = 10^{-3}.$

b. (Intensity of surrounding noise alone)
$86 = 10 \log I_x/10^{-12}.$ Therefore, $I_{x(1)} = 3.98 \times 10^{-4}.$

c. (Intensities of fan alone — by subtraction)
$(1 \times 10^{-3}) - (3.98 \times 10^{-4}) = 6.02 \times 10^{-4}.$

d. (Intensity level of fan alone)
$dB = 10 \log 6.02 \times 10^{-4}/10^{-12}$
$= 87.8.$

Because the preceding computational methods might sometimes be inconvenient, published charts are available to aid with combining decibels. Direct computations are preferable, however, if precise determination of small differences is required.

■ SUMMARY OF DECIBELS FOR SOUND INTENSITY AND SOUND PRESSURE

Earlier in this chapter two steps were suggested for solution of decibel problems. First, select the proper equation. Second, form a ratio and solve the problem. When the problem involves **intensity or power**, use Equation 4.4 — the so-called "10 log equation." When the problem involves **pressure**, use Equation 4.7 — the "20 log equation."

The distinction between power and pressure applies if decibels are used to express the level of some quantity other than sound. For example, if you have three dollars, and someone gives you three more dollars, that represents an increase of 3 dB. In contrast, if a committee comprises three people, and three more members are added, that represents an increase of 6 dB. We might justify use of the 10 log equation in one case, but the 20 log equation in the other, because "money is power," but "people are pressure."

The only confusion that should remain might stem from problems that involve combining sound levels from independent sources. In those instances it is important to keep in mind that unless the relative phases are known, *it is the energies or powers or intensities that should be added, not the pressures.* Thus, it does not matter whether the problem is stated by reference to IL or SPL. *As long as the references are equivalent, dB IL = db SPL, and you must always use Equation 4.4 —* the "10 log equation."

■ PRACTICE PROBLEMS

Recall the two-step procedure for solving decibel problems. (1) Select the proper equation, and (2) form a ratio and solve the problem.

It will always be useful to inspect a problem to see if it involves powers of 2 (3 dB for intensity; 6 dB for pressure) or powers of 10 (10 dB for intensity; 20 dB for pressure). Even though some problems cannot be solved in this way, you will be able to estimate the answers in many cases by using powers of 2 and powers of 10 to set upper and lower limits that bracket the correct answers reasonably closely. Try to solve as many problems as possible "mentally," using powers of 2 and powers of 10, and then use your calculator to check your computations.

Set 1

Convert each of the following intensity ratios to decibels.

a.	1:1	g.	3:1	m.	9:1	s.	1:7	y.	.001:1
b.	10:1	h.	4:1	n.	1:2	t.	1:8	z.	10^{-3}:1
c.	100:1	i.	5:1	o.	1:3	u.	1:9	aa.	20:1
d.	1,000:1	j.	6:1	p.	1:4	v.	1:10	bb.	200:1
e.	10^3:1	k.	7:1	q.	1:5	w.	1:100	cc.	40:1
f.	2:1	l.	8:1	r.	1:6	x.	1:1,000	dd.	400:1

ee.   60:1

ff.   600:1

gg. 2.45×10^0:1

hh. 2.45×10^1:1

ii. $2.45 \times 10^1/10^{-12}$:1

jj. $2.45 \times 10^{-8}/10^{-16}$:1

Set 2

Convert each of the following decibels to intensity ratios.

a. 0	f. 70	k. 23	p. −10	u. 17
b. 10	g. 3	l. 29	q. −20	v. 62
c. 20	h. 6	m. 46	r. −30	w. 91
d. 30	i. 9	n. 56	s. −23	x. 5.4
e. 40	j. 12	o. 76	t. −36	y. 12.6

Set 3

Calculate dB IL re: 10^{-12} watt/m^2 for each of the following values of sound intensity (I_x).

a. 10^{-12}	f. 2×10^{-8}	k. 1×10^{-2}	p. 0.25×10^{-12}
b. 10^{-11}	g. 4×10^{-8}	l. 2×10^{-2}	q. 1.4×10^{-4}
c. 10^{-10}	h. 8×10^{-8}	m. $.5 \times 10^{-2}$	r. 2.8×10^{-4}
d. 10^{-9}	i. 1×10^{-3}	n. $.5 \times 10^{-5}$	s. 1.65×10^{-6}
e. 10^{-8}	j. 4×10^{-3}	o. $.5 \times 10^{-12}$	t. 3.00×10^{-6}

Set 4

Calculate sound intensity (I_x) in watt/m^2 for each of the following values of dB IL re: 10^{-12} watt/m^2.

a. 0	f. 60	k. −10	p. −23	u. 87
b. 10	g. 13	l. −20	q. −26	v. 16.8
c. 20	h. 23	m. −3	r. 41	w. 24.2
d. 30	i. 36	n. −6	s. 62	x. 38
e. 40	j. 49	o. −13	t. 73	y. 47

Set 5

Convert each of the following pressure ratios to decibels.

a.	1:1	g. 3:1	m. 9:1	s. 1:7	y. .001:1
b.	10:1	h. 4:1	n. 1:2	t. 1:8	z. 10^{-3}:1
c.	100:1	i. 5:1	o. 1:3	u. 1:9	aa. 20:1
d.	1,000:1	j. 6:1	p. 1:4	v. 1:10	bb. 200:1
e.	10^3:1	k. 7:1	q. 1:5	w. 1:100	cc. 40:1
f.	2:1	l. 8:1	r. 1:6	x. 1:1,000	dd. 400:1

ee.	60:1	kk.	10^0:1
ff.	600:1	ll.	$10^{-4}/10^{-4}$:1
gg.	10^{-4}:1	mm.	$10^{-3}/10^{-4}$:1
hh.	10^{-5}:1	nn.	$(2 \times 10^{-4})/(2 \times 10^{-4})$:1
ii.	10^{-2}:1	oo.	$(4 \times 10^{-4})/(2 \times 10^{-4})$:1
jj.	10^{-1}:1	pp.	$(10^{-4})/(2 \times 10^{-4})$:1

Set 6

Convert each of the following decibels to pressure ratios.

a.	0	g.	6	m.	26	s.	30
b.	20	h.	12	n.	46	t.	50
c.	40	i.	18	o.	72	u.	44
d.	60	j.	24	p.	−20	v.	17
e.	80	k.	−6	q.	−40	w.	62
f.	100	l.	−12	r.	10	x.	5.5

Set 7

Calculate dB SPL re: 2×10^1 µPa for each of the following values of sound pressure (P_x) in µPa.

a. 2×10^1 g. 4×10^1 m. 1.05×10^6

b. 2×10^2 h. 8×10^1 n. 1×10^5

c. 2×10^3 i. 8×10^4 o. $.5 \times 10^5$

d. 2×10^4 j. 2×10^0 p. 4×10^5

e. 2×10^5 k. 4×10^0 q. 4.25×10^5

f. 10^5 l. 4×10^3 r. 8.5×10^5

Set 8

Calculate sound pressure (P_x) in µPa for each of the following values of dB SPL re: 2×10^1 µPa.

a.   0   f. 40   k. 30   p.   34

b.   6   g. 60   l. 50   q.   72

c.   12   h. 3   m. 43   r.   16.8

d. −6   i. 9   n. 46   s.   −7

e.   20   j. 10   o. 36   t.   −8

Set 9

Calculate dB SPL re: 2×10^{-4} dyne/cm^2 for each of the following values of sound pressure (P_x) in dyne/cm^2.

a. 0.0002   f. 0.002

b. 0.0004   g. 2×10^{-3}

c. 8×10^{-4} h. 4×10^{-2}

d. 2×10^{-4} i. 1×10^{-5}

e. 4×10^{-4} j. 2×10^0

Set 10

Calculate the sound pressure level that results from combining the following uncorrelated sound sources whose levels are given in dB SPL.

a. 20 + 20   d. 20 + 20 + 20   g. 60 + 70

b. 30 + 30   e. 30 + 30 + 30   h. 60 + 66

c. 46.2 + 46.2   f. 46.2 + 46.2 + 46.2   i. 60 + 70 + 80

Set 11

Calculate the total intensity in watt/m^2 that results from combining the following intensities from uncorrelated sources.

a. $10^{-8} + 10^{-8}$ d. $2 \times 10^{-6} + 5 \times 10^{-6}$

b. $10^{-6} + 10^{-6}$ e. $2 \times 10^{-6} + 5 \times 10^{-6} + 2 \times 10^{-6}$

c. $2 \times 10^{-6} + 10^{-6}$ f. $2 \times 10^{-6} + 3 \times 10^{-5}$

Set 12

Calculate the intensity level re: 10^{-12} watt/m^2 that results from combining the intensities in Set 11.

a.   d.

b.   e.

c.   f.

■ ANSWERS TO PRACTICE PROBLEMS

Set 1

Equation 4.4 should be used to convert the intensity ratios to decibels. In each of these problems, the reference is not specified, but the ratio I_x/I_r is known. For example, if the intensity ratio is 12:1,

$$N(dB) = 10 \log 12$$
$$= 10 \times 1.08$$
$$= 10.8 \text{ dB.}$$

Set 1 *(continued)*

a. 0	g. 4.8	m. 9.5	s. −8.5	y. −30
b. 10	h. 6	n. −3	t. −9	z. −30
c. 20	i. 7	o. −4.8	u. −9.5	aa. 13
d. 30	j. 7.8	p. −6	v. −10	bb. 23
e. 30	k. 8.5	q. −7	w. −20	cc. 16
f. 3	l. 9	r. −7.8	x. −30	dd. 26

ee. 17.8	gg. 3.9	ii. 133.9
ff. 27.8	hh. 13.9	jj. 83.9

Notes

(a). 0 dB does not mean "silence." It means only that $I_x = I_r$ and, therefore, that the ratio $I_x/I_r = 1.0$ regardless of the absolute value of I_x.

(b, c, d). You should note that each of these involves powers of 10, and each power of 10 corresponds to 10 dB. Thus, in 1-c the ratio is 100, which is a power of 10 twice (10^2). Because each power of 10 corresponds to 10 dB, the answer is given by 10 dB + 10 dB = 20 dB.

(f). A power of 2, which is 3 dB.

(h). Another power of 2. The ratio 4:1 corresponds to a power of 2 twice (2^2), and each power of 2 is 3 dB. Thus, 3 dB + 3 dB = 6 dB.

(i). Can you see that the ratio 5:1 involves powers of 10 and powers of 2? The ratio 5:1 can be thought of as the ratio 10:1 (+10 dB) divided by the ratio 2:1 (−3 dB), which is 7 dB.

(l). A power of 2 three times (2^3), which therefore involves 3 dB + 3 dB + 3 dB = 9 dB.

(n–z). These are the inverse of the otherwise identical problems that were solved earlier in this set. Because the absolute value of $I_x < I_r$, the answer in decibels will be negative. Solution of such problems is simplified by recalling Log Law 4 (log 1/a = −log a). Thus, for example:

$$10 \log 1/2 = -10 \log 2 = -3 \text{ dB.}$$

(aa–dd).   By now you should quickly see that each involves a combination of powers of 10 (10 dB) and powers of 2 (3 dB). Thus, 400 consists of a power of 10 twice (+20 dB) and a power of 2 twice (+6 dB): $10 \times 10 \times 2 \times 2 = 400$ and the corresponding quantities in decibels are 10 dB + 10 dB + 3 dB + 3 dB = 26 dB.

(ee, ff).   These can only be approximated by powers of 2 and 10. To see how the approximation works, consider the ratio 600:1. You know that 400 ($10 \times 10 \times 2 \times 2$) is 26 dB and that 1,000 ($10 \times 10 \times 10$) is 30 dB. So, the answer for 600 must lie between 26 dB and 30 dB. However, if you think back to problem 1–i, you should be able to set the limits even closer. You solved that 5:1 is 7 dB (10/2). If 5:1 is 7 dB, 500 must be another 20 dB for a total of 27 dB. Therefore, because 600 lies between 500 and 1,000, the answer must lie between 27 and 30. See if you can find a way, still using powers of 2 and 10, to lower the upper limit. (Hint: you should be able to set the upper limit to 29 dB.)

(gg, hh).   Solution of these problems is made easy by recalling two concepts from Chapter 3. First, both problems involve the log of a product. We learned from Log Law 1 that "log ab = log a + log b." Thus, with Problem 1-gg, we need only to add the logs of the two factors: $\log 2.45 + \log 10^0$. You will need a calculator or log table to determine the log of 2.45, but a second concept from Chapter 3 will allow you to determine the log of 10^0 without reference to a log table: "An exponent is a log, and a log is an exponent." Thus, the log of 10 raised to any power is the value of the power. $\log 10^0 = 0$; $\log 10^1 = 1$; $\log 10^2 = 2; \ldots; \log 10^n = n$.

(ii, jj).   These problems represent application of two laws of logarithms and one law of exponents. As a consequence, the problems can be solved in two ways. We will use 1–ii as an example. We can apply Log Law 1, where a = 2.45 and b = $(10^1/10^{-12})$. The log of 2.45 is determined from a calculator or log table, but there are two approaches available for determining the log of the ratio $10^1/10^{-12}$. With the first approach we apply Log Law 2: log a/b = log a − log b. Because we know that an exponent is a log, the log of that ratio is given by the difference between the exponents, $1 - (-12)$, which is 13. From Log Law 1, then the log of the product is 0.4 + 13 = 13.4, which multiplied by 10 = 134 dB. With the second approach we apply Law 2 of exponents, which is a companion to Log Law 2: $X^m/X^n = X^{m-n}$. Therefore,

$$10^1/10^{-12} = 10^{13}$$
$$\log 10^{13} = 13$$
$$\text{and}$$
$$dB = 10 \ (0.4 + 13) = 134 \ dB.$$

Why do both approaches give the same answer? With one we use Log Law 2. With the other we use the second law of exponents. *We get the same answer because a log is an exponent.*

Set 2

Equation 4.4 also should be used to convert each of the decibels to intensity ratios. Note that you are not solving for the absolute intensity, I_x, but just the ratio of the two intensities, I_x/I_r. For example, if dB = 5,

$$5 = 10 \log X$$

$$0.5 = \log X \quad \text{(dividing both sides of the equation by 10)}$$

$$X = 3.16 \quad \text{(the ratio of the unknown } I_x \text{ to the unknown } I_r.)$$

a. 10^0:1 (1:1) f. 10^7 k. 2×10^2 p. 10^{-1} u. 5×10^1

b. 10^1 g. 2   l. 8×10^2 q. 10^{-2} v. 1.58×10^6

c. 10^2 h. 4   m. 4×10^4 r. 10^{-3} w. 1.26×10^9

d. 10^3 i. 8   n. 4×10^5 s. 5×10^{-3} x. 3.47×10^0

e. 10^4 j. 16   o. 4×10^7 t. 2.5×10^{-4} y. 1.82×10^1

Notes

(a–f).   Each of the decibel values is divisible evenly by 10, and each 10 dB of intensity corresponds to a power of 10. Thus, for these five problems, the solutions are a power of 10: the powers of 0, 1, 2, 3, 4, and 7, respectively. A second, but not independent, approach is to recall that when you convert decibels to intensity ratios, the first step is to divide by 10. The result is a log, which in these cases is an integer of 0, 1, 2, 3, 4, and 7 followed by 0.0000. The integers are the characteristics, and they indicate the exponents in scientific notation. Thus, the results are 10^0, 10^1, 10^2, 10^3, 10^4, and 10^7.

(g–j).   Each of these is a value that is evenly divisible by 3, and each 3 dB corresponds to a power of 2. Thus, the answers are 2, 4, 8, and 16.

(k–o).   Each of these involves a combination of powers of 10 and powers of 2. For example, 2–k is 23 dB, and 23 dB consists of 10 + 10 + 3. Each 10 dB is a power of 10, and each 3 dB is a power of 2. Thus, the answer is $10 \times 10 \times 2 = 200 = 2 \times 10^2$.

(p–t).   Each of these involves either a power of 10 or a combination of powers of 10 and powers of 2. However, because the decibel is negative, we know that *the exponent will be negative*. Thus, 10 dB corresponds to 10^1, whereas -10 dB corresponds to 10^{-1}.

(u).   Although you might not see it on first inspection, this problem also can be solved with powers of 10 and 2. Actually, 17 comprises $10 + 10 - 3$. Thus, 17 dB would correspond to a tenfold increase in intensity twice, and a halving of intensity once: $(10 \times 10)/2 = 50$. If the problem had involved 14 dB, could you have used the same approach? Yes. $14 = (10 + 10 - 3 - 3)$. Thus, 14 dB corresponds to: $(10 \times 10)/(2 \times 2) = 25$.

(v, w).   These, too, actually can be worked as combinations of powers of 10 and 2, but it might be quicker to solve them step-by-step with a log table or more quickly with your calculator rather than to spend time seeing if the powers of 10 and 2 rules apply. However, it is surprising how many problems can be solved in that simple way without use of log tables or calculators. Consider 2-v. 62 dB $= 10 + 10 + 10 + 10 + 10 + 3 + 3 + 3 + 3$. So, we have a power of 10 five times (10^5) and a power of 2 four times (2^4). That corresponds to 16×10^5, which is 1.6×10^6 in scientific notation. Can you see how Problem 2-w can be approached in the same way? (Hint: You need to sum 10s and subtract 3s.)

(x, y).   There is no quick solution available for these, but you should be able to determine upper and lower limits to check to see if the answers you calculate are reasonable.

General Comment

We have emphasized that reasonably quick solutions to many problems can be realized by employing powers of 10 (10 dB) and powers of 2 (3 dB). However, because the log of $2 = 3.0103$, not 3.0000, you will sometimes experience a rounding error that might or might not be tolerable, depending on the accuracy that is required. Thus, 3 dB really corresponds to an intensity ratio of 1.9953:1 rather than 2:1, and that probably will not pose any difficulty most of the time. However, look at problem 2–1. For 29 dB the answer was listed as 800:1, but the correct answer (two decimals) is 794.33:1. When greater accuracy is required, you should use the powers of 10 and powers of 2 shortcut only to estimate the answer and to aid you in determining if the answer you calculated is reasonable.

Set 3

Equation 4.4 also should be used for all of these problems. All problems in the set are conceptually identical to those in Set 1. The only difference is that in Set 1 you dealt only with a ratio of intensities (I_x/I_r) where the absolute values of I_x and I_r were unknown. In Set 3, both I_x and I_r are known. The first step, then, is to solve the ratio by reference to Law 2 of exponents $(X^m/X^n = X^{m-n})$, and the exponent in the result is the log of the ratio. For example,

$$dB = 10 \log 10^{-7}/10^{-12}$$
$$= 10 \log 10^{(-7)-(-12)}$$
$$= 10 \log 10^5$$
$$= 10 \times 5$$
$$= 50.$$

a. 0	f. 43	k. 100	p. −6
b. 10	g. 46	l. 103	q. 81.5
c. 20	h. 49	m. 97	r. 84.5
d. 30	i. 90	n. 67	s. 62.2
e. 40	j. 96	o. −3	t. 64.8

Notes

(a–e).   Each involves a power of 10, and by now you should be able to solve these quickly. For example, in 3-c, 10^{-10} is two powers of 10 larger than the reference of 10^{-12}, each power of 10 corresponds to 10 dB, and the answer, therefore, is 20 dB.

(f–h).   These are combinations of powers of 10 and powers of 2.

(m).   This also is a combination of powers of 10 and powers of 2. Therefore, 10^{-2} involves 10 tenfold increases (100 dB). If 10^{-2} is 100 dB, then 0.5×10^{-2} (which is only half as great) must be 3 dB less, or 97 dB.

(q–r).   Problem 3-q cannot be solved by inspection. However, having already solved 3-q, the answer to 3-r must be 3 dB greater than the answer to 3-q because 2.8×10^{-4} is twice as great as 1.4×10^{-4}.

Set 4

Equation 4.4 also should be used for these problems, which are conceptually identical to those in Set 2. The only difference is that in Set 2 you solved only for the intensity ratio (X), whereas in Set 4 you must carry the computation one step further to determine the actual value of I_x.

a. 10^{-12} f. 10^{-6} k. 1.00×10^{-13}

b. 10^{-11} g. 2×10^{-11} l. 1.00×10^{-14}

c. 10^{-10} h. 2×10^{-10} m. 0.50×10^{-12}

d. 10^{-9} i. 4×10^{-9} n. 1.25×10^{-12}

e. 10^{-8} j. 8×10^{-8} o. 0.50×10^{-13}

p. 0.50×10^{-14} u. 5.00×10^{-8}

q. 0.25×10^{-14} v. 4.79×10^{-11}

r. 1.26×10^{-8} w. 2.63×10^{-10}

s. 1.58×10^{-6} x. 6.30×10^{-9}

t. 2.00×10^{-5} y. 5.00×10^{-8}

Notes

(m).   If you followed the step-by-step procedures, you probably obtained 5×10^{-13} for your answer rather than 0.5×10^{-12} that is shown above, but the two are numerically identical. The answer of 0.5×10^{-12} came from inspecting for powers of 2 and 10. We know that 0 dB corresponds to an intensity of 10^{-12}, so -3 dB must correspond to only half as much intensity, or 0.5×10^{-12}. The same explanation applies to Problems 4-n, o, p, and q.

(u–y).   Did you notice that you could solve these by inspection for powers of 10 and 2?

Set 5

Equation 4.7 should be used to convert the pressure ratios to decibels. Each of these problems is identical in concept to those in Set 1, and problems 5-a through 5-ff are identical numerically. The only difference is that now you are presented with pressure ratios rather than intensity ratios, and therefore the log of the ratio is multiplied by 20 rather than by 10. Solution of the two sets of problems is otherwise identical.

Because the two sets of problems are virtually identical, except for the multiplier, there are no explanatory notes to accompany these problems. When in doubt, consult the notes for the corresponding problem in Set 1. However, as a general reminder, the vast majority of the problems can be solved by inspection for powers of 10 and powers of 2, where a power of 10 for pressure corresponds to 20 dB (20 log 10) and a power of 2 for pressure corresponds to 6 dB (20 log 2).

a.	0	g.	9.5	m.	19.1	s.	−16.9	y.	−60
b.	20	h.	12	n.	−6	t.	−18	z.	−60
c.	40	i.	14	o.	−9.5	u.	−19.1	aa.	26
d.	60	j.	15.6	p.	−12	v.	−20	bb.	46
e.	60	k.	16.9	q.	−14	w.	−40	cc.	32
f.	6	l.	18	r.	−15.6	x.	−60	dd.	52

ee.	35.6	kk.	0
ff.	55.6	ll.	0
gg.	−80	mm.	20
hh.	−100	nn.	0
ii.	−40	oo.	6
jj.	−20	pp.	−6

Set 6

Equation 4.7 should be used to convert decibels to pressure ratios. The only difference in solutions of these problems from those encountered with Set 2 is that the first step is to divide by 20 rather than by 10 because the problems involve pressure rather than intensity.

a.	10^0 (1:1)	g.	2	m.	2×10^1	s.	3.16×10^1
b.	10^1	h.	4	n.	2×10^2	t.	3.16×10^2
c.	10^2	i.	8	o.	4×10^3	u.	1.58×10^2

d. 10^3 j. 16   p. 10^{-1} v. 7×10^0

e. 10^4 k.   .5   q. 10^{-2} w. 1.26×10^3

f. 10^5 l.   .25   r. 3.16×10^0 x. 1.88×10^0

Set 7

Equation 4.7 should be used for all of these problems, and all are identical in concept to the problems in Set 5. The only difference is that in Set 5 you dealt only with a pressure ratio (P_x/P_r) where the absolute value of P_x and P_r were not specified. In Set 7, both P_x and P_r are known. The first step, then is to solve the ratio by use of the 2nd Law of exponents $(x^m/x^n = x^{m-n})$, and the exponent in the result is the characteristic in the log of the ratio. For example,

$$dB = 20 \log (3 \times 10^3)/(2 \times 10^1)$$
$$= 20 \log 1.5 \times 10^2$$
$$= 20 \times 2.18$$
$$= 43.6.$$

a.   0   g.   6   m. 94.4

b. 20   h.   12   n. 74

c. 40   i.   72   o. 68

d. 60   j. -20 p. 86

e. 80   k. -14 q. 86.6

f. 74   l.   46   r. 92.6

Notes

Almost all of these problems can be solved by use of powers of 10 (20 dB) and powers of 2 (6 dB).

(a).   In this problem $P_x = P_r$, the ratio is therefore 1:1, the log of 1 is 0.0000, and the answer must be 0 dB.

(a-e).   As you proceed from 7-a through 7-e, you progressively increase by one power of 10 (10^1), which for pressure corresponds to increases of 20 dB. Thus, the answers are 0, 20, 40, 60, and 80 dB SPL.

(f–h).   Problem 7-f is one power of 2 (2^1) *less* than 7-e, which means that the sound pressure level for 7-f must be 6 dB less than the sound pressure level for 7-e. Similarly, you should see powers of 2 relations between 7-g and 7-a, between 7-h and 7-g, between 7-i and 7-d, and so on.

(m).   The value of P_x is only fractionally greater than 10^6. By using powers of 10 and 2 you should see that if P_x were 10^6, SPL = 94 dB (2×10^6 would equal 100 dB, so 1×10^6, which is half as much pressure, must be 6 dB less). If SPL = 94 dB when P_x = 1×10^6, SPL must be only fractionally greater when P_x = 1.05×10^6. Thus, the answer of 94.4 seems reasonable.

Set 8

Equation 4.7 also should be used for these problems, which are identical in concept to those in Set 6. The only difference is that in Set 6 you solved only for the pressure ratio (X), whereas in Set 8 you must carry the computation one step further to determine the actual value of P_x.

a. 2×10^1	f. 2×10^3	k. 6.32×10^2	p. 10^3
b. 4×10^1	g. 2×10^4	l. 6.32×10^3	q. 8×10^4
c. 8×10^1	h. 2.82×10^1	m. 2.82×10^3	r. 1.38×10^2
d. 10^1	i. 5.64×10^1	n. 4×10^3	s. 8.93×10^0
e. 2×10^2	j. 6.32×10^1	o. 1.26×10^3	t. 7.96×10^0

Notes

(a–g).   As with many decibel problems, laborious, step-by-step calculations can be avoided with problems 8-a through 8-g by inspecting to determine if powers of 2 (6 dB) or powers of 10 (20 dB) apply. In 8-a, 0 dB *always* means that $P_x = P_r$; therefore the answer must be 2×10^1. The answer to 8-b must be a power of 2 greater (6 dB) than the answer to 8-a, and therefore is 4×10^{-4}; 8-c is one power of 2 greater than 8-b; 8-d is one power of 2 *less* than 8-a; 8-e is one power of 10 (20 dB) greater than 8-a; 8-f is one power of 10 greater than 8-e; and 8-g is one power of 10 greater than 8-f.

(h, i).   You need to calculate the answer to 8-h, but having done so, the answer to 8-i must be one power of 2 greater than 8-h because the difference between the two is 6 dB.

(j, k, l).   You need to calculate the answer to 8-j, but having done so, you should see that 8-k and 8-l are powers of 10 relative to 8-j.

Set 9

Equation 4.7 should be used for all of these problems. The only difference between these and the problems in Set 7 is that pressure now is expressed in dynes/cm^2 (**cgs** system) rather than µPa, and the reference pressure (P_r) is 2×10^{-4} dyne/cm^2. For example,

$$dB = 20 \log (3 \times 10^{-4})/(2 \times 10^{-4})$$
$$= 20 \log 1.5$$
$$= 20 \times 0.18$$
$$= 3.6.$$

a.	0	f.	20
b.	6	g.	20
c.	12	h.	46
d.	0	i.	−26
e.	6	j.	80

Notes

(a).   The answer to 9-a must be 0 dB because $P_x = P_r$.

(b, c).   The values of P_x in 9-b and 9-c are, respectively, one and two powers of 2 (each power of 2 corresponds to 6 dB) greater than the value of P_x in 9-a.

(d). 2×10^{-4} dyne/cm^2 is the same as 0.0002 dyne/cm^2 in 9-a.

(e–j).   All of the remaining problems in Set 9 involve powers of 2 (6 dB) and/or powers of 10 (20 dB).

Set 10

Even though the uncorrelated noise levels that are being combined are expressed in dB SPL, it is the energies, or powers, or intensities that should be added, not the pressures (See "Combining Sound Intensities from Independent Sources," Chapter 4). If the sources have equal intensity, you can use Equation 4.9:

$$dB_N = dB_i + 10 \log N.$$

For example, if five sources each produce a noise level of 72 dB,

$$dB_N = 72 + 10 \log 5$$
$$= 72 + 10 \ (0.7)$$
$$= 79.$$

If the source intensities are not equal, you must execute three calculations.

1. Calculate the *intensity* in watt/m^2 for each source (Equation 4.4).

2. Add the intensities to determine the value of I_x to be used in the third step.

3. Calculate decibels with Equation 4.4 where $I_r = 10^{-12}$ watt/m^2. The result can be expressed as dB IL or dB SPL; they are synonymous.

For example, if two sources have noise levels of 80 dB SPL and 83 dB SPL:

Step 1:

$80 = 10 \log I_x/10^{-12}$,   Therefore, $I_x = 10^{-4}$.

$83 = 10 \log I_x/10^{-12}$,   Therefore, $I_x = 2 \times 10^{-4}$.

Step 2:

$I_x + I_x = (1 \times 10^{-4}) + (2 \times 10^{-4}) = 3 \times 10^{-4}$.

Step 3:

$dB = 10 \log (3 \times 10^{-4})/10^{-12}$
$= 10 \log 3 \times 10^8$
$= 10 \times 8.48$
$= 84.8 \ (dB\ IL\ or\ dB\ SPL)$.

a. 23   d. 24.8   g. 70.4

b. 33.0   e. 34.8   h. 67

c. 49.2   f. 51   i. 80.5

Notes

(a–f).   Problems 10-a through 10-f involve equal source intensities, which therefore permits you to solve the problems with Equation 4.9. Thus, for 10-a, the answer would be $20 + 10 \log 2 = 23$ dB. For 10-f, $46.2 + 10 \log 3 = 51$ dB.

(g, h, i).   For each of these problems you should use the three-step procedures described above. The solution for 10-i is shown below.

> *Step 1:*
>
> $60 = 10 \log I_x/10^{-12} = 10^{-6}$
>
> $70 = 10 \log I_x/10^{-12} = 10^{-5}$
>
> $80 = 10 \log I_x/10^{-12} = 10^{-4}$
>
> *Step 2:*
>
> 0.01×10^{-4}
>
> $0.1 \;\; \times 10^{-4}$
>
> $+ \; 1.0 \;\; \times 10^{-4}$
> _____
>
> $= 1.11 \times 10^{-4}.$
>
> *Step 3:*
>
> $dB = 10 \log (1.11 \times 10^{-4})/10^{-12}$
>
> $= 10 \log 1.11 \times 10^{8}$
>
> $= 10 \times 8.05$
>
> $= 80.5$

Set 11

In Set 10 you were to calculate the level (dB IL or dB SPL) that resulted from having combined uncorrelated sound sources. In Set 11 you simply execute Steps 1 and 2 of the three-step procedure used in Set 10, because you are asked to determine the *total intensity* in watt/m^2 rather than the *level* in decibels that corresponds to the total intensity.

a. 2×10^{-8} d. 7×10^{-6}

b. 2×10^{-6} e. 9×10^{-6}

c. 3×10^{-6} f. 3.2×10^{-5}

Notes

(f).   The only difficulty, if any, that should be encountered is with 11-f. The key is that you must be certain that both intensities have the same exponent before you add. Thus, for example, $2 \times 10^{-6} = 0.2 \times 10^{-5}$, which when added to $3 \times 10^{-5} = 3.2 \times 10^{-5}$.

Set 12

The procedure used to solve these problems should have been sufficiently mastered that no explanation should be necessary.

a. 43   b. 63   c. 64.8   d. 68.5   e. 69.5   f. 75.1

■ NOTES

1. The proper form for all equations concerning the decibel is "$\log_{10} X$" preceded by a multiplier of either 10 (intensity) or 20 (pressure), where "X" refers to some ratio. However, because the **base** for all calculations of decibels is **10**, the base will frequently be omitted for convenience.
2. The equivalent reference intensity in the **cgs** metric system is 10^{-16} watt/cm^2.
3. The unit of measure in the **cgs** metric system is the **dyne/cm²** or the **microbar**.
4. In most reference texts, the symbol for the speed of sound is **c** rather than **s**. Thus, the equation for characteristic impedance ordinarily is expressed as $Z_c = \rho_o c$. We have elected to use **s** so that we can consistently distinguish between speed (**s**), which is a scalar quantity, and velocity (**c**), which is a vector quantity.
5. The equivalent reference pressure in the **cgs** metric system is **2 × 10⁻⁴ dyne/cm²** or **2 × 10⁻⁴ microbar**. See Table 4–3 for a more complete description of equivalent measures of pressure in the two metric systems.

Complex Waves

All of the sound waves that have been described to this point were of the **sinusoidal** form that appears in panel A of Figure 5-1. Although the sine wave is not the type of vibratory motion that we are likely to experience in our daily lives, it is important to understand it thoroughly because *the sine wave is the fundamental component of other sound waves that will be encountered.*

The other sound waves shown in Figure 5-1 are much more complex in form than the simple sine wave, and they are, indeed, called

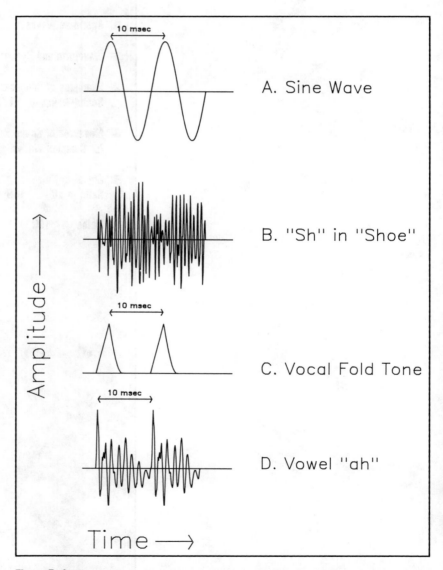

Figure 5-1. Comparison of a sine wave with three complex waves: the /sh/ sound from the word "shoe"; the sound wave created by the vibratory movement of the vocal folds; and the vowel /a/.

complex waves. The wave in panel B is similar to the "sh" sound in the word "shoe," panel C shows one kind of sound wave that results from vibratory motion of the vocal folds during production of a vowel, and panel D shows the same vowel as recorded near the mouth opening rather than deep in the throat just above the vocal folds.

■ FOURIER'S THEOREM

A **complex wave** can be defined as *any sound wave that is not sinusoidal*. That definition, though, does not reveal exactly what a complex wave is, but the following theorem should help. The complex waves in Figure 5–1 — and all other sound waves that are not sinusoidal — *are composed of a series of simple sinusoids that can differ in amplitude, frequency, and phase*. Thus, when two or more sine waves that differ in amplitude, frequency, or phase are added together, a complex wave is produced.

The degree of complexity of a complex sound wave depends on the number of sine waves that are combined and on the specific dimensional values (amplitude, frequency, and phase) of the sinusoidal components. This theorem was first stated by Joseph Fourier, a French mathematician who lived at the time of Napoleon I, and, hence, the series of sine waves that are combined to compose a complex wave is called a **Fourier series** in his honor.

Fourier's theorem has two important implications for the study of complex waves. First, because a complex wave consists of some number of sinusoids of different amplitudes, frequencies, and phases, the nature of any complex wave should not be difficult to comprehend if we understand the concept of simple harmonic motion that is associated with each of the sinusoidal components, and if we recall the relevant dimensions of sine waves: **amplitude, frequency**, and **phase**. Second, we can derive the **Fourier series** by a process called **Fourier analysis**, which means that *any complex waveform can be decomposed or analyzed to determine the amplitudes, frequencies, and phases of the sine waves that compose the complex wave.*

All sound waves can be classified by reference to (1) the presence or absence of **periodicity** in the wave and (2) the degree of complexity of the wave.

■ PERIODIC WAVES

A **periodic wave**, whether sinusoidal or complex, is a wave that *repeats itself at regular intervals over time*. Because the wave repeats itself periodically over time, it also can be called a **periodic time function**. The sine wave in Figure 5–1 provides an obvious example of periodicity because we can see that the characteristics of any one cycle of the wave are duplicated exactly in every other cycle — each cycle in the wave is repeated regularly over time.

Sine waves are not the only forms of wave motion that are characterized by periodicity. The vocal fold wave (panel C) and the vowel (panel D) in Figure 5–1 appear to be reasonably periodic (they are in fact called **quasiperiodic**) because we can verify that all of the features within one "cycle" of vibration are duplicated *almost exactly* during the next and every other cycle. Thus, there are two kinds of **periodic waves**: sinusoidal and complex. A **sinusoidal wave** *is a wave that results from simple harmonic motion and that comes from a relation that contains a sine function.* A **complex periodic wave** *is a periodic wave, but it is not sinusoidal.*

Components of a Complex Periodic Wave

According to Fourier's theorem, any complex periodic wave consists of some number of simple sinusoids that are summed, but the sinusoidal components cannot be selected randomly if the resultant sound wave is to be periodic. Instead, they must satisfy a basic mathematical requirement that is called a **harmonic relation**.

The term **harmonic relation** means that *the frequencies of all of the sinusoids that compose the series must be integral (whole number) multiples of the frequency of the sinusoid with the lowest frequency* in the series. For example, if the sinusoid with the lowest frequency is 100 Hz, the other sinusoidal components of the complex wave must be selected from the frequencies 200, 300, 400, 500 Hz, and so forth, because other frequency values would not satisfy the requirement of being integral multiples of the lowest frequency. Similarly, if the sinusoid with the lowest frequency is 110 Hz, the other sinusoidal components must be selected from the frequencies 220, 330, 440, 550 Hz, and so on.

A Harmonic Series

When a harmonic relation exists among frequency components, the series of frequencies is called a **harmonic series**, and all of the sinusoids in the harmonic series are called **harmonics**. The harmonics are numbered consecutively from lowest to highest frequency: 1st harmonic, which also is called the **fundamental frequency**, (f_o), 2nd harmonic, 3rd harmonic, and so on until we reach the nth harmonic, or the last component in the series.

In the case of the first example above, the 1st harmonic (also called the f_o), = 100 Hz, the 2nd harmonic = 200 Hz, the 3rd harmonic = 300 Hz, and so on. There also is a special circumstance in which the fundamental frequency (1st harmonic) is missing from the series. In that case, all of the higher frequencies in the harmonic series are integral multiples of what is called the repetition rate.

Figure 5–2 shows the waveform of one example of a periodic complex wave that consists of an infinite number of sinusoidal waves. Its

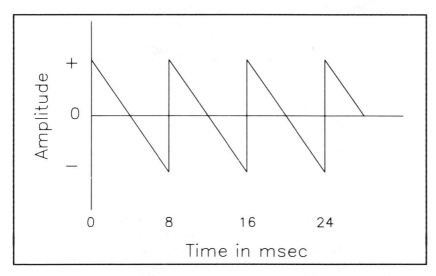

Figure 5-2. A **complex periodic** sound wave that is called a **sawtooth wave** because its shape resembles the teeth of a saw.

periodicity should be apparent, and because it obviously is not sinusoidal, it must be a complex periodic wave. This particular wave is called a **sawtooth wave** because its shape resembles the shape of the teeth of a saw. The sawtooth wave will be of interest to those who become interested in the study of the acoustics of speech because the waveform of the sawtooth wave resembles the waveform of the sound produced by the vibrating vocal folds.

The period of the fundamental frequency (the 1st harmonic) of the sawtooth wave in Figure 5-2 is 8 msec, which means that f_0, the fundamental frequency, is 125 Hz (Equation 1.12). All components — the **harmonics** — of the sawtooth wave are odd and even whole number (integral) multiples of the fundamental frequency. Thus, if the fundamental frequency is 125 Hz, the harmonic components would be: 125 (f_0 x 1), 250 (f_0 x 2), 375 (f_0 x 3), 500 (f_0 x 4), 625 (f_0 x 5), and so on for an infinity of odd and even multiples.

We see in Table 5-1 that the lowest frequency, 125 Hz, is called the fundamental fequency, f_0, and it also is called the 1st harmonic. The remaining components are labeled the 2nd harmonic, 3rd harmonic, 4th harmonic, and so on.

Partials and Overtones

You occasionally will find that the components in a complex periodic wave are called **partials** or **overtones** instead of **harmonics**. Table 5-1 also shows the relations among these different labels.

We can see from the entries in the table that the designations of **harmonic** and **partial** are synonymous *as long as all components are*

Table 5–1. Fundamental frequency, harmonics, partials, and overtones in a complex periodic sound wave.

Frequency	Harmonic	Partial	Overtone
125 (f_0)	1	1	
250	2	2	1
375	3	3	2
500	4	4	3
625	5	5	4
750	6	6	5

exact integral multiples of the fundamental frequency: the 1st harmonic (also the fundamental) is the 1st partial, the 2nd harmonic is the 2nd partial, and so on. The word, **overtone**, which might, for example, be encountered in the musical literature, derives from the fact that the complex wave can be described as consisting of a fundamental frequency, or fundamental tone, and a series of other tones whose frequencies lie *over* the fundamental. Thus, the 2nd harmonic is the 1st overtone, the 3rd harmonic is the 2nd overtone, and so on.

Summary

If the complex wave is to be periodic, the sinusoidal components *must be integral multiples of the fundamental frequency*. Thus, if f_o = 100 Hz, the other components must be selected from 200 Hz, 300 Hz, 400 Hz, and so forth. When that occurs, the partials are indeed harmonics, and the sound wave is exactly periodic. In that circumstance, at the end of one cycle of vibration (10 msec), we will have completed one cycle of the 1st harmonic (100 Hz; T = 10 msec), two cycles of the 2nd harmonic (200 Hz; T = 5 msec), three cycles of the 3rd harmonic (300 Hz; T = 3.33 msec), four cycles of the 4th harmonic (400 Hz; T = 2.5 msec), and so on.

Summation of Sine Waves

As more and more sine waves are added (summed) in the harmonic series, the shape of the resultant complex wave changes. The left side of Figure 5–3 shows four sine waves (S_1, S_2, S_3, and S_4) that have different frequencies and amplitudes, but identical **starting phases** (180°).

The exact frequency of each wave to be summed is unimportant, but an appropriate frequency relation among the four components is maintained; the three higher frequencies must be harmonics of the lowest one — the fundamental frequency. Notice, however, that not all harmonics are present in this example. In fact, we have used only the *odd integral multiples* so that we have the 1st (f_o), 3rd, 5th, and 7th harmonics. Thus, if the frequency of S_1 were 1000 Hz, the frequencies of

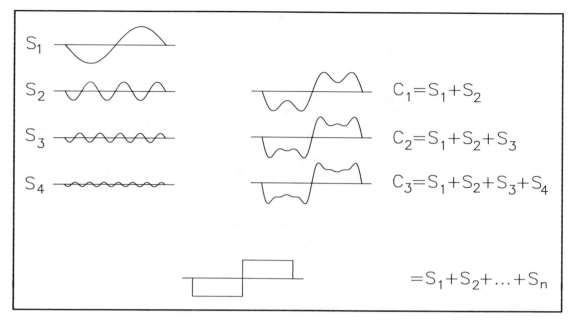

Figure 5-3. Summation of sine waves to form complex waves. The sine waves at the left (S₁ through S₄) are added progressively to form the complex waves (C₁ through C₃) at the right. At the bottom, a **square wave** is created by summation of an infinite number of sine waves of *appropriate* **amplitudes, frequencies,** and **starting phases**.

the other sinusoids would be 3000, 5000, and 7000 Hz; if the frequency of S_1 were 400 Hz, the frequencies of the other sinusoids would be 1200, 2000, and 2800.

At the right of Figure 5-3 we show what happens when the sinusoidal components are summed progressively to form three different complex waves (C_1, C_2, and C_3). The complex wave at the top of the figure (C_1) results from $S_1 + S_2$. Wave C_1 is not a sinusoid — it is complex — and it is composed of two sinusoids that differ in amplitude and frequency.

Although the **starting phases** of the two components of C_1 are identical, it should be apparent that the **instantaneous phases** of the two sinusoidal components vary from moment to moment because of their different frequencies. If the two sinusoidal components had any other values of frequency and amplitude, the complex wave that results would be different from the one shown as C_1 because the resultant wave depends on all of the specific dimensions of the sine waves that compose it.

Wave C_2 looks different from wave C_1 because its shape results from summation of three sinusoids, $S_1 + S_2 + S_3$. Wave C_3 contains all four sinusoidal components. You might notice that the complex waves at the right are becoming more and more "square" in shape as more and more sine waves are added. At the bottom of Figure 5-3 we show what happens if we combine an infinite number of odd-numbered integral multiple sinusoids (1×, 3×, 5×, 7×, 9×, + ... + n×). If, for example, the lowest frequency were 100 Hz, the other components would be 300, 500, 700 Hz, and so on. A complex wave with a perfectly square shape is created by summing an infinity of sinusoids with frequencies that are odd integral multiples of the fundamental frequency and that have appropriate relative amplitudes and identical starting phases.

Figure 5–4 provides another example of summation of sine waves to form a resultant periodic complex wave. In this case, we have added the first three of *both odd and even* integral multiples of the fundamental (f_o); all **starting phases** = 0° in this example. The two resultant waves, C_1 and C_2, look rather different from the resultant waves seen

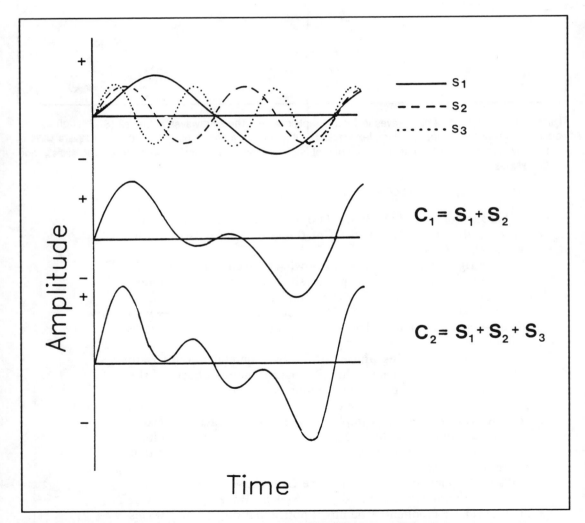

Figure 5–4. Summation of sine waves to form a different **complex periodic wave**. Because the shape of this complex wave is different from those shown previously, the parameter values for amplitude, frequency, and starting phase of the sinusoidal components must also be different.

previously in Figure 5–3 because both odd and even harmonics are included rather than just odd.

When an infinity of odd harmonics with appropriate relative amplitudes and starting phases is summed, the result is the square wave that was shown in Figure 5–3. However, when an infinity of odd and even harmonics with appropriate relative amplitudes and starting phases is summed, the result is a sawtooth wave such as that shown in Figure 5–2. In fact, with only three components, and a bit of imagination, you can see that the resultant wave in Figure 5–4 is beginning to assume a sawtooth kind of shape.

In the two examples cited thus far, the **starting phase** was identical for the individual components. However, variations in the resultant wave also will occur if we vary the starting phase of the components while holding their amplitudes and frequencies constant, as is illustrated in Figure 5–5.

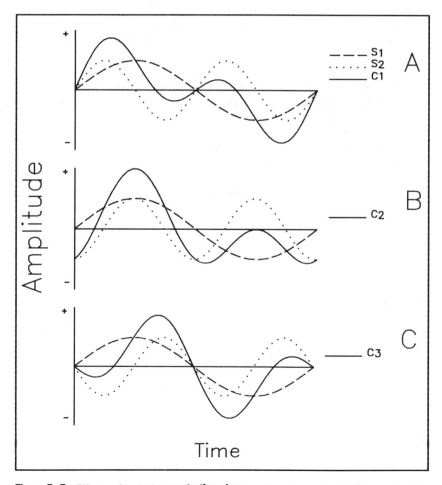

Figure 5–5. Effects of variation in **starting phase** on the shape of a complex wave that results from summation of sine waves.

In panel A of Figure 5–5, the two components (dashed and dotted lines) have identical starting phases (0°) and we can see the shape of the complex wave (solid line) that results from summation. The resultant wave in panel B is different from the one in panel A because the starting phase of S_1 has remained at 0°, but the starting phase for S_2 has been shifted from 0° to 270°. In panel C, S_1 again remains at 0°, but the starting phase of S_2 is now 180°. Thus, with these changes in starting phase of one of the components, three different complex periodic waves have been produced.

■ APERIODIC WAVES

The principal distinguishing characteristic of complex periodic waves is their regularity over time, or **periodicity**. They repeat themselves indefinitely. The **aperiodic wave** is a second category of waveform, and its name derives from a lack of periodicity. Thus, it is very difficult, and in the extreme case impossible, to predict what the wave will look like during one time interval from knowledge of its characteristics during another time interval of equal duration.

The vibratory motion of an aperiodic wave is **random**, and therefore unpredictable, and vibratory motions of this type are called **random time functions**. In acoustics, this is called an **aperiodic sound wave**. The sound wave shown in Figure 5–6 is an aperiodic, or random, wave, and you should see that it is virtually impossible (except by chance) to identify any two time intervals during which the characteristics of the vibratory motion are identical in all respects.

We encounter aperiodic sound waves daily. Familiar examples are the noises from aircrafts, automobiles, or speed boats. Each of those

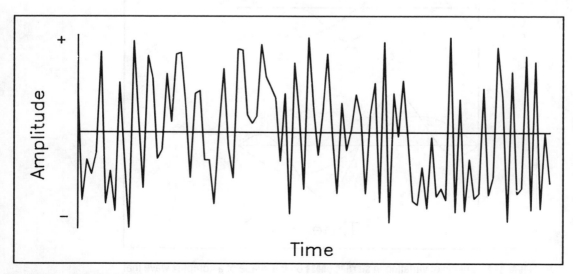

Figure 5–6. An **aperiodic** sound wave.

sounds is characterized by random vibratory motion — aperiodicity — but that does not mean that all aperiodic sounds are unpleasant. The water cascading down the side of the mountain produces an aperiodic sound wave, but under the right circumstances it might produce a very satisfying sensation. Many of the sounds of speech ("sh" in "she"; "s" in "see"; "f" in "foolish"; "th" in "three"; and so on) are characterized by random vibratory motion, but we usually don't think of such sounds as "noise."

■ WAVEFORM AND SPECTRUM

Waveform

Each picture of periodic (both sinusoidal and complex) and aperiodic waves that has been shown to this point has focused on the **waveform**. By that we mean, we have plotted changes in one variable (pressure, velocity, acceleration, displacement, etc.) *as a function of time*. The waveform defines, for example, the distribution of instantaneous amplitudes of a sinusoidal or complex wave over time.

Return to the waveforms for the sawtooth wave in Figure 5–2 and the square wave in Figure 5–3. We can identify the **fundamental period** of each wave, and from that we can calculate the **fundamental frequency**. However, unless we happen to remember that the square wave consists of all odd harmonics and that the sawtooth wave consists of all odd and even harmonics, we would have no way of knowing what **frequencies** other than the fundamental frequency were present by visual examination of the waveform.

We also cannot determine the **amplitudes** or the **starting phases** of the sinusoidal components by visual inspection of the waveform. We shall see subsequently that both the square wave and the sawtooth wave must satisfy very specific requirements relative to both the amplitudes and starting phases of the components, but the point we wish to emphasize now is that visual inspection of the waveform will not reveal sufficient details about these important dimensions of the sinusoidal components.

Amplitude Spectrum

A graphic alternative to the **waveform** is the **amplitude spectrum in the frequency domain**, which often is shortened to just **amplitude spectrum**. Whereas the waveform shows instantaneous magnitudes such as amplitude as a function of time, the **amplitude spectrum** *shows amplitude (in either absolute or relative values) as a function of* **frequency**.

In Figure 5–7 the waveforms of the sawtooth and square wave are shown at the left and their respective amplitude spectra are shown

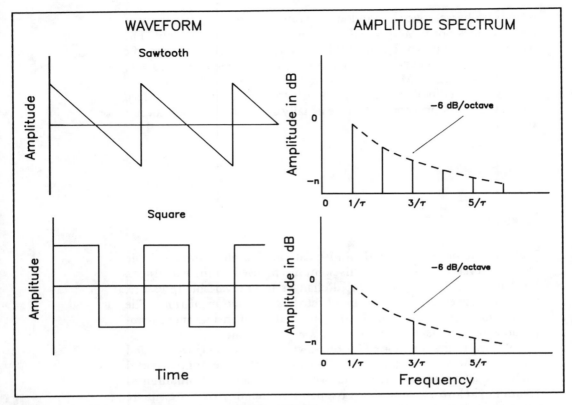

Figure 5–7. A comparison of **waveforms** and **amplitude spectra** for sawtooth and square waves, both of which are complex periodic waves. The spectrum is called a **line spectrum**.

at the right. The amplitude spectrum is shown by plotting relative amplitude in dB as a function of frequency. The location of each vertical line along the horizontal axis indicates the frequency of that component, and the height of each line is proportional to its relative amplitude; 0 dB represents the amplitude of the component with the greatest energy, and all other amplitudes therefore are shown as negative because their amplitudes are shown in dB relative to the amplitude of the fundamental.

The **envelope** of the amplitude spectrum in Figure 5–7 is shown by a dashed line that connects the peaks of each of the vertical lines. We can see that the square wave has energy at all odd harmonics and the sawtooth wave has energy at all odd and even harmonics, just as was described.

Inspection of amplitude spectra reveals information that, although present in the waveform, was not readily apparent from visual inspection of waveforms. You might have noticed that when the sinusoidal components in Figure 5–3 were summed to create a square wave, the amplitudes of the components decreased with increasing frequency. That also can be seen in the amplitude spectrum for the square wave in Figure 5–7, and now the relation among the amplitudes of the components can be seen. For the square wave, the **spectral envelope** in the frequency domain *decreases at a rate of 6 dB per octave*, which is the same as saying that the spectral envelope has a slope of −6 dB per octave.

The Octave

An **octave** refers to a *doubling in frequency* (2f). Thus, 250 Hz is one octave above 125 Hz, and 500 Hz is one octave above 250 Hz and two octaves above 125 Hz. An octave always refers to a *frequency ratio of 2:1 or 1:2, not to a frequency difference*. Thus, 2000 Hz is one octave above 1000 Hz and 200 Hz is one octave above 100 Hz because, in both cases, a ratio of 2:1 exists. The fact that the frequency difference is 1000 Hz in one case, but 100 Hz in the other, is irrelevant.

The white keys on a piano correspond to the musical notes that are designated "A,B,C,D,E,F,G,A." The lowest note is A_1, which has a frequency of 27.5 Hz. Seven white keys to the right of A_1 is A_2, which has a frequency of 55 Hz. Thus, A_2 is one octave above A_1. At the extreme right of the keyboard is A_8, which has a frequency of 3520 Hz. Thus, A_8 is one octave above A_7, which has a frequency of 1760 Hz, and seven octaves above A_1.

Another example of octave relations can be seen by returning to Table 5–1 where the harmonic components of a complex periodic wave are listed. There we see that the 2nd harmonic is one octave above the 1st harmonic, and conversely, the 1st harmonic is one octave below the 2nd. The 4th harmonic is one octave above the 2nd and two octaves above the 1st, and so forth. In each case, the frequency ratio was either 2:1 or 1:2.

Line Spectra

The amplitude spectra in Figure 5–7 are called **line amplitude spectra**, or just **line spectra**, because the sinusoidal components of the complex periodic waves can be represented by a *set of lines*; the location of a particular line in the frequency domain (horizontal axis) identifies the frequency of that component, and the height of the line along the amplitude scale (vertical axis) identifies the amplitude.

With a line spectrum, *energy is present only at frequencies represented by the vertical lines*. Even though, for example, the spectral envelope is shown by a line that connects the harmonics of the sawtooth wave, *there is no energy at frequencies between two adjacent components*.

Continuous Spectra

The random, or aperiodic, waveform of the noise in Figure 5–6 is shown again in Figure 5–8 along with its amplitude spectrum. The result is called a **continuous amplitude spectrum**, or just **continuous spec-**

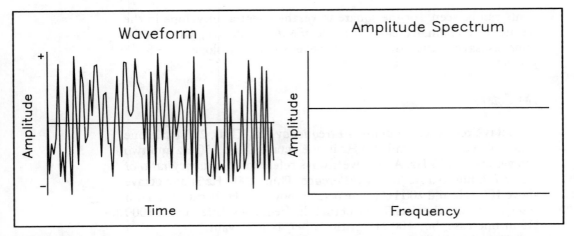

Figure 5-8. Waveform and amplitude spectrum for a complex aperiodic wave. The spectrum is called a **continuous spectrum**.

trum, in contrast to the line spectrum shown previously.

A **continuous spectrum** is one in which *energy is present at all frequencies between certain frequency limits*. Thus, the complex aperiodic wave does not result from summation of a harmonic series — odd and/or even multiples of the fundamental frequency — but rather there is energy present at all frequencies between some lower and upper limits.

In the case of the noise shown in Figure 5-8, energy is present at all frequencies and the spectral envelope has a slope of 0 dB. In other words, an identical amount of energy is present at all frequencies throughout the range. However, equal energy at all frequencies is not a requirement for all aperiodic waveforms, and subsequently we shall describe different types of aperiodic waveforms and their corresponding amplitude spectra.

Phase Spectra

In addition to the **amplitude spectrum** of a sound wave, we can also describe what is called the **phase spectrum in the frequency domain**, or just the **phase spectrum**. Whereas the amplitude spectrum describes relative amplitude as a function of frequency, the **phase spectrum** defines *the starting phase as a function of frequency*. The combination of the amplitude spectrum and the phase spectrum defines the waveform completely in the frequency domain.

■ EXAMPLES OF COMPLEX SOUND WAVES

Examples of several different complex signals, both periodic and aperiodic, are shown in Figure 5-9 and are compared with the familiar sine

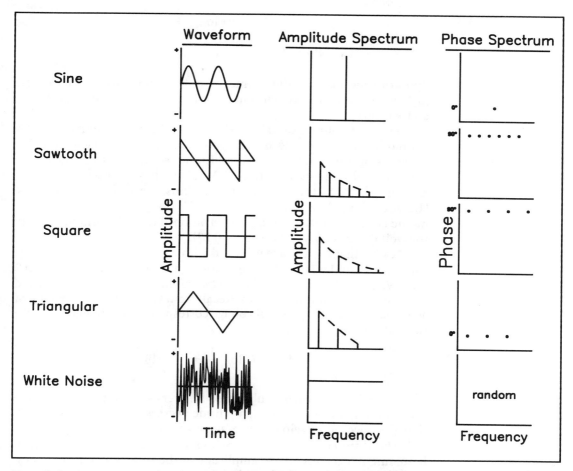

Figure 5–9. A comparison of waveforms, **amplitude spectra**, and **phase spectra** for a sine wave, sawtooth wave, square wave, triangular wave, and white noise.

wave. The panels at the left show the **waveforms**, the middle panels show the **amplitude spectra**, and the panels at the right show the **phase spectra**. The waveform of the sine wave should be thoroughly familiar by now with no further discussion.

Sawtooth Wave

A **sawtooth wave** is a complex periodic wave with energy at all, odd and even, integral multiples of the fundamental frequency. We can see from Figure 5–9 that the amplitudes of the sinusoidal components decrease with increasing frequency. Specifically, the amplitudes decrease as the inverse (the reciprocal) of the harmonic number. The relative amplitude, in decibels, for each component frequency is given by:

Equation 5.1
$$dB = 20 \log_{10} \frac{1}{h_{i,}}$$

where h_i is the harmonic number.

By **harmonic number** (h_i) we mean 1st harmonic (h_1), 2nd harmonic (h_2), and so on to the nth harmonic. Thus, **h** always is an integer: 1, 2, 3, and so forth.

The first column of Table 5–2 lists the first nine harmonics of a sawtooth wave generated by an appropriate waveform generator. For purposes of illustration, we will arbitrarily set the rms voltage of the fundamental frequency, f_o, to be 2 V. The voltage of each of the harmonics is listed in the second column. Thus, the 2nd harmonic is 1 V ($1/2 \times 2 = 1$ V), the 3rd harmonic is 0.67 V ($1/3 \times 2 = 0.67$), the 4th harmonic is 0.5 V ($1/4 \times 2 = 0.5$), and so on until the 9th harmonic where the voltage is 0.22 V ($1/9 \times 2 = 0.22$).

Notice that the voltage is halved with each doubling of frequency. Thus, between the 1st and 2nd harmonics, the voltage decreases from 2 V to 1V. The voltage also is halved between the 2nd and 4th, the 3rd and 6th, and 4th and 8th harmonics. Recall from Chapter 4 that halving of acoustic pressure or electrical voltage corresponds to a change in amplitude of −6 dB:

$$dB = 20 \log \frac{1}{2} = -6 \text{ dB}.$$

Therefore, because each doubling of frequency corresponds to an octave, and for each octave the amplitude decreases by 6 dB, we can say that the spectral envelope has a slope of −6 dB per octave.

The third column of Table 5–2 expresses the amplitude of each harmonic in decibels re: the amplitude of the fundamental frequency. Thus, for example, with the aid of Equation 5.1 we can calculate that the level of the 5th harmonic is −14 dB:

$$dB = 20 \log \frac{1}{5} = -14 \ (-13.98) \text{ dB}.$$

Table 5–2. Amplitudes (in voltage) of sinusoidal components of a **sawtooth** wave in which the amplitude of the fundamental frequency is 2 V.

Harmonic Number	rms voltage	$20 \log_{10} 1/h_i$
1 (f_0)	$1/1 \times 2 = 2$	0
2	$1/2 \times 2 = 1$	−6
3	$1/3 \times 2 = .67$	−9.5
4	$1/4 \times 2 = .50$	−12
5	$1/5 \times 2 = .40$	−14
6	$1/6 \times 2 = .33$	−15.6
7	$1/7 \times 2 = .29$	−16.9
8	$1/8 \times 2 = .25$	−18.1
9	$1/9 \times 2 = .22$	−19.1

It is important to recognize that the *absolute amplitude* (voltage in this case because the sawtooth wave is an electrical signal) for each harmonic listed in column two of Table 5-2 *depends upon the absolute voltage of the fundamental frequency.* You might wish to try a few calculations and confirm that if the voltage of the fundamental of the sawtooth waveform were 1 V rather than 2 V, the voltages of the eight higher harmonics would be: 0.5 V; 0.33 V; 0.25 V; 0.2 V; 0.17 V; 0.14 V; 0.13 V; and 0.11 V.

We have seen, then, with those calculations that the absolute voltage of each of the harmonics in the sawtooth wave does, indeed, depend upon the absolute voltage of the fundamental. However, the relative amplitude, in decibels, for each of the harmonics in a sawtooth wave *is independent of the voltage of the fundamental frequency.* In other words, the level of the 2nd harmonic will always be −6 dB, the level of the 3rd harmonic will always be −9.5 dB, and so on.

If you continue with your computations by calculating $20 \log_{10} 1/h_i$ (Equation 5.1) for each of the calculations that you just made for the case where $\mathbf{f_o} = 1$ V, you should obtain the same answers for a fundamental frequency of 1 V (subject to rounding error) that appear in the third column of Table 5-2 for a fundamental frequency of 2 V. For example, the relative level of the 5th harmonic still is −14 dB.

What does the amplitude spectrum of a sawtooth wave "look like?" It is a **line spectrum** because energy exists only at discrete frequencies that are integral multiples of the fundamental or lowest frequency. However, the shape of the **spectral envelope** depends on your choice of how to plot the amplitudes as a function of frequency. For example, in panel A of Figure 5-10 the voltage of each harmonic (from column two of Table 5-2) is plotted as a function of harmonic number. The scales for both the y-axis and x-axis are linear, and the resulting spectral envelope is curvilinear.

In panel B of Figure 5-10, the amplitude scale is logarithmic because we have plotted relative amplitudes in decibels re: the amplitude of the fundamental frequency $(\mathbf{f_o})$. In addition, frequency also is plotted on a logarithmic scale. The resulting spectral envelope is now linear. However, you should see that in either case, panel A or panel B, the spectral envelope has a slope of −6 dB per octave because for each doubling of frequency, the amplitude decreases by 6 dB.

In summary, a **sawtooth wave** is *a complex periodic wave with energy at odd and even integral multiples of the fundamental frequency with a spectral envelope slope of −6 dB per octave.* In Figure 5-9, each of the sinusoidal components (harmonics) of the sawtooth wave has a starting phase of 90°. The starting phases could just as well be, for example, 180°, or 0°, or 270°. However, it is essential that the starting phases of all frequency components be identical.

Square Wave

A **square wave** also is a complex periodic wave, but it has energy only at *odd integral multiples of the fundamental frequency.* We can see

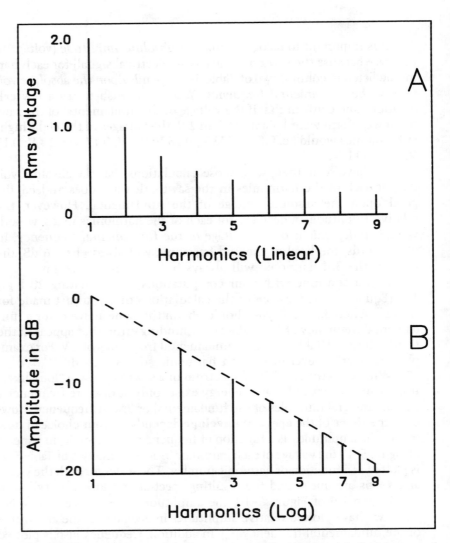

Figure 5–10. Amplitude spectra for a sawtooth wave. In panel A, the measure of amplitude is rms voltage, and the resultant **spectral envelope** is curvilinear. In panel B, the measure of amplitude is decibels, and the resultant spectral envelope is linear.

from Figure 5–9 that the amplitudes of the sinusoidal components decrease with increasing frequency, just as they did with the sawtooth wave. Moreover, we shall see that the slope of the spectral envelope of a square wave is identical to the slope of the envelope for a sawtooth wave, because the amplitudes of the frequency components also decrease as the reciprocal of the harmonic number.

The first column of Table 5–3 lists five odd harmonics (1, 3, 5, 7, and 9) of a square wave. As with the sawtooth wave, we will arbitrarily set the voltage of the fundamental frequency to be 2 V for purposes of comparison. We can see that the decrease in voltage for each of the harmonics is identical to the decrease seen for the *same harmonics* in Table

Table 5–3. Amplitudes (in voltage) of sinusoidal components of a **square** wave in which the amplitude of the fundamental frequency is 2 V.

Harmonic Number	rms voltage	$20 \log_{10} 1/h_i$
1 (f_0)	$1/1 \times 2 = 2$	0
3	$1/3 \times 2 = .67$	-9.5
5	$1/5 \times 2 = .40$	-14
7	$1/7 \times 2 = .29$	-16.9
9	$1/9 \times 2 = .22$	-19.1

5–2 for the sawtooth wave. For example, the level of the 5th harmonic is -14 dB re: the level of the fundamental frequency for both the square wave and the sawtooth wave.

With the aid of Equation 5.1 you might wish to perform another set of computations with a voltage other than 2 V for the fundamental. Your answers for absolute voltage should differ from those in the second column in Table 5–3, but you should obtain the same answers in decibels that appear in the third column, regardless of the voltage of f_0. Thus, for example, if the voltage of the fundamental frequency is 3 V, the voltage of the 5th harmonic is 0.6 V, but its relative level in decibels is still -14 dB. It therefore is reasonable to conceptualize a square wave as being a sawtooth wave that is devoid of even harmonics. We should reason, therefore, that the slope of the square wave also is -6 dB per octave.

In summary, a **square wave** is defined as *a complex periodic wave with energy at odd integral multiples of the fundamental and a spectral envelope slope of -6 dB per octave.* The amplitude spectrum of a square wave is a **line spectrum**. In the example shown in Figure 5–9, each of the components has a starting phase of 90°, but that is not a requirement. Those who read other introductory reference books or chapters will encounter what, at first glance, might appear to be inconsistencies. Hirsh (1952), for example, shows all components of the square wave to have 0° starting phase, whereas Yost and Nielson (1977) show all starting phases to be 90°.

Figure 5–11 should clarify any confusion. In panel A, starting phases are 0°, and the corresponding waveform begins its first excursion upward (with an infinitely steep slope) from 0°. In panel B, starting phases = 90°, and only half of the first positive-going excursion of the waveform is shown, which means in this case the waveform also begins at 90°. However, regardless of the starting phase chosen, we still are faced with the restriction that the starting phase must be identical for each frequency component.

Triangular Wave

The **triangular wave** shown in Figure 5–9 is a complex periodic wave with energy at odd integral multiples of the fundamental frequency.

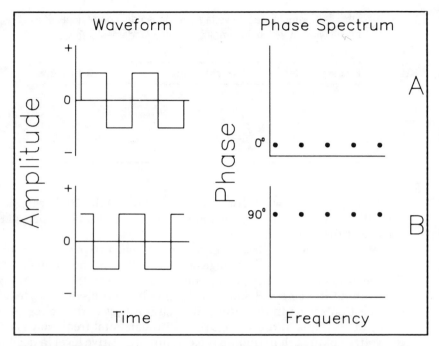

Figure 5–11. A comparison of waveforms and phase spectra for two square waves with different **starting phases**, 0° in panel A and 90° in panel B.

Because the exact same statement was made when we introduced the square wave, we must look for other explanations to account for the differences in the shapes of the two waveforms.

The first column of Table 5–4 lists the first five harmonics of a triangular wave for which the amplitude of the fundamental frequency again arbitrarily has been set at 2 V for easy comparison with our earlier calculations for sawtooth and square waves. It should be apparent that the amplitudes of the frequency components of the triangular wave decrease at a greater rate than was seen for either the sawtooth wave or the square wave, in which the amplitudes decrease as the reciprocal of the harmonic number.

The amplitudes of a triangular wave decrease as the reciprocal of the *square* of the harmonic number (rather than decrease as the reciprocal of the harmonic number itself, as with the sawtooth and square waves), and the relative amplitudes in decibels are given by:

Equation 5.2

$$dB = 20 \log_{10} \frac{1}{h_i^2},$$

where h_i is the harmonic number.

Consider, for example, the 3rd harmonic. For a sawtooth wave or square wave, we have seen that the amplitude of the 3rd harmonic is −9.5 dB re: the amplitude of the fundamental frequency because:

$$dB = 20 \log \frac{1}{3} = -9.5 \text{ dB}.$$

Table 5–4. Amplitudes (in voltage) of sinusoidal components of a **triangular** wave in which the amplitude of the fundamental frequency is 2 V.

Harmonic Number	rms voltage	$20 \log_{10} 1/h_i^2$
$1(f_0)$	$1/1^2 \times 2 = 2$	0
3	$1/3^2 \times 2 = .22$	-19.1
5	$1/5^2 \times 2 = .08$	-28
7	$1/7^2 \times 2 = .04$	-33.8
9	$1/9^2 \times 2 = .025$	-38.2

In contrast, the level of the 3rd harmonic of a triangular wave is -19.1 dB re: the level of the fundamental frequency because:

$$dB = 20 \log \frac{1}{3^2} = -19.1 \text{ dB.}$$

Thus, the slope of the spectral envelope of a triangular wave is twice as steep, -12 dB per octave, as it is for the sawtooth wave and the square wave.

Therefore, a **triangular wave** is defined as *a complex periodic wave with energy at odd integral multiples of the fundamental and a spectral envelope slope of -12 dB per octave*. The amplitude spectrum of a triangular wave also is a line spectrum because its waveform is periodic. Triangular and square waves are both characterized only by odd harmonics, but the slope of the envelope is -6 dB for the square wave and -12 dB for the triangular wave. For the example shown in Figure 5–9, all frequency components have a starting phase of 0°.

Pulse Train

Panel A of Figure 5–12 shows what is called a **pulse train**, a repetitious series of rectangularly shaped "pulses" of some width (duration, P_d) that occur at some regular rate. For the example in the figure, the interval between the onset of one pulse and the onset of the next pulse is 10 msec. That defines the *period* (T) of the pulse train[1]. By taking the reciprocal of the period ($1/T$), we calculate the frequency of the pulse train, which for the example in the figure would be 100 Hz. This is called the **pulse repetition frequency**.

It should be apparent that the pulse train is a complex periodic waveform, and therefore, there can only be energy at *harmonics* of the pulse repetition frequency: 100 Hz, 200 Hz, 300 Hz, and so on. Panel B of Figure 5–12 shows the amplitude spectrum of the pulse train with frequency plotted on a linear scale. First, note that the component with the greatest amplitude corresponds to *0 Hz*, which refers to what is called a *dc* (direct current) component of the signal. Recall from Chapter 2 that direct current means that current is flowing only in a single

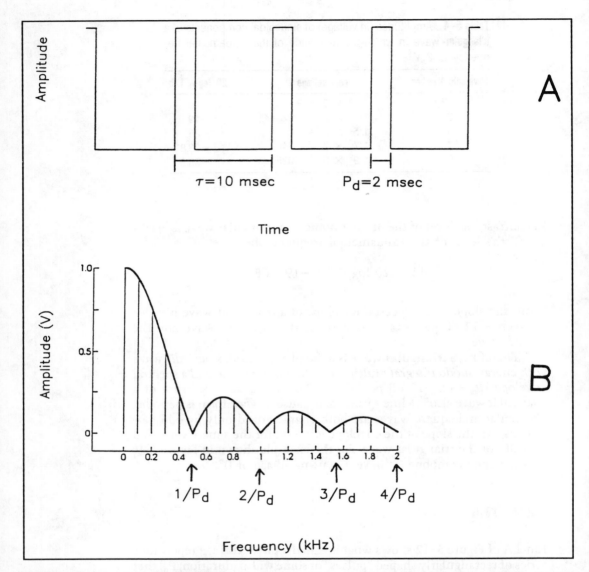

Figure 5–12. Panel A shows a **pulse train** with period = 10 msec and pulse duration (**P$_d$**) = 2 msec. Panel B shows the amplitude spectrum corresponding to the waveform in panel A. **Harmonics** are present at integral multiples of the pulse repetition frequency (100 Hz), and nulls are present at integral multiples of the reciprocal of pulse duration. Adapted from *Signals and systems for speech and hearing* (pp. 138–139) by S. Rosen and P. Howell, 1991: Academic Press, Inc., San Diego, CA. Copyright 1991 by Academic Press Limited. Printed with permission.

direction, either positive or negative, in contrast to alternating current that alternates back and forth (sinusoidally) in positive and negative directions.

Second, notice the irregularly shaped spectral envelope with lobes and valleys in panel B of Figure 5–12. Each valley or "null" occurs at integral multiples of the reciprocal of the pulse duration, **P$_d$**. Thus, we should expect to find nulls at frequencies corresponding to $1/P_d$, $2/P_d$, $3/P_d$, and so on. The duration of each pulse in the figure is 2 msec, and therefore, the first null appears at 500 Hz ($1/0.002 = 500$ Hz), the next null appears at 1000 Hz ($2/0.002 = 1000$ Hz), and so on.

The relation among the starting phases of the frequency components is more complicated than the relation observed for the sawtooth, square, and triangular waves. The components within the first lobe below the first null at 500 Hz have a starting phase of 0°, the components within the second lobe between the first and second nulls (500 Hz and 1000 Hz) have a starting phase of 180°, and the pattern continues to alternate in this fashion from lobe to lobe as frequency increases. We shall see subsequently that it is important to emphasize that the amplitude spectrum of a pulse train is a **line spectrum**.

White, or Gaussian, Noise

White, or **Gaussian**, **noise**, which also was shown in Figure 5–9, is defined as *an aperiodic waveform with equal energy within any frequency band 1 Hz wide* (from $f - 0.5$ Hz to $f + 0.5$ Hz) *and with all phases present in a random array*. It is called **white noise** to be analogous to white light, which is characterized by equal energy at all light wavelengths.

The reason white noise is also called **Gaussian noise** is somewhat more complicated. A random time function can be described by what is called a **cumulative probability distribution**, which reveals *the percentage of the total time that any instantaneous value of the waveform's amplitude is less than some specified value*. Such a distribution for white noise is shown at the left of Figure 5–13. The slope of such a cumulative probability distribution is called a **probability density function**. For white noise, it takes the form shown at the right of Figure 5–13.

Those who have had an elementary course in descriptive statistics undoubtedly will recognize such a function as a **normal curve**, and the amplitudes (and phases) of white noise are distributed normally. A normal distribution is also called a **Gaussian** distribution in honor of Karl Friedrich Gauss, a German mathematician, astronomer, and physicist. Therefore, white noise, which is characterized by a normal probability density function, also can be called **Gaussian noise**.

The amplitude spectrum of white noise is a continuous spectrum. You can see in Figure 5–9 that the spectral envelope is a line drawn parallel to the baseline, because white noise has the same amount of energy in every frequency band that is 1 Hz wide regardless of the value of f. We will discuss the slope of the envelope of white noise (and introduce "pink" noise) in more detail in Chapter 6 after the concepts of **pressure spectrum level** and **octave band level** have been presented.

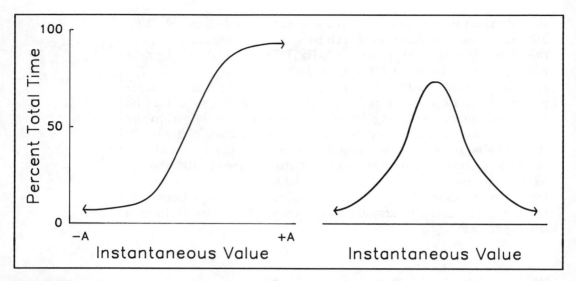

Figure 5–13. At the left is the *cumulative probability distribution* of **white noise**, which shows the percentage of total time that any instantaneous amplitude is less than some specified value. At the right is the *probability density function* for white noise, which is a plot of the slope of the function at the left. Because the probability density function assumes the shape of a normal curve, which also is called a Gaussian curve, **white noise** also is called **Gaussian noise**.

A Single Pulse

Panel A of Figure 5–14 shows the waveform of a single pulse that has the same width (duration = 2 msec) as each rectangular pulse in the pulse train that was shown in Figure 5–12. Is the waveform periodic or aperiodic? We must not be deceived because the shape of the waveform appears to be "regular" instead of random as we saw for white noise; that is irrelevant. The concept of *periodicity* means that an event occurs periodically over time. If there is only a single event (a single pulse), it cannot conceivably occur periodically.

Recall that the period of the pulse train is defined by the interval from the onset of one pulse to the onset of the next successive pulse. From that perspective, the "period" of a single pulse is infinity. If a single pulse is not periodic, we must consider it to be an aperiodic signal, and we therefore should expect that the amplitude spectrum is a **continuous spectrum** rather than a line spectrum.

Look again at the amplitude spectrum of the *pulse train* in Figure 5–12. It is a line spectrum with energy at harmonics of the pulse repetition frequency. For the example in Figure 5–12, the harmonics are spaced at 100 Hz intervals because the period of that pulse train is 10 msec (f = 1/.01 = 100 Hz).

Although it might be difficult to conceive of what would happen if the period were increased from 10 msec to infinity, we can, with a few examples, progress in that direction. If the period were increased from 10 msec to 20 msec, the pulse repetition frequency would decrease

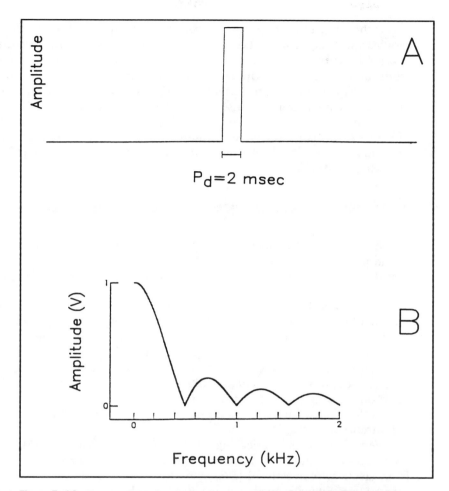

Figure 5–14. The waveform and spectrum of a **single rectangular pulse**. Nulls appear at integral multiples of the reciprocal pulse duration, just as they did for a pulse train in Figure 5–12. However, in this case the spectrum is a **continuous spectrum** in contrast to the line spectrum observed previously for a pulse train because a single pulse *cannot* be periodic. Adapted from Signals and systems for speech and hearing (pp. 143–144) by S. Rosen and P. Howell, 1991: Academic Press, Inc., San Diego, CA. Copyright 1991 by Academic Press Limited. Printed with permission.

from 100 Hz to 50 Hz (f = 1/.02 = 50 Hz), and the harmonics would be spaced twice as closely together at intervals of 50 Hz.

Recall from Chapter 1 that each time the period is doubled, frequency is halved. Therefore, for a complex wave, each time the period is doubled, the spacing between harmonics is halved. For example, if we continue to double the period to 40 msec, 80 msec, 160 msec, 320 msec, and so on, the intervals between harmonics in the amplitude spectrum progressively decrease to 25 Hz (f = 1/.04), 12.5 Hz (f = 1/.08), 6.25 Hz (f = 1/.16), 3.125 Hz (f = 1/.32), and so on.

If this process were continued to infinity, the spacing between harmonics would continue to become smaller and smaller. At infinity, the spacing between harmonics would equal 0, and the result would be a continuous spectrum of the sort shown in panel B of Figure 5–14.

The *shape of the spectral envelope* is the same as was shown previously for the pulse train because the width of the single pulse in Figure 5–14 is the same (2 msec) as the width of each of the pulses in the train of Figure 5–12. Thus, the envelope shows nulls at frequencies that correspond to integral multiples of the reciprocal of the pulse width ($1/P_d$, $2/P_d$, $3/P_d$, and so on).

■ MEASURES OF SOUND PRESSURE FOR COMPLEX WAVES

In Chapter 2 we described several alternative metrics by which the sound pressure of a *sine wave* could be described, and we emphasized that the various equations introduced in Chapter 2 *applied strictly only to the sine wave*. Table 5–5 contains the sine wave equations shown previously, in addition to the modifications to those equations that are required for calculating the rms, mean square, FW_{avg}, and peak sound pressure for square waves and for typical aperiodic waveforms.

It is apparent that different equations must be used for different waveforms. This introduces a problem in measurement of sound pressure. Although measurement techniques are beyond the scope of this book, one example can emphasize the importance of knowing the kind of waveform on which a measurement is being performed before the measurement is made.

Very often, an acoustical signal is converted (transduced) into an electrical signal and then various measurements are performed. Voltage is an electrical correlate of (analogous to) acoustical sound pressure. Thus, a transduced acoustical sine wave is an electrical waveform with sinusoidally fluctuating voltages over time. Measures of voltage are then performed with the aid of a voltmeter, which registers **rms** voltage.

Rms voltage is analogous to rms sound pressure. But, one type of voltmeter is called an "average-responding meter" and another type is called a "true rms meter." The average-responding meter actually "reads" the peak value of the voltage and then performs a computation

Table 5–5. Measures of sound pressure for sine, square, and random waveforms. **A** refers to the peak or **maximum amplitude** as defined in Chapter 2.

Metrics	Types of Waveforms		
	Sine Wave	Square Wave	Random Wave
rms	$A/\sqrt{2}$	A	~0.3 A
mean square	$A^2/2$	A^2	~0.1 A
FW_{avg}	$2A/\pi$	A	~ .25 A
peak	A	A	A

to convert the peak reading to an rms reading by dividing the peak value by $\sqrt{2}$. A true rms meter, on the other hand "reads" the rms directly, thereby avoiding any necessity for conversion. There is no problem as long as the waveform is sinusoidal.

What happens if an average-responding meter is used to measure the rms voltage of a square wave? Suppose the peak value is 1 V. We can see from Table 5–5 that the rms value also is 1 V for a square wave. However, the average-responding meter does not "know" that it is responding to a square wave. It will read the peak value of 1, divide the reading by $\sqrt{2}$, and register that the rms voltage is an erroneous 0.707.

The same measurement problem will occur with other complex waveforms. One must either know the appropriate conversions or purchase a more sophisticated and expensive measuring instrument that requires no conversion.

■ SIGNAL-TO-NOISE RATIO IN dB

Without exception, we listen to signals in the presence of some form of background noise. The relation between signal level and noise level is quantified by the **signal-to-noise ratio (S/N)** in dB. A positive S/N ratio means that signal level exceeds noise level, a negative S/N ratio means that noise level exceeds signal level, and an S/N ratio of 0 dB means that signal level and noise level are equal to each other. Suppose, for example, that a signal with SPL = 70 dB is presented against a background noise with SPL = 66 dB. In that case,

$$dB\ S/N = 70/66 = +4\ dB.$$

If the S/N ratio truly is *a ratio*, why do we solve for decibels by *subtracting* noise level from signal level rather than dividing signal level by noise level? Recall Log Law 2 from Chapter 3, which states that the log of some ratio is equal to the difference between the logs of the factors.

A decibel is (ten times) a log, and therefore we simply subtract the denominator from the numerator rather than divide the numerator by the denominator. If, on the other hand, signal intensity and noise intensity were each expressed in watt/m^2, then division would be the appropriate operation. In the example cited above, the *intensity* of the signal is 10^{-5} watt/m^2 (Equation 4.4) and the intensity of the noise is 4×10^{-6} watt/m^2. In that case,

$$dB\ S/N = 10\ \log\ 10^{-5}/(4 \times 10^{-6}),$$
$$= 10\ \log\ 0.25 \times 10^1,$$
$$= +4\ dB.$$

Obviously, it is easier to simply subtract decibels.

■ **NOTES**

1. Some authors such as, for example, Yost and Nielson (1977), use the symbols **P** for **period** and **T** for **pulse duration**. For the sake of consistency, we will continue to use **T** for **period** and we have adopted the symbol P_d for **pulse duration**; the subscript **d** serves to distinguish P_d from **P**, which we have used as a symbol for **pressure**.

■

Resonance and Filtering

Sound waves, whether sinusoidal or complex, that are produced by vibratory motion often are weak, uninteresting, and perhaps lacking in "richness." Consider, for example, the complex periodic waveform at the left of Figure 6-1 that is produced by the vibrating vocal folds during, for example, vowel production. Imagine that a microphone is placed in the throat immediately above the vocal folds. That location would permit us to record the sound produced by the motion of the folds in a way that would minimize the effects of supralaryngeal cavities on the sound wave.

The waveform is approximately sawtooth in shape and, perceptually, the result sounds similar to a "buzz."[1] The amplitude spectrum at the right of Figure 6-1 shows that there is a fundamental frequency, f_o, and a series of harmonics that are odd and even integral multiples of the fundamental. An important feature of the vocal fold spectrum is that the envelope is fairly smooth in the sense that there are no regions of sharp prominence.

Most of the energy is located in the lower frequencies, and the amplitudes of the harmonics fall off in a smooth, regular fashion with increasing frequency. With natural vocal production, those amplitudes decrease at a rate of approximately 12 dB per octave. Recall, of course, from Chapter 5 that if this were a perfect sawtooth, all harmonics would be present and the slope would be -6 dB/octave. If it were a perfect triangular wave, only the odd harmonics would be present, but the slope would be -12 dB/octave.

We would have an extremely limited vowel component of our language system if the sound wave shown in Figure 6-1 was all that was available for human vowel production. Basically, the system would have only three principal parameters that could be varied to produce a set of vowels with which to communicate. We could vary the amplitude to produce a series of tokens that would differ perceptually in loudness;

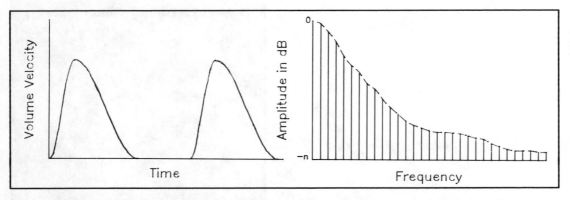

Figure 6-1. The waveform and amplitude spectrum of a sound produced by the vibrating vocal folds. The waveform is approximately sawtooth in shape. The spectrum is a line spectrum with energy at odd and even integral multiples of the fundamental frequency, f_o, and with a spectral envelope slope of approximately -12 db/octave.

we could vary the fundamental frequency to produce a series of tokens that would differ in perceived pitch; and we could vary the duration. However, we would not be able to form the series of vowels that actually compose an important part of the phonological system to which we have become accustomed. To compensate for this situation, the sound wave produced by the vocal fold source — and all other sound waves as well — can be "reinforced" or altered by a process called **resonance**, or **filtering**.

The sounds produced by stringed instruments also need to be "enhanced," rather than rely simply on the vibrating strings alone to produce the desired sound waves. This is accomplished by use of what some call a "mechanical amplifier," known as a sounding board. It is more properly called a **resonator**, because it does not truly amplify sound waves, yet a resonator such as a sounding board "reinforces" the sound waves emanating from the vibrating strings.

■ RESONANCE

We will begin by attempting to gain an intuitive understanding of what is meant by the word "resonance," and examine what takes place when a system is "set into resonance." The next step, then, will be to learn *why* resonance occurs.

One easy way to demonstrate the phenomenon of resonance is to strike a tuning fork and hold the vibrating tuning fork in the air medium. The sound wave that results is approximately sinusoidal. It will be characterized by a certain frequency of vibration that is governed by the **mass** and **stiffness** of the fork. As we learned in Chapter 2, the frequency with which a specific fork vibrates is called its **natural frequency**, and that frequency of vibration will give rise to the perception of a certain pitch. Frequency of vibration will not change as the fork continues to vibrate.

The sound wave will also be characterized by a certain amplitude of vibration that will depend upon the force applied to the fork when it is struck, and the amplitude of vibration will give rise to the perception of loudness. We learned previously that the amplitude of vibration will diminish over time because of **resistance**, and the decay of amplitude over time is called **damping**.

Once the loudness of the tone has become noticeably softer, touch the stem of the fork to a wooden table or some other hard surface. That hard surface is also a system that is characterized by **mass** and **stiffness** and therefore it too can be *forced into vibratory motion*. However, we shall subsequently see that the hard surface does not engage in **free vibration** at its own **natural frequency**. Instead, it is forced to vibrate by a force imparted to it by the vibrating tuning fork.

When the tuning fork is held against the hard surface, you should observe that the sound immediately becomes louder. It is important to emphasize that even though the loudness becomes perceptually greater when the fork is held against the hard surface, *no energy is added to the sound wave.* The sound wave that results from touching the stem of the fork to the table does have greater **power** and greater **intensity**, but not greater **energy**.

Power is *the amount of energy per second,* and an increase in power can be realized by either an increase in energy, *or a decrease in time of vibration.* In this case, the greater power that results from touching the vibrating fork to a hard surface is gained at the expense of a shorter time of vibration. The duration of vibration is shorter when the fork is held against the hard surface than if the fork were left to vibrate only in the surrounding air medium.

The Principle of Resonance

The general principle of resonance that is demonstrated by applying the vibrating tuning fork to a hard surface is:

> When a periodically vibrating force is applied to an elastic system, the elastic system will be forced to vibrate with the frequency of the applied force. Furthermore, the nearer the frequency of the applied force to the **natural frequency** of the elastic system, the greater will be the resulting amplitude of vibration.

A Comparison of Two Elastic Systems

In Figure 6–2 we can examine the amplitude spectra that result from driving two elastic systems that have different characteristics. Instead of assembling a large array of tuning forks that span a wide frequency range, we will generate sine waves of variable frequency with an electronic device called an "audio oscillator," or "sine wave generator."

Sine waves of variable frequency *but constant amplitude* are directed to each of the two different systems represented in the figure. Each system will be forced to vibrate at the frequencies of the applied forces, that is, at the frequencies produced by the sine wave generator. We then can examine, separately for each driving frequency, the amplitudes of vibration *at the outputs of the elastic systems.* Finally, we can plot the results that are shown in Figure 6–2. In that plot, 0 dB has been assigned to the amplitude of the frequency that produces the greatest magnitude of vibration.

Let us first consider the example at the left of Figure 6–2. When the driving frequency is 100 Hz, the elastic system is forced to vibrate with a frequency of 100 Hz; when the driving frequency is 200 Hz, the elastic system vibrates at 200 Hz; and so on. This is an example of **forced vibration** because the elastic system is *forced* to vibrate at the frequency of the applied force. As we move through higher and higher frequencies, the elastic system always vibrates with the frequency of the force applied. In other words, *the process of resonance does not change the frequency of vibration.* This is consistent with the first part of the

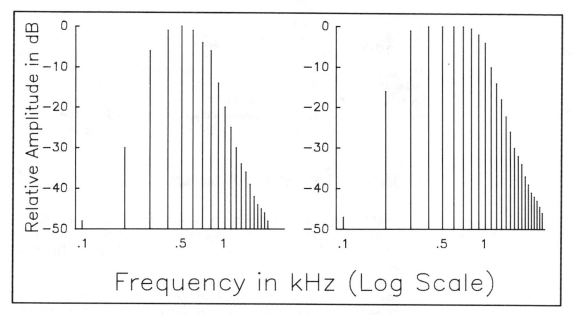

Figure 6–2. An illustration of the **principle of resonance**. Sine waves with different frequencies are applied with equal amplitudes to two resonant systems. The resonant system is forced to vibrate at the *frequency of the applied force*, and the nearer the frequency of the applied force to the **natural** or **center frequency, f_c,** of the resonant system, the greater will be the amplitude of vibration. As a consequence, the resulting amplitudes of vibration of the resonant system vary as a function of frequency. The system at the left is a **narrowly tuned** system with a fairly well-defined f_c, whereas the system at the right is **broadly tuned** because maximum amplitude of vibration occurs over a fairly wide range of frequencies.

principle of resonance that was stated previously: When a periodically vibrating force is applied to an elastic system, the elastic system will be forced to vibrate with the frequency of the applied force.

Return now to the lowest driving frequency, 100 Hz, and look at the amplitude of vibration that results at the output of the elastic system. In this example, the resulting amplitude is almost 50 dB lower than the largest amplitude that is achieved, which occurs at 500 Hz. At 200 Hz, the amplitude of vibration is greater than at 100 Hz.

As we move from 100 Hz to higher and higher frequencies, we see that the amplitude of vibration continues to *increase* until it reaches a maximum, in this case when f = 500 Hz. Then, as the frequency of the applied force continues to increase beyond 500 Hz, the amplitude of vibration *diminishes* in a manner that is symmetric (in log frequency) with the increase that was observed for the lower frequencies.

The driving frequency that produces the greatest amplitude of vibration of the elastic system, 0 dB, corresponds to the **natural frequency (f_c)** of the elastic system, which in the case of the example at the left of the figure is 500 Hz. That outcome is in agreement with the second part of the principle of resonance: The nearer the frequency of the applied force to the **natural frequency** of the elastic system, the greater will be the resulting amplitude of vibration.

The right side of Figure 6–2 shows a different outcome when the same driving frequencies are applied to a different elastic system. The second system also is forced to vibrate at the driving frequencies, but the principal difference between the response of this system and the one at the left of the figure is that maximum amplitude (0 dB) is realized for several driving frequencies, not just one. We shall see later that the elastic system on the left can be called a more **narrowly tuned** system, and the one on the right can be called a more **broadly tuned** system.

A "Shattering" Example of Resonance

You might have seen a television commercial sponsored by a maker of one brand of audio tape that shows a drinking glass shatter when the recorded voice of Ella Fitzgerald is reproduced near the glass. The glass, as with any other system that has mass and stiffness, has a **natural frequency**, which also is called a **resonant frequency**.

In accordance with the principle of resonance, the glass is forced to vibrate at the frequency of the applied force (the driving frequency), which in this case is determined by the fundamental frequency, f_o, of Fitzgerald's singing voice. When the fundamental frequency (sometimes referred to as the "fundamental pitch") of her voice reaches the resonant, or natural, frequency of the glass, the amplitude of vibration increases until the vibration of the glass becomes so great that it finally breaks.

■ RESONANCE AND FILTER CURVES

Figure 6–3 shows the same process described above, but in a slightly different fashion. Frequency of applied force again is shown on the abscissa and resulting amplitude of vibration of the elastic system in dB is shown on the ordinate. However, in this case, there are no tuning forks or other sources of sound. There is, in fact, no sound. Instead, the curve that is shown represents *the relative amplitude of forced vibrations as a function of frequency that would be realized if driving forces were applied to the elastic system.*

From inspection of the curve in Figure 6–3, you can determine the relative amplitude of vibration resulting for any frequency of vibration that is applied to the system as long as all of the driving frequencies are applied with exactly the same force. If the force of application were increased for all of the frequencies, would the curve be displaced upward? *No.* It is true that the amplitude of response would be increased by an identical amount (to some upper limit) for each frequency, but because the ordinate is scaled in *relative amplitude*, where 0 dB refers to the amplitude of the frequency with the greatest energy, the curve would appear exactly as it does in Figure 6–3.

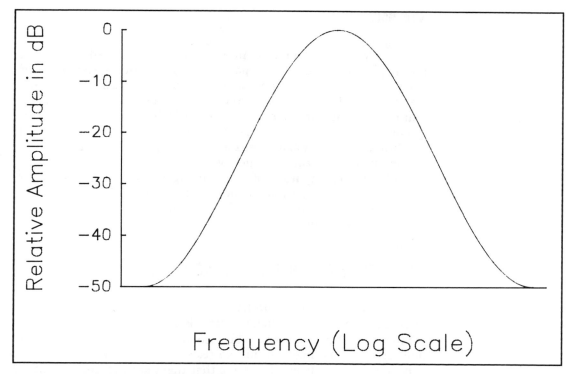

Figure 6–3. A **resonance curve**, or **filter curve**. The curve shows the relative amplitude of vibration as a function of frequency for a resonator. The curve also can be called a **transfer function**.

The curve in Figure 6–3 can be called a **resonance curve** because it behaves in a manner consistent with the definition of resonance stated earlier: The system vibrates at the frequency of the applied force, and the amplitude of vibration depends on the proximity of the frequency of the applied force to the natural frequency of the elastic system.

The curve in Figure 6–3 also can be called a **filter curve**, which is simply emphasizing a different aspect of the same phenomenon. Look first at the frequency that corresponds to the **natural frequency** of the system — the peak of the curve. The amplitude of vibration is greatest at that point and therefore corresponds to 0 dB.

As we move from the natural frequency in either direction the system is less responsive to the frequencies that are lower or higher than the natural frequency, and the corresponding amplitudes of vibration are less than the amplitude at the natural frequency. Thus, we can say that *the system responds differentially, or selectively, as a function of frequency*, and it therefore can be called a **frequency-selective system**. Frequencies that are remote from the natural frequency are said to have been filtered.

Summary

When an elastic system is set into resonance, it is forced to vibrate at the frequencies of the forces applied to it. The elastic system has mass and stiffness, and those properties determine what is called the **natural frequency**, or **resonant frequency**, of the system. When an elastic system is driven by a frequency that corresponds to its own **natural frequency**, we obtain the greatest amplitude of vibration. Finally, the amplitudes of vibration are less for frequencies that are either lower or higher than the natural frequency.

Why is the amplitude of vibration greatest when the driving frequency equals the natural frequency of the system? To explain this phenomenon, we will review and expand on **acoustic impedance** introduced in Chapter 2.

■ ACOUSTIC IMPEDANCE AND RESONANCE

The **impedance** of a system has two components. One is an energy-dissipating component called **resistance**. The magnitude of resistance is independent of frequency. The second is an energy-storage component called **reactance**, and unlike resistance, reactance is frequency dependent. Recall from Chapter 2 that there are two components of reactance, **mass reactance**, which increases with increasing frequency ($X_m \propto f$), and **compliant reactance**, which decreases with increasing frequency ($X_c \propto 1/f$). **Impedance** (Z) is the complex sum of its components: R, X_m, and X_c.

Effects of Impedance on a Resonance Curve

Figure 6–4 shows a sample of resonance curves. The characteristics (shapes) of each of the different curves *are determined by the impedance of the system being driven*. Importantly, the shape of each curve and its location in the frequency domain reflect the relative contribution of the three components of **impedance** to the total opposition to transfer of energy: **resistance, mass reactance**, and **compliant reactance**.

If no resistance is present, which is the so-called ideal case, maximum transfer of energy occurs, and the response of the system is infinite at the natural frequency. That circumstance is represented by the dashed resonant curve in the figure with the arrows pointing upward. Consider next resonance curve A with the sharp peak. **Resistance** now is present, which serves to limit the maximum amplitude of vibration relative to the "ideal" or lossless case where there is no dissipation of energy. Curve A is frequency selective and the location of the peak of the curve along the frequency axis corresponds to the **natural frequency** of the system. The greatest amplitude of vibration occurs at the

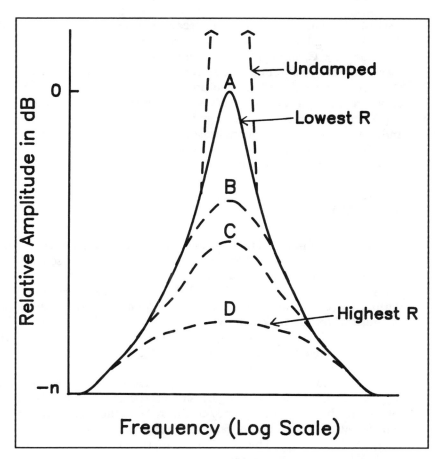

Figure 6–4. A series of resonance curves. The dashed curve reflects the response of a theoretically lossless system with no resistance. From curve A through curve D, resistance increases, which produces two obvious effects on the shape of the curve: (1) the maximum amplitude of response decreases and (2) the system becomes more broadly tuned.

natural frequency because that is the frequency at which the least **impedance** is encountered.

At the **natural frequency** (f_c), $X_m = X_c$, and the impedance, the total opposition to transfer of energy, is determined entirely by the **resistance**. When the driving frequency equals the natural frequency of the system, we say the system has been *set into resonance*. The amplitude of vibration is less for frequencies below f_c, and for those frequencies the system is called **compliance**, or **stiffness, dominant**. By that we mean, the relative contribution of **compliant reactance** to **impedance** is greater than the contribution of **mass reactance**. The response of the system also diminishes with increasing frequency above f_c, and for those frequencies the system is called **mass dominant** because the contribution of **mass reactance** to impedance is greater than the contribution of **compliant reactance**.

Curves B, C, and D in Figure 6–4 show the effects of progressively increasing the **resistance** of a system. The **natural frequency** is unchanged because there has been no change in the **mass reactance** or **compliant reactance**. However, as **resistance** (which is frequency independent) *increases*, more energy is dissipated, damping is increased, and the system becomes more broadly tuned. Stated conversely, as the resistive component of impedance *decreases*, the system becomes less damped and more narrowly tuned.

Admittance

When we have discussed the concept of impedance, we have, in a sense, emphasized the "negative." By that we mean, we have focused on opposition to motion or transfer of energy. Thus, we say that the transfer of energy to an elastic system is **impeded** at frequencies remote from the natural frequency, and *the more remote the **driving frequency** from the **natural frequency** of the system, the greater is the impedance.* The result is a reduction in the response of the system as the driving frequency becomes progressively lower or higher than the natural frequency of the system.

We can just as easily emphasize the inverse, or (musically speaking) "accentuate the positive" by saying, the closer the driving frequency to the natural frequency of the system, the greater will be the transfer of energy to the system. In a sense we are saying that more energy will be accepted by, or *admitted* to, the elastic system when the driving frequency equals the natural frequency.

Admittance is inversely proportional to **impedance** (Z) and the appropriate symbol for **admittance** therefore is Z^{-1}. Thus, the ordinate in Figure 6–4 could have been labeled **admittance** (instead of "relative amplitude in dB"). The unit of measure of **impedance** is the **ohm**, whereas the unit of measure of **admittance** is the **mho**.

System Tuning

Figure 6–5 shows two resonance curves. The curve at the left of the figure reflects what is called a **narrowly tuned system**, whereas the curve at the right reflects a **broadly tuned system**. A narrowly tuned system *can be forced to vibrate*, but only over a *very narrow range of frequencies*. A tuning fork and the wires or strings of stringed musical instruments are examples of narrowly tuned systems and they vibrate freely at their own natural frequencies when energized.

We have, for convenience, discussed sources of sound such as the tuning fork or string separately from resonant systems, which might convey the erroneous impression that a source of sound cannot be set into resonance. Both the source of sound and the resonant system are

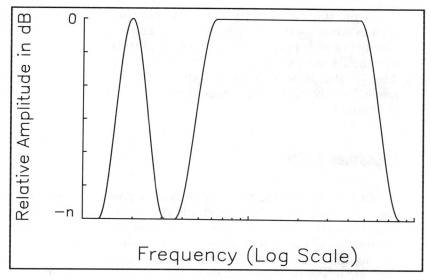

Figure 6–5. Comparison of two resonance systems, one that is narrowly tuned with low damping (left) and one that is broadly tuned with high damping (right).

characterized by **resistance** and **reactance**. Hence, they both are characterized by some amount of impedance. The tuning fork and the string *are indeed resonant systems*. Thus, when the string is plucked or the fork is struck, each vibrates freely at its own **natural frequency**, which corresponds to the frequency at which the **mass reactance** equals the **compliant reactance**.

The tuning fork also can be forced to vibrate if it is tightly coupled to another tuning fork, but to transfer energy efficiently from one fork to another requires that the two forks have nearly identical frequency, because the response curve for each reflects very narrow tuning. That is because the impedance increases (and admittance decreases) rapidly as we descend or ascend in frequency from the natural frequency.

In contrast to a narrowly tuned system, a **broadly tuned system**, such as that shown at the right of Figure 6–5, can be forced to vibrate by external forces over a wide range of frequencies. In addition to the table surface we cited previously, other familiar examples of broadly tuned systems include the diaphragms of microphones, earphones, loudspeakers, and our own eardrums.

Systems that are **narrowly tuned** always are associated with little **resistance**, which means that such systems have little **damping**. That circumstance allows free vibrations to continue for some considerable amount of time, and, thus, narrowly tuned systems are efficient *generators of sound*.

On the other hand, systems that are **broadly tuned** are always associated with a higher **resistance**, which means that they have much higher **damping**. Therefore, the free vibrations that occur after the external force is removed are very brief in duration, and broadly tuned systems are efficient *transducers of sound*.

If you think about it for a moment, you should want a transducer such as a loudspeaker to be broadly tuned so that it will respond efficiently to a wide range of frequencies with little loss in amplitude. You also should want a transducer to be highly damped so that it does not "ring" — that is, so that the transducer does not continue to vibrate freely for any appreciable amount of time after the external force is removed.

Impedance Matching

When a force is applied to an elastic system, power is transferred from the source (the "driver") to the elastic system (the "load"), and the system is forced to vibrate. We know by now that the maximum amplitude of vibration of the system will be achieved when the frequency of the driving force corresponds to the natural frequency of the system. In that circumstance, mass reactance equals compliant reactance, and resistance is the only component of impedance. At the natural frequency of the system, therefore, **impedance** $(\mathbf{Z})$ is minimal and, of course, **admittance** $(\mathbf{Z^{-1}})$ is maximal.

Transfer of power from the driver to the load is optimal when the impedance of the source equals the impedance of the load (the elastic system). When the strings of a piano are set into vibration, their motion forces the sounding board (a resonator) of the piano to vibrate. As we stated previously, the sounding board *does not amplify the sound produced by the vibrating string*. Instead, it serves to improve the match of the impedance of the driver (the vibrating string) and the surrounding air mass. As a consequence, more sound power is delivered to the air.

The concept of impedance matches or mismatches will be encountered again in Chapter 8 when we discuss sound wave reflection.

■ FREQUENCY-SELECTIVE SYSTEMS: FILTERS

The effects of a frequency-selective system — a filter — on a driving signal that is directed to its input are illustrated in Figure 6–6. Each vertical line (the total length of solid and dashed portions) in the figure represents the relative amplitude with which each frequency was applied to the filter, and the array of vertical lines defines the **amplitude spectrum** of the complex periodic signal that is applied to the system, the driving signal. The absolute amplitude of each frequency is unimportant, but it is important for our purpose now to ensure that all frequencies of vibration be applied with exactly the same amplitude.

The resonance, or filter, curve shows the amplitude with which the system will vibrate for each of the various frequencies that is applied. Thus, the length of each solid vertical line that lies *under* the curve shows the resulting amplitude of vibration of the resonant system. The greatest amplitude of response, of course, is realized at the **natural**

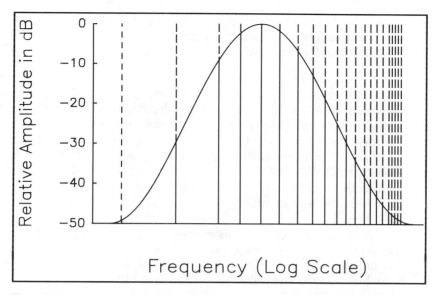

Figure 6–6. The effects of a resonator, or filter, on the amplitude spectrum of sine waves directed to the system. The total length of each line (solid plus dashed) represents the relative amplitude of each frequency that is directed to the resonator. The length of each solid line *under the curve* represents the relative amplitudes of the input frequencies after they have been selectively attenuated by the resonator, or filter.

frequency of the system where $X_m = X_c$. Frequencies remote from the natural frequency are said to be **filtered**; their amplitudes are diminished relative to the amplitude at the natural frequency because of **mass reactance** and **compliant reactance**, each of which varies with frequency. Stated differently, the mismatch of impedances increases as the frequency of the driver departs, up or down, from the natural frequency.

The curve in Figure 6–6 also can be called a **system transfer function**. That simply means that the curve (a resonance, or filter, curve) describes the way in which the sound wave will be altered or transferred (amplitudes changed as a function of frequency) by application of the external forces to the elastic system.

We emphasize that the *curve* in Figure 6–6 *is not a sound wave*. It simply shows the way in which the amplitude spectrum of a sound wave will be altered if the sound wave is applied to the elastic system and forces it to vibrate. In Figure 6–6, then:

1. The line spectrum represented by the equal-length vertical lines (sum of solid and dashed) is the **amplitude spectrum** of the sound wave that is applied to the elastic system;
2. The curve is the **transfer function** (not a sound wave) of the elastic system that shows how the amplitude spectra of sound waves will be altered when applied to the elastic system; and

3. The lengths of the lines (solid) under the curve show the **amplitude spectrum** of the sound wave that results from application of the external forces to the elastic system.

The curve in Figure 6–7 is identical to the one in Figure 6–6. However, in this case, the signal that is applied to the elastic system is **white noise**. White noise, as you recall, has *equal energy at all frequencies* and the **amplitude spectrum** is a **continuous spectrum**. Thus, all frequencies in the white noise signal are applied to the elastic system with equal force, and that is represented by the horizontal line drawn parallel to the baseline that intersects the ordinate at 0 dB. The curve, as before, shows the system transfer function or filter characteristics, and it reveals the way in which the system will respond when the forces are applied.

Because the signal in this example is white noise, the curve also shows the continuous amplitude spectrum of the altered, or filtered, sound wave. The array of frequencies no longer is characterized by equal amplitude; the noise has been filtered by a frequency-selective device. In point of fact, the sound wave at the output of the filter is no longer white noise. Instead, it is properly called a **frequency-limited white noise** or a **band-limited white noise**. It is called a band-limited white noise to signify that it was a white noise signal that was applied to the system, but that the output was restricted to some smaller band of frequencies.

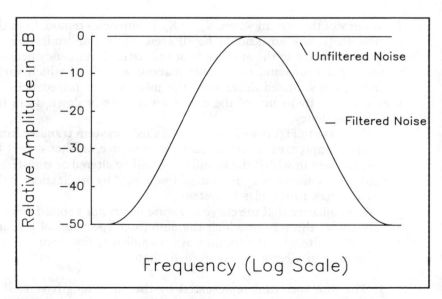

Figure 6–7. The solid line parallel to the baseline shows the envelope of white noise that is directed to a resonator, or filter. The curve is the system transfer function of the filter. The area under the curve shows the distribution of amplitude as a function of frequency at the output of the resonator, or filter. The result is called **band-limited white noise** because the output signal was restricted to some smaller band of frequencies.

■ PARAMETERS OF A FILTER (SYSTEM TRANSFER FUNCTION)

Figure 6–8 displays two filter curves, or system transfer functions. Filter curves such as those shown in the figure have five principal parameters: (1) the **natural frequency**, which also is called the **center frequency**, f_c; (2) the **upper cutoff frequency** (f_U); (3) the **lower cutoff frequency** (f_L); (4) the **bandwidth** (**BW** or Δf); and (5) the **attenuation rate**, which also is called the **rejection rate**.

Natural, or Center, Frequency (f_c)

The **natural frequency**, or **center frequency**, f_c, specifies the frequency that will result in a maximum amplitude of vibration. The center frequency depends upon the mass and elastic properties of the system if we are referring to an acoustical system[2] and, as we learned previously, corresponds to the frequency at which $X_m = X_c$.

The two curves in Figure 6–8 have different f_cs, and f_c is one important parameter that allows us to distinguish one filter from another. It might appear at first glance that the difference in f_c for the two curves is the only distinguishing characteristic, but after reading the subsequent section on "constant bandwidth filters" you should return to Figure 6–8 and try to discover another way in which the two curves differ.

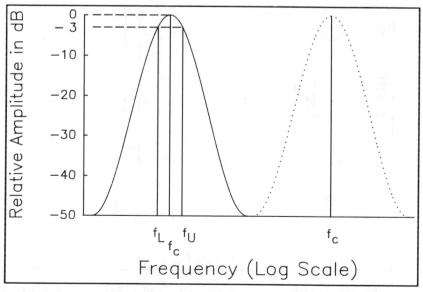

Figure 6–8. Two filter curves with different center frequencies, f_c.

Upper Cutoff Frequency (f_U)

A second parameter is called the **upper cutoff frequency**, f_U. We know that frequencies above f_c are attenuated, and we describe this by saying that the higher frequencies are filtered, that is to say, their amplitudes are attenuated.

At what frequency does the filtering begin? Consider the two examples in Figure 6–9. Both curves (system transfer functions) have exactly the same f_c, but the response of the two systems is different for frequencies above (and below) f_c. Actually, the filtering begins almost immediately above f_c and progresses continuously from there on. However, a convention has been adopted to describe the "upper limit" of the filter by designating a single frequency as the point above f_c where filtering is said to commence.

By that convention, the **upper cutoff frequency**, f_U, is defined as the **3-dB down point** or as the **half-power point**. More specifically, f_U is that frequency *above* f_c for which the amplitude of response is 3 dB less than the amplitude at maximum, f_c. It is called the **half-power point** because it is that frequency for which the power in the resulting sound wave is one-half the power existing in the wave for f_c. It is called the **3-dB down point** because halving of acoustic power corresponds to -3 dB:

$$10 \log_{10} \frac{1}{2} = -3 \text{ dB}.$$

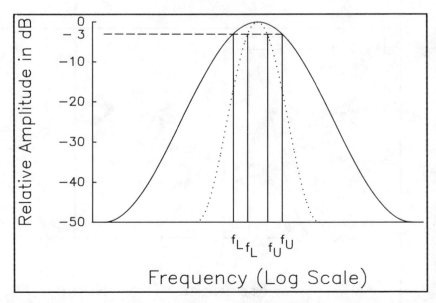

Figure 6–9. Two filter curves with the same center frequency, f_c, but different upper cutoff frequencies, f_U, lower cutoff frequencies, f_L, and bandwidths, Δf.

Lower Cutoff Frequency (f$_L$)

A third parameter of the filter is the **lower cutoff frequency, f$_L$**. By convention, f$_L$ is defined as that frequency *below* f$_c$ for which the amplitude of response is 3 dB less than the amplitude of response at maximum, f$_c$. f$_L$, like f$_U$, is also the half-power point because it is that frequency below f$_c$ for which the power in the resulting wave is one half the power existing in the wave for f$_c$.

Bandwidth (Δf or BW)

A fourth parameter is the **bandwidth, BW or Δf**, of the filter. Δf is defined as the width of the band of frequencies that are "passed" by the filter:

$$\Delta f = f_U - f_L.$$ **Equation 6.1**

Thus, bandwidth refers to the width of the band of frequencies between the lower and upper cutoff frequencies, and it defines the range of frequencies over which energy is *passed* by the filter. It can also be called the **passband** of the system to emphasize the band of frequencies that is passed by the filter. The two filter curves in Figure 6–9 have the same f$_c$, but different upper (f$_U$) and lower (f$_L$) cutoff frequencies and different bandwidths (Δf).

Return to Figure 6–4 and examine the resonance curves again. We said previously that as we moved from curve A to curve D, resistance progressively increased and the systems reflected broader tuning. Now we should see that the degree of tuning can be quantified by expressing the bandwidth, Δf. Thus, curve D in Figure 6–4 has a wider bandwidth than curve A.

Attenuation Rate (in dB/Octave)

The fifth parameter describes the *slope* of the skirts of the filter curve. It is referred to variously as: the **attenuation rate**, the rate with which the amplitude of response is attenuated as a function of frequency; the **roll-off rate**, the rate with which the response of the system "rolls off" on either side of f$_c$; and the **rejection rate**, the rate with which energy for frequencies on either side of f$_c$ is rejected. All three terms are synonymous. They all are measures of the slope of the curve on either side of f$_c$, and the unit of measure is **dB/octave**.

The two curves in Figure 6–10 have the same f$_c$. However, the attenuation rates for the two filters are different. The response (relative amplitude in dB) at 1000 Hz for filter A is -10 dB re: the response for f$_c$, and one octave lower (500 Hz), the response for filter A is -20 dB. Thus,

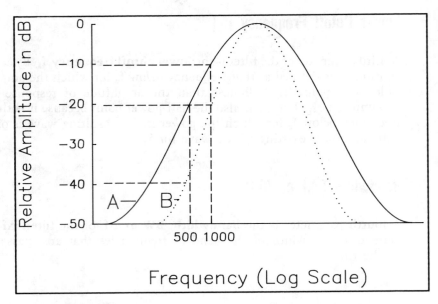

Figure 6–10. Two filter curves with the same center frequency, f_c, but different **attenuation rates**.

the **attenuation rate** over this linear portion of the curve for filter A is 10 dB/octave. For filter B, which has a steeper slope, the response at 1000 Hz is −20 dB, the response at 500 Hz is −40 dB, and the attenuation rate, therefore, is 20 dB/octave. Thus, attenuation rate is a parameter that distinguishes filter A from filter B, and filter B can be described as being a "more selective" filter than filter A. Because it is more selective, that is to say, it is more narrowly tuned, we know that it offers less resistance to the transfer of energy.

◼ IDEAL VERSUS REALIZED FILTERS

Consider a filter with the following characteristics: f_c = 1000 Hz; f_L = 800 Hz; f_U = 1200 Hz; Δf = 400 Hz; and **attenuation rate** = 24 dB/octave. We would describe such a filter as one that (1) rejects energy below 800 Hz and above 1200 Hz; (2) passes energy in a band 400 Hz wide that is centered on the natural frequency of 1000 Hz; and (3) rejects energy outside the passband (800-1200 Hz) at the rate of 24 dB/octave.

The filter just described can be envisioned as having a rectangular shape, and an **ideal rectangular filter** would take the form of the rectangle in Figure 6–11. All energy between 800 (f_L) and 1200 Hz (f_U) is passed by the ideal filter, all energy below 800 Hz and above 1200 Hz is rejected, and the filter slopes are infinity. Analog filters that are likely to be encountered will be more of the form shown by the bell-shaped curve in Figure 6–11. Because the slopes in the figure are 24 dB/octave rather than infinity, the analog filter in Figure 6–11 has fallen short of the ideal filter.

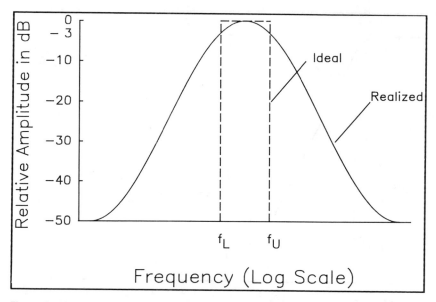

Figure 6–11. A comparison of an analog filter curve (solid line) with an **ideal rectangular filter** (dashed line) with infinitely steep attenuation rates.

When we specify the lower cutoff frequency, the upper cutoff frequency, and the bandwidth of the real filter, we are describing the *real filter* as if it were an **ideal rectangular filter**. However, because the slope of the real filter is not infinity, specification of the **attenuation rate** provides a measure of the amount by which the real filter *departs* from the ideal filter. Filter B in Figure 6–10 is more nearly ideal than filter A because it has the steeper slope. If another filter were chosen with an attenuation rate of 72 dB/octave rather than 10 or 20 dB/octave, it would be even more nearly ideal. Thus, the steeper the attenuation rate, the more the real filter approximates the ideal filter.

■ TYPES OF FILTERS

There are four common types of filters: **low-pass, high-pass, band-pass**, and **band-reject**. We will provide a brief description of each type and also specify the parameters that are necessary to describe each type of filter.

Low-Pass Filter

The **low-pass filter** is one that passes energy *below* some designated upper cutoff frequency. The two defining parameters are f_U and **attenuation rate**. Figure 6–12 shows four low-pass filters. The two curves at the left have the same attenuation rates, but different upper

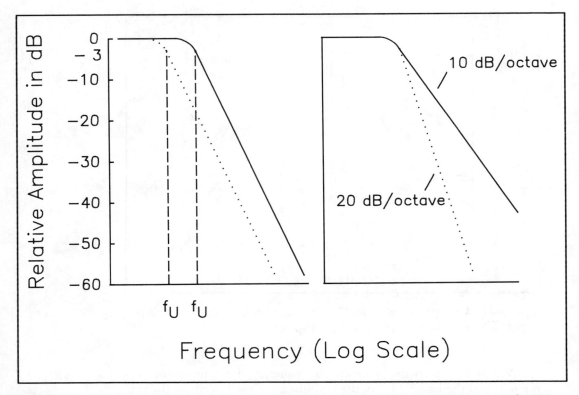

Figure 6–12. Four low-pass filter curves, filters that pass energy *below* some upper cutoff frequency, f_U. The two at the left have the same attenuation rates, but different upper cutoff frequencies, f_U. The two at the right have the same upper cutoff frequencies, but different attenuation rates.

cutoff frequencies. The two curves at the right have the same upper cutoff frequencies, but different attenuation rates. However, in each case, energy for frequencies above f_U is rejected.

High-Pass Filter

A **high-pass filter** is one that passes energy *above* some designated lower cutoff frequency. The two relevant parameters are f_L and **attenuation rate**. Figure 6–13 shows four high-pass filters that differ in terms of the values of those two parameters. In each case, energy for frequencies below f_L is rejected.

Band-Pass Filter

A **band-pass filter** is one that *passes energy in some specifiable band of frequencies* between a lower cutoff frequency and an upper cutoff fre-

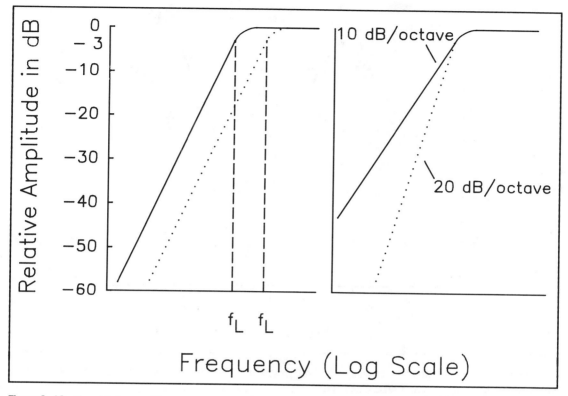

Figure 6–13. Four high-pass filter curves, filters that pass energy above some lower cutoff frequency, f_L. The two at the left have the same attenuation rates, but different lower cutoff frequencies, f_L. The two at the right have the same lower cutoff frequencies, but different attenuation rates.

quency. All five parameters are relevant: f_L, f_c, f_U, Δf, and **attenuation rate**. Figure 6–14 shows four band-pass filters that are characterized by differences in those five parameters.

A band-pass filter may be thought of as reflecting the combined effects of low-pass and high-pass filtering as is illustrated in Figure 6–15. The low-pass filter (solid line) passes energy below a designated **upper cutoff frequency**, which specifies f_U for the band-pass filter. The high-pass filter (dotted line) passes energy above a designated **lower cutoff frequency**, which specifies f_L for the band-pass filter. The bandwidth of the band-pass filter is given by the difference between the upper and lower cutoff frequencies, $f_U - f_L$. Finally, the slope of the low-pass filter curve determines the upper slope of the band-pass filter (the rate of attenuation above f_c), and the slope of the high-pass filter determines the lower slope of the band-pass filter (the rate of attenuation below f_c). Although those two slopes could be different from one another, they are almost always identical.

A word of caution is in order when we say that "a band-pass filter is the combined effect of low-pass and high-pass filtering." That is true

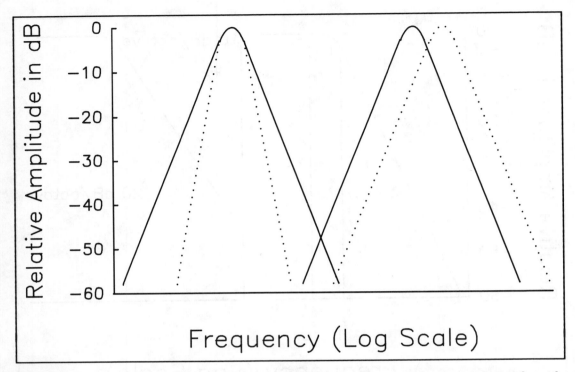

Figure 6–14. Four band-pass filter curves, filters that pass energy in a band of frequencies between f_L and f_U, that differ in f_c, f_L, f_U, Δf, and **attenuation rate**.

only if we use what is called a *series, or cascade,* system. By that we mean, a signal is directed to the input of a low-pass filter with an appropriate f_U. Then, the output of the low-pass filter is directed to the input of a high-pass filter with an appropriate f_L. Under that circumstance, the signal at the output of the second filter will have been band-passed. Of course, the procedure could be reversed (high-pass followed by low-pass) as long as the output of the first filter is sent to the input of the second filter for additional processing.

Band-Reject Filter

A **band-reject filter**, which also is called a **band-stop filter** or a **notch filter**, is one that *rejects, rather than passes, energy for frequencies between the upper and lower cutoff frequencies.* Such filters are usually quite narrow, and all five parameters are useful in helping distinguish among various band-reject filters.

Figure 6–16 contains two band-reject filter curves that differ in f_c and, therefore, by definition that differ in f_U and f_L. However, it should be apparent that the meaning of f_c for a band-reject filter is different

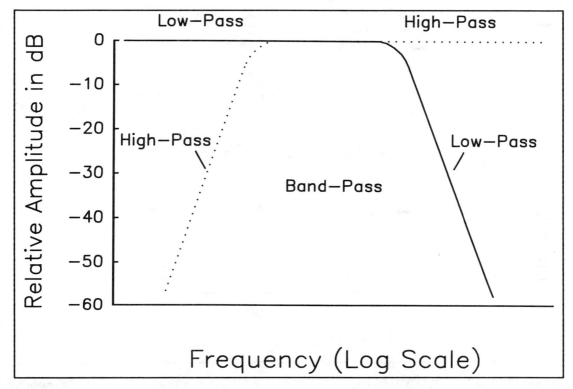

Figure 6–15. An illustration of how a band-pass filter represents the combined effects of a low-pass filter and a high-pass filter that are connected "in series."

from the meaning of f_c for a band-pass filter. Although the two filter curves in Figure 6–16 appear to have the same bandwidth, we shall see subsequently that such is not really the case; the curve at the right, in fact, has a wider bandwidth. Band-reject filters will probably be encountered less frequently than the other three types, but they are important for such applications as measuring distortion.

A **band-reject filter** also represents the combined effects of low-pass and high-pass filtering. However, in this case the two filters are operated in *parallel*, rather than in *series*. By that we mean, a signal is directed simultaneously (in parallel) to the inputs of each of the two filters, one low-pass and one high-pass. When the outputs of the two filters are summed, the result is a signal that has been band-rejected.

■ TWO TYPES OF BAND-PASS FILTERS

The band-pass filters that were shown in Figure 6–14 can be one of two types: a **constant bandwidth filter** or a **constant percentage bandwidth filter**.

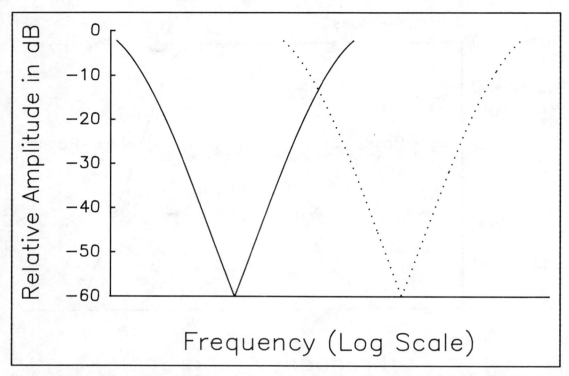

Figure 6–16. A comparison of two band-reject filter curves, filters that reject energy over a band of frequencies.

Constant Bandwidth Filter

A **constant bandwidth filter** is one in which the *bandwidth, Δf, is independent of the center frequency, f_c.* By that we mean that the bandwidth and the center frequency can be varied independently of one another. Consider the examples in Figure 6–17.

Two constant bandwidth filters are shown, and each will serve as the transfer function for a **white noise** signal, an aperiodic sound wave that has equal energy at all frequencies (the spectral envelope has a slope of 0 dB). **X** represents the amplitude spectrum of the unfiltered noise; **Y** represents the amplitude spectrum of the noise as modified by the filter with the lower f_c; and **Z** represents the amplitude spectrum of the noise as modified by the filter with the higher f_c. For filter **Y**, $f_c =$ 1000 Hz and Δf = 500 Hz.

If we were to measure the intensity of the white noise signal *at the input to the filter* (that is, the unfiltered white noise), we would observe some level that we will call **X_{dB}**. At the output of filter **Y** we would observe only a portion of the original spectrum because only a portion of the signal has been passed by the filter; energy at frequencies below f_L and above f_U has been rejected.

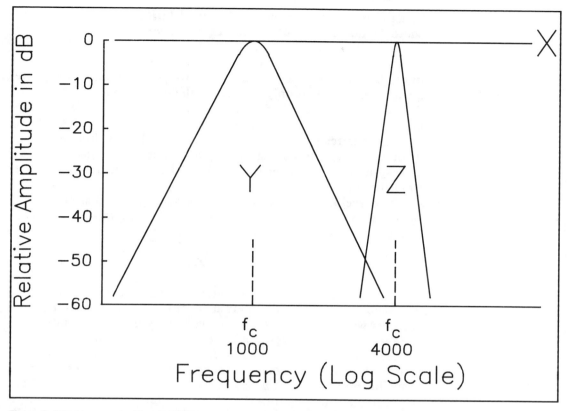

Figure 6–17. Two **constant bandwidth** filter curves in which the bandwidth is independent of the center frequency. The curves labeled **Y** and **Z** show how the amplitude spectrum of white noise, **X**, is modified differently by the two different filters. The curve at the right *appears* to have a more narrow bandwidth because frequency is plotted on a logarithmic scale, but the two bandwidths in reality are identical.

The level at the output of this filter, then, can be called some level Y_{dB}, and

$$Y_{dB} < X_{dB},$$

because some of the energy in **X** (the original unfiltered signal) has been filtered. If some of the energy that was present at the *input* of the filter is rejected and therefore is not present at the output of the filter, the output level Y_{dB} must be less than the input level X_{dB}. The signal at the input to the filter has a theoretical bandwidth of infinity because it is white noise, but the output signal has been *band limited* by a filter with a center frequency of 1000 Hz and a bandwidth of 500 Hz.

Consider, now, what would happen if f_c were raised from 1000 Hz to 4000 Hz, which is shown as filter **Z** in Figure 6–17. Even though f_c has been raised by a factor of 4, we can preserve a bandwidth of 500 Hz because the filter is *a **constant bandwidth filter** in which the bandwidth is independent of the center frequency.*

Filter **Z** *appears* to have a smaller bandwidth than filter **Y**, but that is because frequency is represented on a log scale. On a log scale, the linear distance occupied by 500 Hz (the bandwidth) around a center frequency of 4000 Hz is only one-fourth the linear distance occupied by 500 Hz (the bandwidth) around a center frequency of 1000 Hz. Thus, because f_c is raised by a factor of 4, filter **Z** has the appearance of being only one-quarter as wide as filter **Y**, but the two bandwidths are, in fact, identical. (Return now to Figure 6–8, as suggested previously, and see if f_c was the only parameter that distinguished one of the filter curves from the other.)

The level Z_{dB} at the output of filter **Z** will be less than the level at the input to the filter X_{dB} because, as before, the input signal has been filtered. Thus, $Z_{dB} < X_{dB}$. However, the critical factor is that:

$$Y_{dB} = Z_{dB}.$$

Why are the output levels from the two different filters identical? The bandwidths of the two filters are identical, and as long as the input signal is white noise, which has equal energy in all frequency bands 1 Hz wide, the output level of the filters will remain constant as f_c is changed to any value *as long as the bandwidth does not change.* Of course, you can have a constant bandwidth filter with the capability of providing many different Δf's, and the wider the Δf, the greater will be the energy at the output of the filter. The important characteristic of the **constant bandwidth filter** is that Δf *does not vary automatically* with changes in f_c. The two parameters f_c and Δf can be adjusted independently of each other.

Constant Percentage Bandwidth Filter

The distinguishing feature of a **constant percentage bandwidth filter** is that Δf is always some *constant percentage* of f_c. The concept of a constant percentage bandwidth filter is not unlike the concept of a sales tax. For example, if your state levies a 6% sales tax, that means that the dollar value of tax owed increases as your purchase price increases. If the purchase price is $10, you pay $0.60 of tax. If the purchase price increases by a factor of 4 to $40, your tax also increases by a factor of 4 to $2.40. The purchase price and the sales tax are not independent; the tax is a constant percentage of the purchase price. The same relation exists between Δf and f_c with a constant percentage bandwidth filter. As f_c increases by some factor, Δf increases by the same factor.

Look next at the two filters, **Y** and **Z**, in Figure 6–18. As in Figure 6–17, a white noise signal is directed to the input of the filters, the amplitude spectrum of the unfiltered noise is represented by **X**, and the level of the noise at the input is some value X_{dB}. For filter **Y**, $f_c = 1000$ Hz, and, for this example,

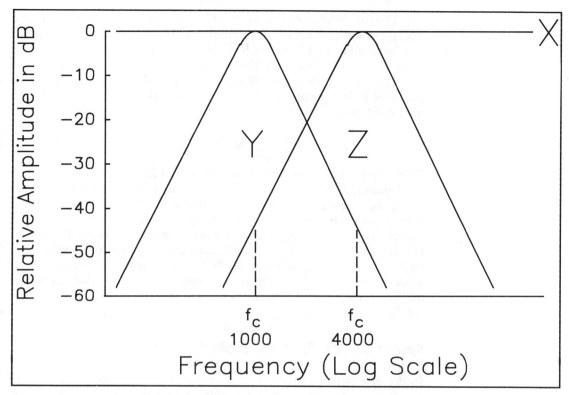

Figure 6–18. Two **constant percentage bandwidth** filter curves in which the bandwidth is a constant percentage of the center frequency. The curves labeled **Y** and **Z** show how the amplitude spectrum of white noise, **X**, is modified differently by the two filters. The two curves *appear* to have the same bandwidth because frequency is plotted on a logarithmic scale, but the bandwidth of the curve at the right is four times greater because its center frequency is four times higher.

$$\Delta f = 0.707 \ (f_c) = 707 \ Hz,$$

which means that the bandwidth has a value that is 70.7% (which would be a very high sales tax) of the value of the center frequency. The level at the output of filter **Y** will be some value Y_{dB}, and as before,

$$Y_{dB} < X_{dB},$$

because the signal has been filtered.

Now, suppose we insert filter **Z** with a center frequency of 4000 Hz to replace filter **Y** with a center frequency of 1000 Hz. Because the filter is a **constant percentage bandwidth filter** whose bandwidth will always be some constant percentage of the center frequency, and because the center frequency of filter **Z** is four times higher than the center frequency of filter **Y**, the bandwidth of filter **Z** will be four times as great as the bandwidth of **Y**:

$$\Delta f = 0.707 \ (f_c) = 2828 \ Hz.$$

The bandwidths of filter **Z** and filter **Y** *appear* to be identical in the figure, but again, that is because frequency is represented on a log scale. The bandwidth of filter **Z** is four times as great as the bandwidth of filter **Y**, but on a log scale they occupy the same linear distance.

The level at the output of filter **Z**, **Z_{dB}**, will of course be less than the level at the input, **X_{dB}**, because the signal has been filtered. The important point is that:

$$Z_{dB} > Y_{dB}.$$

That relation exists because the bandwidth of **Z** is four times as great as the bandwidth of **Y**. The white noise signal is characterized by equal energy per cycle at the input to the filter, and filter **Z** passes that equal energy per cycle over a frequency range of 2828 Hz, whereas filter **Y** passes that equal energy per cycle over a frequency range of only 707 Hz. Subsequently, we will describe how much greater the level of **Z_{dB}** will be than the level of **Y_{dB}** *in decibels*, but the impatient reader might wish to try to solve the problem in advance by recalling the discussion on "combining sound intensities from independent sources" in Chapter 4.

Common Constant Percentage Bandwidth Filters

In the preceding example, a percentage of 70.7 was used, but actually any value is acceptable, just as different local and state governmental bodies levy different amounts of sales tax. However, there are a few common percentages that will be encountered with constant percentage bandwidth filters. One of the most common is called a **1-octave (1/1) filter**.

For a **1-octave filter**,

Equation 6.2 $\Delta f = 0.707 \, f_c.$

Thus, the bandwidth (Δf) of a 1-octave filter is always 70.7% of the center frequency (f_c). Why is it called a **1-octave filter**? Recall that an octave is a doubling of frequency ($f_2 = 2f_1$). For a 1-octave filter, *and only for a 1-octave filter*,

Equation 6.3 $f_L = 0.707 \, f_c$

and

Equation 6.4 $f_U = 1.414 \, f_c.$

Therefore, from Equations 6.3 and 6.4, we can see that the upper cutoff frequency for a 1-octave filter is *1 octave* (2f) higher than the lower cutoff frequency.

Table 6–1 shows how the parameters of a constant percentage bandwidth filter change with changes in f_c. You should see from the

Table 6–1. Lower cutoff frequency (f_L), upper cutoff frequency (f_U), and bandwidth (Δf) for various values of the center frequency (f_c) for a one-octave filter.

f_c	f_L	f_U	$\Delta f = f_U - f_L$
100	70.7	141.4	70.7
200	141.4	282.8	141.4
1,000	707	1,414	707
2,000	1,414	2,828	1,414
10,000	7,070	14,140	7,070

table that as f_c increases by some factor, f_L, f_U, and Δf increase by the same factor. For example, if f_c increases by a factor of 2 from 100 Hz to 200 Hz, the values of the other three parameters also increase by a factor of 2.

Figure 6–19 shows the 1-octave filter from Table 6–1 with a center frequency of 1000 Hz. As you look at the filter curve, the center frequency appears to be at the "center" of the passband, and in fact it is located at what is called the "geometric center." However, that should not lead you to believe that the center frequency is the common arithmetic mean of the upper and lower cutoff frequencies. The arithmetic mean of 707 Hz and 1414 Hz is 1060.5 Hz, but we indicate in the table that the center frequency is 1000 Hz, not 1060.5 Hz. That apparent discrepancy exists because, for a constant percentage bandwidth filter, the center frequency is the *geometric mean*, not the common arithmetic mean, of the upper and lower cutoff frequencies. Thus,

$$f_c = \sqrt{f_L \times f_U},$$

Equation 6.5

which states that the geometric mean of two numbers is the square root of the product of the two numbers.

There are other common constant percentage bandwidth filters in addition to the 1-octave filter. They include, for example, a **1/2 octave filter**, a **1/3 octave filter**, and a **1/10 octave filter**. Because a constant percentage bandwidth filter can, in principle, be any fractional value in addition to unity (1/1), the general expression is: **1/n octave filter**. Each is a constant percentage bandwidth filter, and the defining characteristic that is common in all such filters is that *the bandwidth is always some constant percentage of the center frequency*. The exact constant percentage varies with the value of **n** that specifies the fraction of an octave that characterizes the filter.

Calculation of Parameters of Constant Percentage Bandwidth Filters

The equations for calculating the important parameters of a constant percentage bandwidth filter are:

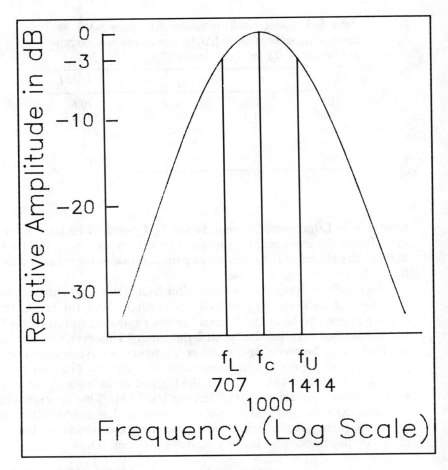

Figure 6–19. Parameters of a 1-octave (1/1) filter curve.

Equation 6.6 $f_L = \dfrac{f_c}{2^{1/2n}}$ $= \text{antilog}_{10}\,(\log_{10}\,f_c - .3/2n);$

Equation 6.7 $f_U = 2^{1/n}f_L$ $= \text{antilog}_{10}\,(\log_{10}\,f_c + .3/2n);$

and

Equation 6.8 $\Delta f = f_U - f_L.$

Table 6–2 shows how the lower and upper cutoff frequencies and the bandwidth vary as different fraction-octave filters are employed. Each row in the table represents a different constant percentage bandwidth filter, and, in this example, each of the four filters has the same center frequency, 1000 Hz. For the 1-octave, 1/2 octave, 1/3 octave, and 1/10 octave filters in Table 6–2, the upper cutoff frequency is always 1 octave, 1/2 octave, 1/3 octave, and 1/10 octave, respectively, higher than the lower cutoff frequency.

Table 6–2. Parameters of various constant percentage bandwidth filters. The center frequency is a constant 1000 Hz.

1/n	f_c	f_L	f_U	Δf	%
1/1	1000	707	1414	707	.707
1/2	1000	844	1190	346	.346
1/3	1000	891	1122	231	.231
1/10	1000	966	1035	69	.069

■ SPECIFICATION OF LEVEL AT THE OUTPUT OF FILTERS

We have learned that the sound pressure level of a signal is reduced at the output of a filter (low-pass, high-pass, band-pass, or band-reject) relative to the level of the signal at the input to the filter. The level at the output is reduced because the filter attenuates the energy *selectively as a function of frequency*. Energy at some frequencies is passed by the filter, whereas energy at other frequencies is rejected.

We will now describe methods for calculating the actual amount by which signal level is reduced by filtering. Although any sound wave can be filtered, it will be convenient to use **white noise** in most of our examples. White noise, as you recall, is characterized by *equal energy per cycle*. That means simply that energy is present at all frequencies of vibration (to reasonable upper and lower frequency limits), and that the level or intensity *within any frequency band that is 1 Hz wide* (from $f-0.5$ Hz to $f+0.5$ Hz) is exactly the same, regardless of the value of f.

The calculations will be much simpler for white noise than for other complex sound waves, but the principles that will be described are applicable for specification of the level of other types of sound waves that are filtered. Before we consider the equations that will be used to accomplish that task, it will be useful to become familiar with a new concept and a new form of decibel notation called the **pressure spectrum level**, L_{ps}.

Pressure Spectrum Level

Pressure spectrum level, L_{ps}, (commonly called just **spectrum level**) is defined as *the sound pressure level in a frequency band of unit width* (1 Hz), centered at some particular frequency, f. L_{ps} is expressed in decibels, and it refers to the level in any frequency band that is 1 Hz wide, regardless of the frequency upon which that band is centered. For a white noise signal, we could identify an infinity of frequency bands that satisfy that definition, and they need not be integers: for example, $f = 300$ Hz, ± 0.5 Hz; $f = 1300$ Hz, ± 0.5 Hz; $f = 5000$ Hz, ± 0.5 Hz; $f = 425.5$ Hz, ± 0.5 Hz; and so forth.

We stated previously that for a white noise signal, the level or intensity within any frequency band that is 1 Hz wide is exactly the same, regardless of the value of f. That is the same as saying that white noise has a pressure spectrum level *slope* of 0 dB; L_{ps} is constant for all values of f.

L_{ps} is given by:

Equation 6.9

$$L_{ps} = SPL_{wb} - 10 \log \frac{\Delta f_{wb}}{\Delta_o f}$$

where L_{ps} is expressed in **dB SPL**,

SPL_{wb} refers to the sound pressure level in some wide-band signal,

Δf_{wb} refers to the bandwidth of the wide-band signal,

and

$\Delta_o f$ is a reference bandwidth equal to unity (1 Hz).

Because the denominator in the ratio in Equation 6.9 is 1, and the log of $1 = 0$, Equation 6.9 for L_{ps} can be simplified to become:

Equation 6.10

$$L_{ps} = SPL_{wb} - 10 \log \Delta f_{wb}.$$

Suppose a white noise signal with a bandwidth of 10,000 Hz has an overall level of 80 dB SPL re: 20 µPa. What is the pressure spectrum level?

$$L_{ps} = 80 - 10 \log 10,000 = 40 \text{ dB SPL}.$$

The reference pressure for pressure spectrum level is the same as the reference pressure used to express the sound pressure level of a sinusoid or of any complex periodic or aperiodic sound wave: 20 µPa (**MKS**) or 2×10^{-4} dyne/cm^2 or microbar (**cgs**). Thus, for the example above, the overall level is 80 dB SPL re: 20 µPa and the pressure spectrum level is 40 dB SPL re: 20 µPa.

To conceptualize pressure spectrum level, simply imagine that the white noise signal is filtered with an **ideal rectangular filter** with a bandwidth of 1 Hz that is centered at any desired frequency (f). The level at the output of the rectangular filter is called the **pressure spectrum level**. For the example above, $L_{ps} = 40$ dB SPL, and, because the wide-band signal is white noise, we will measure precisely that same pressure spectrum level of 40 dB SPL for any frequency band that is 1 Hz wide regardless of the value of f.

Suppose we do not know the overall level of a signal, but we are given its bandwidth and pressure spectrum level. We can then calculate the overall level of the signal by rearranging Equation 6.10 to read:

Equation 6.11

$$SPL_{wb} = L_{ps} + 10 \log \Delta f_{wb}.$$

For example, suppose the pressure spectrum level of a white noise signal with a bandwidth of 8000 Hz = 45 dB SPL. What is the overall level of the noise?

$$SPL_{wb} = 45 + 10 \log 8000 = 84 \text{ dB SPL}.$$

We have emphasized that with a white noise signal, the level or intensity within any frequency band that is 1 Hz wide (from $f-0.5$ Hz to $f+0.5$ Hz) is exactly the same, regardless of the value of f. We can think of each of those frequency bands as being an *independent sound source* and, by definition for white noise, each of those frequency bands or independent sound sources has exactly the same level or intensity as any other frequency band.

Recall from Equation 4.9 in Chapter 4 that the total intensity level resulting from combining some number of independent sound sources, each of which has equal intensity, is given by:

$$dB_N = dB_i + 10 \log N,$$

where **i** refers to the SPL of one of the sources

and

N refers to the number of sources that are combined.

We can now rewrite Equation 4.9 and rename the terms in the equation, so that it can be applied to the problem of specifying the level of filtered white noise:

$$SPL_{wb} = L_{ps} + 10 \log \Delta f_{wb},$$

where Δf_{wb} is the bandwidth of the signal

and

L_{ps} is the **pressure spectrum level**.

The bandwidth of the signal (Δf_{wb}) is analogous to "the number of sources being combined" (**N**), and the pressure spectrum level (L_{ps}) is analogous to the "sound pressure level of one of the equal sources" (**i**). The result is Equation 6.11, which we have seen previously.

In summary, if we know the bandwidth and overall level of the white noise signal, we can calculate the pressure spectrum level with Equation 6.10 by *subtracting* 10 log Δf_{wb} from the overall level. If, on the other hand, we know the bandwidth and the pressure spectrum level, we can calculate the overall level with Equation 6.11 by *adding* 10 log Δf_{wb} to the pressure spectrum level, L_{ps}.

Sample Problems

Problem 1: A white noise signal has a bandwidth of 9000 Hz and an overall level of 72 dB SPL. What is the pressure spectrum level? Use Equation 6.10.

$$L_{ps} = 72 - 10 \log 9000 = 32.5 \text{ dB SPL}.$$

Problem 2: A white noise signal has a bandwidth of 10,000 Hz and an overall level of 34 dB SPL. What is the pressure spectrum level? Use Equation 6.10.

$$L_{ps} = 34 - 10 \log 10,000 = -6 \text{ dB SPL}.$$

What do we mean by saying that the pressure spectrum level in decibels is a *negative* 6 dB? The answer is the same as it was in Chapter 4. Negative decibels simply mean that the sound pressure of the signal of interest is *less* than the *reference sound pressure*, which for dB SPL is 20 µPa.

Problem 3: A white noise signal has a bandwidth of 7000 Hz and a pressure spectrum level of 51 dB SPL. What is the overall level? Use Equation 6.11.

$$SPL_{wb} = 51 + 10 \log 7000 = 89.5 \text{ dB SPL}.$$

Problem 4: A white noise signal has a bandwidth of 6000 Hz and a pressure spectrum level of -12 dB SPL. What is the overall level? Use Equation 6.11.

$$SPL_{wb} = -12 + 10 \log 6000 = 25.8 \text{ dB SPL}.$$

Specification of Level at the Output of Filters: The More General Case

In the previous section we learned that we can calculate the pressure spectrum level from our knowledge of the bandwidth and the overall level of a signal (Equation 6.10) or, conversely, we can calculate the overall level of a signal from our knowledge of its bandwidth and pressure spectrum level (Equation 6.11). Let us now consider the more general case of how to calculate the level of any narrow-band signal (**nb**), not just one that is 1 Hz wide, from our knowledge of the overall level of a wide-band signal (**wb**) and, conversely, how to calculate the level of a wide-band signal (**wb**) from our knowledge of the level of a narrow-band signal (**nb**).

In Figure 6–20 we represent a white noise signal with a bandwidth that, because of filtering, becomes progressively more narrow as you move from the top of the figure where the bandwidth is 10,000 Hz to the bottom of the figure where the bandwidth is 1 Hz. It does not matter what type of filter is used (low-pass, high-pass, or band-pass) because our equations only have two parameters: level and bandwidth.

With Equation 6.12 we can calculate the level for any narrow-band signal (**nb**) from our knowledge of (1) the level of a wide-band signal

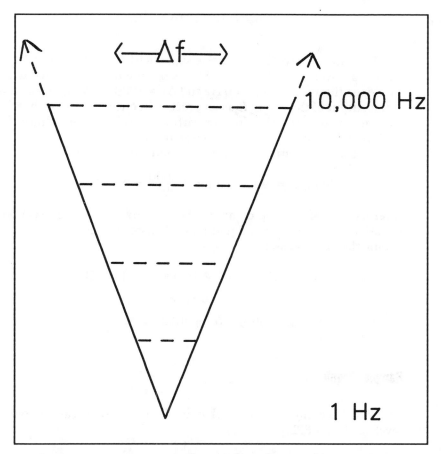

Figure 6–20. Geometric representation of the changing bandwidth of a white noise signal in which the bandwidth becomes progressively more narrow as a consequence of filtering. At the top, the unfiltered bandwidth is infinity. At the bottom, the bandwidth is unity (1 Hz).

(**wb**) and (2) the bandwidths of both the wide-band and the narrow-band signal:

$$\text{SPL}_{nb} = \text{SPL}_{wb} - 10 \log \frac{\Delta f_{wb}}{\Delta f_{nb}}.$$

Equation 6.12

You should see that Equation 6.12 is essentially the same as Equation 6.10 for pressure spectrum level. The only differences are that now the narrow-band signal is not restricted to a bandwidth of 1 Hz and, because of that, the denominator in the ratio can be any value, not just "1."

By rearranging Equation 6.12, we obtain Equation 6.13 which will enable us to reverse the process and calculate the level for any wide-band signal from our knowledge of (1) the level of the narrow-band signal and (2) the bandwidths of both the wide-band and the narrow-band signals:

Equation 6.13

$$SPL_{wb} = SPL_{nb} + 10 \log \frac{\Delta f_{wb}}{\Delta f_{nb}}.$$

Suppose we have a white noise signal with a bandwidth of 10,000 Hz and an overall level of 90 dB SPL. Next, the noise is filtered with a band-pass filter with f_c = 2000 Hz and Δf = 1000 Hz. What is the level at the output of the filter? You can proceed in one of two ways, but first you should recognize that for this particular problem, the value of f_c is irrelevant because f_c does not appear in Equation 6.12.

By use of Equation 6.12, we compute that:

$$SPL_{1000} = 90 - 10 \log \frac{10,000}{1000} = 80 \text{ dB SPL.}$$

Alternatively, if we first compute the **pressure spectrum level** with Equation 6.10, we can use Equation 6.11 instead of Equation 6.12 and obtain the same answer:

$$L_{ps} = 90 - 10 \log 10,000 = 50 \text{ dB SPL}$$

and then

$$SPL_{wb} = 50 + 10 \log 1000 = 80 \text{ dB SPL.}$$

Sample Problems

The signal is white noise with a bandwidth of 12,000 Hz and an overall level of 95 dB SPL.

Problem 1: What is the level at the output of a band-pass filter with Δf = 1200 Hz? With Equation 6.12, we determine that:

$$SPL_{1200} = 95 - 10 \log \frac{12,000}{1200} = 85 \text{ dB SPL.}$$

Although it is perfectly appropriate to use Equation 6.12, when there are a series of problems to solve, it might be more convenient to first calculate the **pressure spectrum level** with Equation 6.10 and then use Equation 6.11 for the rest of the problems. That approach enables us to avoid the necessity of repeated division. For example,

$$L_{ps} 95 - 10 \log 12,000 = 54.2 \text{ dB SPL}$$

and then

$$SPL_{1200} = 54.2 + 10 \log 1200 = 85 \text{ dB SPL.}$$

Either approach should produce the same answer, but using pressure spectrum level saves the step of computing the ratio that is required when using Equation 6.12. It also is advantageous to have alternative approaches to solving a problem because it provides you with an independent check on the correctness of your solution.

Problem 2: What is the level at the output of a 1-octave filter with f_c = 2000 Hz? Note that Δf was not given and, therefore, must be calculated by use of Equation 6.2.

$$\Delta f = 0.707 \times 2000 = 1414 \text{ Hz}$$

and then

$$SPL_{1414} = 54.2 + 10 \log 1414 = 85.7 \text{ dB SPL}$$

or

$$SPL_{1414} = 95 - 10 \log \frac{12,000}{1414} = 85.7 \text{ dB SPL.}$$

Because 85.7 dB SPL is the level at the output of a 1-octave filter, it is referred to as the **octave-band level**. This problem provides a good illustration of why it might be easier to solve some of these problems by first computing the **pressure spectrum level** because, in this instance, it saves us from dividing 12,000 by 1414.

Problem 3: What is the level at the output of a low-pass filter with f_U = 1200 Hz? Note that Δf was not given. However, you should know that for a low-pass filter, $\Delta f = f_U$. Therefore,

$$SPL_{1200} = 54.2 + 10 \log 1200 = 85 \text{ dB SPL}$$

or

$$SPL_{1200} = 95 - 10 \log \frac{12,000}{1200} = 85 \text{ dB SPL.}$$

Problem 4: What is the level at the output of a high-pass filter with f_L = 1200 Hz? As with problem 3, Δf was not given. However, unlike problem 3 with a low-pass filter, the value of f_L for a high-pass filter does not equal the bandwidth. The white noise signal that we are dealing with has an upper limit of 12,000 Hz. If that signal is high-pass filtered with a lower cutoff frequency of 1200 Hz, that means that energy below 1200 is attenuated, and all that remains is the energy between the cutoff frequency of 1200 Hz and the upper limit of the unfiltered noise, 12,000 Hz. Thus, to find the bandwidth of the filtered noise, we subtract f_L from the bandwidth of the unfiltered noise [$\Delta f = \Delta f_{unfiltered} - f_L = 10,800$ Hz]. Therefore,

$$SPL_{10,800} = 54.2 + 10 \log 10,800 = 94.5 \text{ dB SPL,}$$

or

$$SPL_{10,800} = 95 - 10 \log \frac{12,000}{10,800} = 94.5 \text{ dB SPL.}$$

Problem 5: Suppose we were to remove exactly half of the energy in the white noise by some filter. It does not matter what type of filter is used as long as the result is a bandwidth of 6000 Hz. For example, we might use a low-pass filter with f_U = 6000 Hz, a high-pass filter with f_L = 6000 Hz, or a band-pass filter with Δf = 6000 centered on some frequency of our choosing. For each of those examples, the resulting bandwidth is the same, 6000 Hz. By how much will signal level be decreased at the output of the filter relative to signal level at the input? The answer must be the same as it was in Chapter 4. If the bandwidth is narrowed to one-half of its original value, the energy or power or intensity of the signal is halved, and if the intensity is reduced to one-half of its original value, the **level of intensity** will decrease by 3 dB, because:

$$dB = 10 \log \frac{1}{2} = -3 \text{ dB}.$$

Thus, signal level will be decreased by 3 dB from 95 dB SPL to 92 dB SPL. We can confirm that answer by using the procedures described for the first four problems.

$$SPL_{6000} = 54.2 + 10 \log 6000 = 92 \text{ dB SPL},$$

or

$$SPL_{6000} = 95 - 10 \log \frac{12,000}{6000} = 92 \text{ dB SPL}.$$

Does the Type of Filter Affect the Pressure Spectrum Level?

As long as our concern is restricted to **white noise**, type of filter (low-pass, high-pass, band-pass, or band-reject) or bandwidth of the filter, does not affect the **pressure spectrum level**. To illustrate this, suppose we have a white-noise signal with a level of 92 dB SPL and a bandwidth of 20,000 Hz. The **pressure spectrum level** (Equation 6.10) is 49 dB SPL:

$$L_{ps} = 92 - 10 \log 20,000 = 49 \text{ dB SPL}.$$

Next, suppose the noise is directed to the input of a **1-octave filter** (a **constant percentage bandwidth filter**) with f_c = 1000 Hz. What will be the **pressure spectrum level** at the output of the 1-octave filter?

$$\Delta f = 0.707 \times 1000 = 707 \text{ Hz}$$

and then

$$SPL_{707} = 92 - 10 \log \frac{20,000}{707} = 77.5 \text{ dB SPL}.$$

Finally, calculate L_{ps} from your knowledge of the level of the signal at the output of the 1-octave filter. The answer must be the same as computed above from knowledge of the bandwidth and level of the un-filtered signal, 49 dB SPL:

$$L_{ps} = 77.5 - 10 \log 707 = 49 \text{ dB SPL.}$$

The answer of 49 dB SPL is identical to what we calculated before the 1-octave filter was inserted, and that is as it must be. **Pressure spectrum level** is *the sound pressure level in any band 1 Hz wide*. It does not matter which of the infinite number of frequency bands of the noise we had in mind when we calculated the spectrum level. After all, they each had exactly the same amount of energy — and hence the same sound pressure level — which for a unit bandwidth is called the **pressure spectrum level**.

In summary, **pressure spectrum level** *is* **pressure spectrum level**, and neither the type of filter nor the location of the filter along the frequency axis will alter that basic fact.

■ ANOTHER LOOK AT SELECTED TYPES OF NOISE

We will return to a consideration of a **white noise** signal and expand on what was learned in Chapter 5.

White Noise

We know that **white noise** has energy present at all frequencies (to reasonable upper and lower frequency limits) and that the level or intensity within any frequency band that is 1 Hz wide from $f-0.5$ Hz to $f+0.5$ Hz is exactly the same, regardless of the value of f. Figure 6–21 shows the amplitude spectrum of such a noise.

In panel A of the figure, the ordinate is **pressure spectrum level** in dB SPL and the abscissa is frequency (log scale). For this example, $L_{ps} =$ 45 dB SPL. As stated previously, because L_{ps} is a constant, the **envelope** of the amplitude spectrum is a straight line that is parallel to the horizontal axis. However, we must emphasize that such a slope only occurs if the unit of measure on the ordinate is pressure spectrum level. Thus, we can say that **white noise** has a **pressure spectrum level slope** of 0 dB, which is another way of saying that the pressure spectrum level for white noise does not change as a function of frequency.

Next, let us direct that same white noise to the input of a **1-octave filter** and calculate the levels at the output of the filter for each of several center frequencies, f_c (e.g., 100, 200, 400, 800, 1000, 2000, 4000, and so on). The results are shown in panel B of Figure 6–21. The ordinate now is **octave-band level** in dB SPL. We use **octave band level** in this case because we are plotting *the level in a frequency band that is exactly one octave wide* ($f_U = 2f_L$).

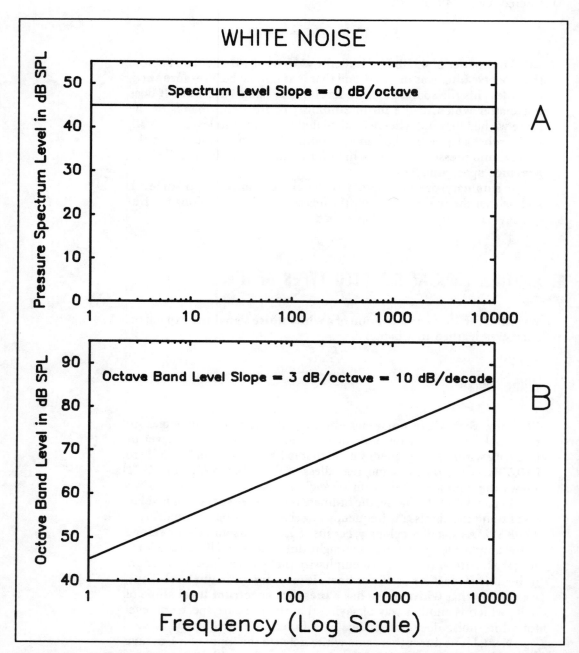

Figure 6–21. Amplitude spectra of white noise. In panel A, the ordinate is **pressure spectrum level, L_{ps}**, and the envelope has a spectrum level slope of 0 dB/octave. In panel B, for the same signal, the ordinate is **octave band level**, and the envelope has an octave band level slope of +3 dB/octave or + 10 dB/decade.

When f_c = 100 Hz, the octave-band level is 63.5 dB SPL because:

$$\Delta f = 70.7 \text{ Hz.}$$

Then,

$$\mathbf{L_{ps}} = 45 \text{ db SPL} \qquad \text{(With Equation 6.10)}$$

and

octave band level = 45 + 10 log 70.7 = 63.5 dB SPL.
(With Equation 6.11)

With each subsequent increase of f_c by a factor of 2:1, the bandwidth also increases by 2:1, twice as much energy is passed by the filter, and the level at the output increases successively by 3 dB. Thus, the level is 66.5 for f_c = 200 Hz, 69.5 for f_c = 400 Hz, and so on. Correspondingly, with each increase of f_c by a factor of 10:1, the bandwidth increases by 10:1, ten times as much energy is passed by the filter, and the level at the output increases by 10 dB. Thus, if the level for f_c = 100 Hz is 63.5 dB SPL, the level for f_c = 1000 Hz is 73.5 dB SPL.

We observed in panel A of Figure 6–21 that white noise has a **pressure spectrum level slope** of 0 dB. It is equally appropriate to say that white noise has an **octave-band level slope** of +3 dB/octave or +10 dB/ decade (decade = 10:1) because the octave band level increases by 3 dB with each doubling of f_c (and hence of bandwidth) and increases by 10 dB with each tenfold increase of f_c (and hence of bandwidth).

Now, look carefully at panel B of Figure 6–21. We have stated that the **pressure spectrum level** (the sound pressure level in a frequency band 1 Hz wide) is 45 dB SPL for the white noise in the figure. Also observe the values for octave band level as a function of frequency: 1000 Hz = 73.5 dB; 100 Hz = 63.5 dB; 10 Hz = 53.5 dB; and *1 Hz = 43.5 dB*. If **pressure spectrum level** *really is* **pressure spectrum level**, how can it be that $\mathbf{L_{ps}}$ = 45 dB, but according to the octave-band level calculations, the level is 43.5 dB when f_c = 1 Hz? There is no discrepancy. The pressure spectrum level is 45 dB SPL just as we calculated, and the octave-band level is 43.5 dB SPL when the filter has a center frequency of 1 Hz. But, if f_c = 1 Hz, Δf = 0.707 Hz, and thus the octave band level is less than the spectrum level, and specifically the octave band level is:

$$SPL_{0.707} = 45 + 10 \log .707 = 43.5 \text{ dB SPL.}$$

Pink Noise

Consider next the noise that is shown in Figure 6–22, which is called **pink noise**. In panel A the ordinate again is pressure spectrum level and the abscissa is frequency (log scale). It should be obvious from examination of the spectral envelope that this noise has very different characteristics from those for white noise shown in Figure 6–21. In this case, the noise has a **pressure spectrum level slope** of −3 dB/octave

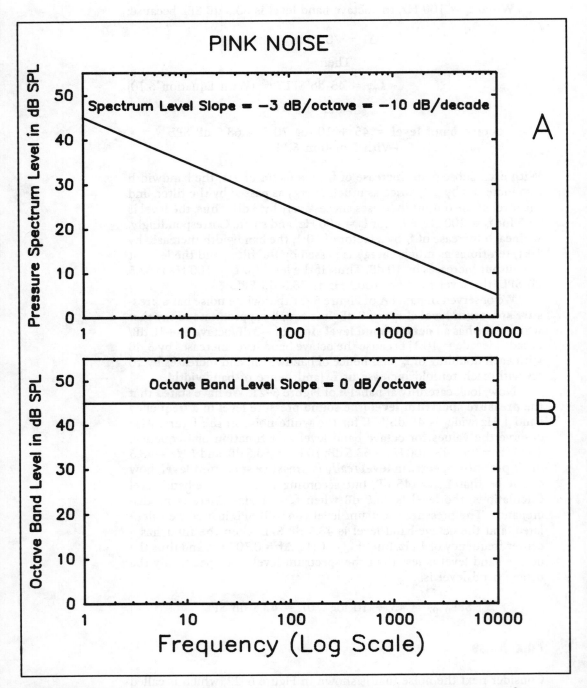

Figure 6–22. Amplitude spectra of pink noise. In panel A, the ordinate is pressure spectrum level, L_{ps}, and the envelope has a spectrum level slope of −3 dB/octave or −10 dB/decade. In panel B, for the same signal, the ordinate is octave band level, and the envelope has an octave band level slope of 0 dB/octave.

and, from the lower panel, an **octave-band level slope** of 0 dB. In other words, for this noise the output level from the 1-octave filter is the same regardless of where in the spectrum the filter is centered.

If f_c = 1000 Hz (Δf = 707 Hz) and the level at the output is, for example, 45 dB SPL, then, when f_c is doubled, the bandwidth is doubled to become 1414 Hz, but the output level, by definition, remains the same. If the bandwidth is doubled, energy is passed at twice as many frequencies. However, if energy is passed at twice as many frequencies, but the octave-band level remains the same, we must conclude that the energy level per unit bandwidth decreases as frequency increases. That is what accounts for a negative **pressure spectrum level slope** of −3 dB/octave or −10 dB/decade.

We can legitimately construct a large array of "acoustic colors" such as red, magenta, and so forth by simply manipulating the pressure spectrum level slopes of the acoustic noises in accordance with standards that have been adopted.

■ PRACTICE PROBLEMS

Set 1

For each of the problems in this set, assume that you are dealing with a white noise that has the following characteristics:

bandwidth (Δf) = 10,000 Hz

overall SPL = 90 dB re: 20 µPa

1. L_{ps} =

2. Calculate the SPL at the output of each of the following filters.

    a. Band-pass filter: Δf = 200 Hz; f_c = 400 Hz

    b. Band-pass filter: Δf = 400 Hz; f_c = 400 Hz

    c. Band-pass filter: Δf = 1000 Hz

    d. Low-pass filter: f_U = 1000 Hz

    e. High-pass filter: f_L = 9000 Hz

    f. One-octave filter: f_c = 1000 Hz

    g. One-octave filter: f_c = 500 Hz

Set 2

1. When you analyze a white noise with a constant percentage bandwidth filter at several different values of f_c, the SPL at the output of the filter increases at a rate of _____ dB/octave or _____ dB/decade.

2. If L_{ps} = 40 dB SPL

   a. What is the value of the *sound pressure* in a band that is 1 Hz wide?

   b. What is the value of the *sound pressure* in a band that is 10,000 Hz wide?

Set 3

For each of the problems in this set, assume that you are dealing with a white noise that has the following characteristics:

bandwidth (Δf) = 5000 Hz
overall SPL   = 80 dB re: 20 µPa

1. L_{ps} =

2. Calculate the SPL at the output of each of the following filters.

   a. Band-pass filter: Δf = 200 Hz; f_c = 400 Hz

   b. Band-pass filter: Δf = 400 Hz; f_c = 400 Hz

   c. Band-pass filter: Δf = 1000 Hz

   d. Low-pass filter: f_U = 1000 Hz

   e. High-pass filter: f_L = 4000 Hz

   f. One-octave filter: f_c = 500 Hz

■ ANSWERS TO PRACTICE PROBLEMS

Set 1

1. 50 dB   (L_{ps} = SPL_{wb} − 10 log Δf = 90 − 10 log 10,000.)

2. a. 73 dB (SPL$_{wb}$ −10 log 10,000/200 or L$_{ps}$ + 10 log 200: *Note:* f$_c$ is irrelevant; bandwidth was specified.)

b. 76 dB (f$_c$ is still irrelevant.)

c. 80 dB

d. 80 dB (The key to solution of this problem is bandwidth.)

e. 80 dB (The bandwidth is the same as in 2-d.)

f. 78.5 dB (With a 1-octave filter you must calculate bandwidth: $\Delta f = f_c \times .707$.)

g. 75.5 dB (Either use the same procedure that you employed in 2-f or realize that this bandwidth is 1/2 as wide as that in 2-f, which means that the output in 2-g will be 3 dB less than that in 2-f.)

Set 2

1. 3 dB/octave
and
10 dB/decade

2. a. 2×10^3 (40 dB = 20 log P$_x$/(2 × 10²); P$_x$ = 2 × 10³.)

b. 2×10^5 (If L$_{ps}$ = 40 dB, then SPL$_{10,000}$ = 80. Now, solve for P$_x$.)

Set 3

1. 43 dB (L$_{ps}$ = SPL$_{wb}$ − 10 log Δf.)

2. a. 66

b. 69

c. 73

d. 73

e. 73

f. 68.5

■ NOTES

1. The ordinate in Figure 6–1 is labeled "volume velocity," which refers to the particle velocity of air molecules flowing through an area of one cubic meter per second (m³/sec) in the **MKS** system.

2. In an electrical system, inductive reactance and capacitive reactance are the relevant determinants of the natural frequency. Inductive reactance is the electrical equivalent of mass reactance, and capacitive reactance is the electrical equivalent of compliant reactance. In a volume system, such as the vocal tract — the cavity that extends from the vibrating vocal folds at the lower end to the mouth opening at the upper end — the natural frequency will depend upon the length of the tube and whether the tube is open at both ends, or open at only one end and closed at the other.

Distortion

Suppose a sound wave is delivered to some system, an amplifier for example, and we then compare the waveform at the output of the amplifier with the waveform at the input. If the system reproduces the shape of the waveform faithfully, the signal is said to be *undistorted*. **Distortion**, on the other hand, means that the shape of the waveform has been altered in some way. Three types of distortion will be described: **frequency distortion; transient distortion,** and **amplitude distortion**.

■ FREQUENCY DISTORTION

Amplitude Response of a System

Panel A of Figure 7–1 illustrates a method for evaluating a system (e.g., a tape recorder, amplifier, loudspeaker, etc.) to determine what is called its **amplitude response**, which sometimes is called the **frequency response** of the system. Sinusoidal signals from a signal generator are directed to the input of the system. Frequency of the sine waves is varied over the frequency range of interest, and *the amplitude of the sine waves at the input must be kept constant.*

With the aid of an appropriate measuring device, we then measure the amplitudes of each of the sine waves at the output of the system. When the output amplitudes are plotted as a function of frequency, we have defined the **amplitude response** of the system. If the system reproduces all frequencies with the same amplitude, the output amplitude spectrum would appear as is shown in panel B of Figure 7–1.

A more realistic output amplitude spectrum is shown in panel C of Figure 7–1. Energy in the low frequency and high frequency regions has been attenuated because the system *could not reproduce all frequencies with the same relative amplitude.* In Chapter 6 we said that the input signal had been filtered, and now we say that *if filtering has occurred,* the signal has undergone **frequency distortion**. A more severe example of **frequency distortion** is shown in panel D of Figure 7–1.

System Transfer Function

The three curves in Figure 7–1 also describe what is called the **system transfer function.** Thus, the system transfer function, or **amplitude response**, reveals the extent to which a signal can be expected to undergo frequency distortion. For example, if you examine the specifications for a moderately priced audio tape recorder, you might see that the recorder has an amplitude response (the specifications probably will refer instead to "frequency response") such as that shown by the curve in panel C of Figure 7–1. The system has a relatively flat passband that extends from approximately 100 Hz to 10,000 Hz. Energy for frequen-

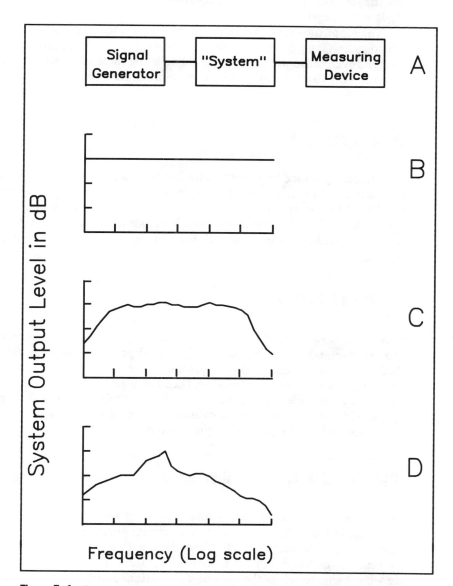

Figure 7–1. Panel A represents the electrical components that might be used for evaluation of a "system." Sinusoidal signals of constant amplitude and varying frequency are directed to some device, the "system," and the amplitudes of the various sine waves are then measured at the output of the device. Panels B, C, and D show three examples of amplitude response (frequency response) that might be measured for different systems. The response in panel B shows the absence of frequency distortion (a hypothetical construct), whereas the responses in C and D show different magnitudes of **frequency distortion** because the systems could not reproduce all frequencies with equal amplitudes.

cies that lie outside the passband, below 100 Hz and above 10,000 Hz, is attenuated.

The amplitude response of a system is described more completely by also specifying just how flat the response is *within the passband.* For example, even if the width of the passband is the same for two different systems, one that is flat ±0.5 dB is more linear than one that is flat ±5 dB.

Linear Systems

Systems that produce frequency distortion are **linear systems**. A linear system is one in which only the amplitudes (and phases) of the signal are altered by the system. In summary, the **amplitude response** of a linear system describes the way in which signals that are directed to the input will evidence **frequency distortion** in the signal observed at the output.

■ TRANSIENT DISTORTION

When sine waves were introduced from a strictly theoretical perspective in Chapter 2, it was convenient to treat their durations as infinite. Under that circumstance the amplitude spectrum of any sine wave would be a line spectrum. However, because duration of sine waves is finite, the amplitude spectrum is not a line spectrum; it *cannot* be represented by a single line whose location along the abscissa identifies the frequency and whose height on the ordinate specifies the amplitude.

Effects of Sine Wave Duration on the Amplitude Spectrum

Figure 7–2 shows the effects of sine wave duration on the amplitude spectrum. In panel A, the sine wave has infinite duration, and its amplitude spectrum, therefore, is a line spectrum with a single line that corresponds to the frequency of the sine wave, 1000 Hz. In panel B, we can see what happens when the duration is shortened to 100 msec and becomes what is called a **tone burst**. Energy is spread to other frequencies, both above and below the frequency of the sine wave. The amplitude spectrum is a **continuous spectrum**. We also can see lobes and nulls in the spectrum with a pattern that is similar, but not identical, to the pattern seen in Chapter 5 for a single rectangular pulse. The nulls occur at *integral multiples of the reciprocal of the duration,* in this case at 10-Hz intervals (1/.1 = ±10 Hz; 2/.1 = ±20 Hz; etc.) Unlike the amplitude spectrum for the single rectangular pulse, nulls occur on either side of the frequency of the sine wave (1000 Hz).

In panel C of Figure 7–2 we see what happens as duration of the sine wave decreases further, from 100 to 4 msec. In both B and C, the

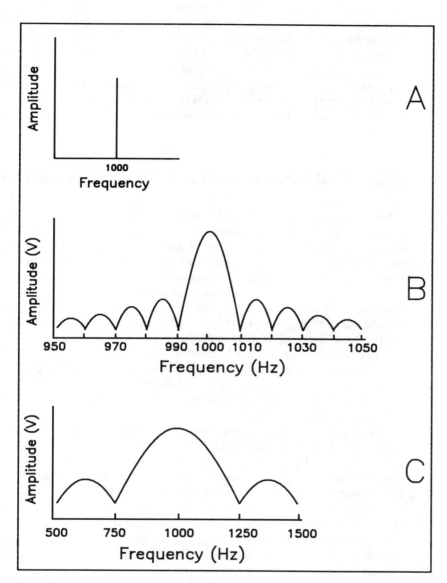

Figure 7–2. Effects of signal duration on the amplitude spectrum of a sinusoid. In panel A, duration is infinite and the amplitude spectrum is a line spectrum with energy at a single frequency. In panel B, duration is 100 msec, and energy is spread to other frequencies to produce a continuous spectrum. In panel C, duration is shortened to 4 msec, which also produces a continuous spectrum. The nulls in panels B and C occur at different frequencies because their locations in the frequency domain are given by integral multiples of the reciprocal of duration. Adapted from *Signals and systems for speech and hearing* (pp. 188–189) by S. Rosen and P. Howell, 1991: Academic Press, Inc., San Diego, CA. Copyright 1991 by Academic Press Limited. Printed with permission.

nulls appear at the appropriate frequency locations. Thus, for example, when duration = 100 msec, the first nulls are at ±10 Hz (1/.1 = 10 Hz), but the first nulls increase in frequency to ±250 Hz when duration is shortened to 4 msec (1/.004 = 250 Hz). It should be apparent that the width of each band of energy or lobe (between adjacent nulls) is inversely proportional to duration. Shortening the duration from 100 msec to 4 msec represents a factor of 1:25, and the consequence is to widen each band of energy by a factor of 25:1 (from 10 Hz at 100 msec to 250 Hz at 4 msec).

Effects of Rise and Decay Time on the Amplitude Spectrum

When a sine wave (or other signal) of fairly long duration, say a second or two, is turned on, its maximum amplitude is not allowed to be attained instantly. Instead, the amplitude is made to rise over time from zero to some maximum or steady-state value, as is shown in panel A of Figure 7–3, and then remains steady-state for a duration of our choosing. Similarly, when the tone burst is turned off, the amplitude does not instantly drop to zero; it decays over time from maximum to zero. The dashed curve in panel A of the figure defines the **amplitude envelope** (in the time domain) of the waveform.

Because the signal must be turned on and off, an amplitude spectrum is created that is more complex than that of a theoretical sine wave, as is shown in panel B of Figure 7–3. Energy is spread to other frequencies, and the amplitude spectrum is a **continuous spectrum** rather than a line spectrum.

Initiating and terminating a signal produces what are called *transients,* which are sometimes called "on-transients" when the signal is turned on and the amplitude is rising, and "off-transients" when the signal is turned off and the amplitude is decaying. The process of creating *transients* can be called **transient distortion**.

The amount of transient distortion varies as a function of the time required for the amplitude to rise from zero to maximum or to decay from maximum to zero. The longer the duration over which the signal is rising or decaying, the rise–decay time, the narrower will be the frequency band over which energy is spread in both directions from the frequency of the driving signal. Thus, slowly rising and slowly decaying signals are characterized by less transient distortion than signals for which the amplitude rises and decays very quickly.

If the rise or decay is very short, an audible "clicking" sound will be heard. Audiologists test people's hearing by use of an instrument called an *audiometer,* which is a device that generates sine waves at various frequencies with variable sound pressure levels. By manipulating those two variables, the audiologist can determine the lowest sound pressure levels at which an individual can just detect sine waves of various frequencies. But, the sine waves must be turned on and off, and we want to be certain that we are determining how well the person hears the sine waves, not the audible clicks that are produced by switching the signal

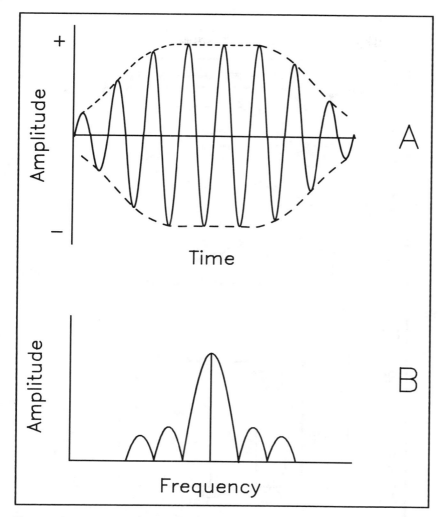

Figure 7–3. Transient distortion. Effects of rise–decay time of the waveform (panel A) on the amplitude spectrum (panel B) of a sine wave. The result is a continuous spectrum and reflects what is called **transient distortion**.

on and off too rapidly. To ensure that transient distortion is minimized, the *American National Standards Institute* has adopted standards for manufacturers to meet by specifying minimum "rise times" and "decay times" for audiometers.

■ AMPLITUDE DISTORTION

All systems can be described by what is called an *input–output function* such as the one shown by the rising curve in panel A of Figure 7-4. Output amplitude on the ordinate is plotted as a function of input ampli-

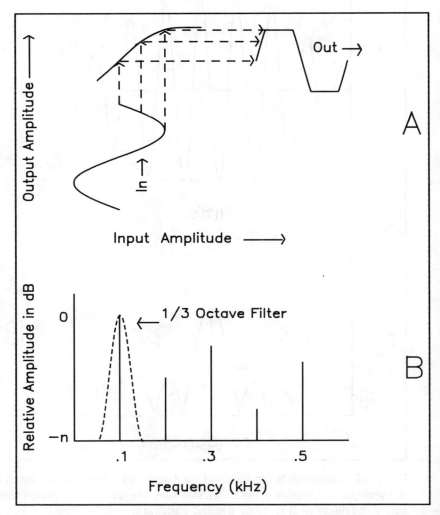

Figure 7–4. Amplitude distortion. Panel A shows an input–output function that reflects output amplitude on the ordinate as a function of input amplitude on the abscissa. Output amplitude is *proportional* to input amplitude over the linear portion of the function. At the right of panel A we see a sine wave that has been "peak clipped" because the input amplitude exceeded the range of linearity of the function. Panel B shows the amplitude spectrum of a sinusoid that results from operating on the non-linear portion of the function. The result is called **amplitude distortion** because the amplitude of the input waveform has been modified, **nonlinear distortion** because the modification is attributable to operating on the nonlinear portion of the input–output function, or **harmonic distortion** because the output signal contains energy at harmonics of the fundamental driving frequency at the input.

tude on the abscissa. If we confine our attention initially to that portion of the function that is *linear* (a straight line), we see that as the amplitude of the signal at the input to the system is increased (from left to right in the figure), we achieve a *proportional* increase in output amplitude. If, for example, the input amplitude is increased by 3 dB, the output amplitude also is increased by 3 dB.

We should not infer that the level of the output signal equals the level of the input signal. Indeed, it need not. Output level could equal input level, but it also could be greater than the input level (amplification) or less than the input level (attenuation). That is why we emphasize that changes in input level produce *proportional* changes in output level. The proportional changes occur only over that portion of the curve where the input–output function is *linear*.

Nonlinear Systems

Notice, though, that as we continue to increase the input amplitude from left to right, we reach a point where the input–output function becomes *nonlinear*, and in that region changes in input amplitude do not produce the proportional changes in output amplitude that occurred over the linear portion of the function. Thus, when we are operating on the nonlinear portion of the function, a 3–dB increase in input amplitude will result in *less* than a 3–dB increase in output amplitude. At the extreme, further increases at the input produce no increase (or even a decrease) in output amplitude. When input level has been increased so much that we are operating on the nonlinear portion of the input–output function, we are said to be "overdriving" or "overloading" the system.

The effect of "overdriving the system" on the waveform also is shown in panel A of Figure 7–4. A large-amplitude sine wave is directed to the input of the system. Many of the *instantaneous amplitudes* of the sine wave lie within the linear portion of the curve, the boundaries shown by dashed vertical lines. However, we can see that those instantaneous amplitudes *at and near the maximum amplitude* extend beyond the dashed lines and they, therefore, lie on the nonlinear portion of the curve. For those amplitudes, the output will not be proportional to the input. Instead, those instantaneous amplitudes will be reduced at the output, and the shape of the output waveform (pointing toward the right) will be altered relative to its sinusoidal shape at the input.

In the example in the figure, the shape has been altered by virtue of the fact that the "peaks" of the sine wave have been "clipped off," and this process therefore is called *peak clipping*. However, peak clipping is not the only form of amplitude distortion that can occur. For example, when the center of the waveform is removed and only the positive and negative peaks are preserved, amplitude distortion occurs due to what is called "center clipping." Moreover, peak clipping itself can be symmetrical (positive and negative peaks distorted similarly) or asymmetrical. As you might expect, the resultant amplitude spectrum varies with the type and severity of amplitude distortion that is produced.

The waveform of the signal has been altered, and therefore we know that the signal has been distorted. Because the *amplitude* of the waveform is the parameter that has been altered, this form of distortion is called **amplitude distortion**. The distortion to the waveform occurred because we overdrove the system. That is to say, we were operating on the *nonlinear portion* of the input–output function, and this form of distortion, therefore, also can be called **nonlinear distortion**. **Amplitude distortion** and **nonlinear distortion** are synonymous.

Effects of Amplitude, or Nonlinear, Distortion on the Amplitude Spectrum

If the waveform is altered by amplitude, or nonlinear, distortion, what happens to the amplitude *spectrum?* The input signal in panel A of Figure 7–4 is a sine wave. The output waveform remains periodic, *but it is not sinusoidal.* We learned in Chapter 5 that any waveform that is not sinusoidal is a *complex waveform.* Thus, a sine wave that undergoes nonlinear, or amplitude, distortion becomes a complex *periodic* waveform.

We should expect, from what we learned in Chapter 5, that the complex periodic waveform at the output of a nonlinear system should have energy at *harmonics* of the fundamental frequency, which is the frequency of the driving sine wave at the input. That is the outcome that occurs when a sine wave undergoes **amplitude**, or **nonlinear, distortion**. Therefore, this form of distortion also can be called **harmonic distortion** because the output signal contains energy at *harmonics* of the fundamental driving signal.

Panel B of Figure 7–4 shows the amplitude spectrum of the sine wave in panel A that has undergone harmonic distortion. The fundamental frequency of the complex periodic wave is the same as the frequency of the input sine wave but, in addition, we see that there is energy at *harmonics* of the fundamental, and the amplitudes $(A_1$–$A_5)$ of five such harmonics are shown in the figure.

Percentage Harmonic Distortion

The magnitude of harmonic distortion usually is expressed in *percentage.* If we return to our mythical purchase of an audio tape recorder, the specifications might say, for example, that you should expect not in excess of 1% harmonic distortion. Unfortunately, it might not be intuitively obvious what "1% harmonic distortion" means. To gain a better understanding of that concept, we will attempt what might be called a "logical derivation" of an equation rather than a mathematical one.

Look again at the amplitude spectrum of the signal that has undergone harmonic distortion in panel B of Figure 7–4. Suppose we are dealing with a sine wave produced by a sine wave generator and directed to some electronic device, such as an amplifier. In this case, our unit of measure of amplitude is *voltage* rather than sound pressure. With the aid of an instrument called a wave analyzer, we can measure the voltage (amplitude) of each of the harmonics in the output signal. A wave analyzer is an electronic instrument that is a combination of a voltmeter (an instrument that measures electrical voltage) and a narrowly tuned band-pass filter with a variable f_c. Thus, one can "tune" the filter (i.e., adjust the center frequency to a desired value) and then measure "only" the voltage of the signal that is passed by the filter.

Suppose, for example, that the wave analyzer contains a 1/3 octave filter centered on the fundamental frequency of the signal, such as that shown by the dashed filter function in panel B of Figure 7–4. If the frequency of the input sine wave is 1000 Hz, we set f_c of the wave analyzer to 1000 Hz. The bandwidth of the filter will be 231 Hz (Equations 6.6, 6.7, and 6.8). Thus, virtually all of the voltage "read" by the voltmeter will be that voltage associated only with the fundamental frequency of 1000 Hz because voltages associated with the higher harmonics will be well above the passband of the analyzing filter. The voltage of the fundamental frequency is recorded and the measurement process is then repeated several times, each time with the filter tuned to a different center frequency to isolate each of the harmonics of interest.

The input signal in Figure 7–4 contains energy only at the fundamental frequency. We shall refer to the voltage of the fundamental (V_1) as reflecting the *desired energy* in the signal. However, the output signal contains energy at the desired frequency and, in addition, it contains *undesired energy* at higher harmonics (limited to four higher harmonics for convenience) of the fundamental, and these voltages are referred to as V_2, V_3, V_4, and V_5. The total energy in the output signal is equal to the sum of the *desired energy* in the fundamental frequency and the *undesired energy* that is contained in the other four harmonics of the fundamental frequency. We can conceive of **harmonic distortion** as the *proportion of total energy that is undesired energy*, which if multiplied by 100, would be expressed as **percentage harmonic distortion**. Thus, by reference to the voltages of the fundamental and the higher harmonics in the output signal, we find that:

$$\text{Percentage Harmonic Distortion} = \frac{f\ (V_2,\ V_3,\ V_4,\ V_5)}{f\ (V_1,\ V_2,\ V_3,\ V_4,\ V_5)} \times 100,$$

where **f** is some undefined function,

and **V** refers to the voltage of some particular harmonic.

Recall from Chapter 4 that we do not ordinarily sum acoustic pressures because we seldom have knowledge of the relative phases, and the same restriction must apply to their electrical analogs, voltages. We can only sum the energies or powers or intensities, which is why the "equation" above does not contain a "+" and therefore is unusable in its present form. We also learned in Chapter 4 that energy, power, or intensity is proportional to the square of pressure ($W \propto P^2$), and electrical energy or power, therefore, also is proportional to the square of voltage ($W \propto V^2$). If we square each of the voltages in the numerator and denominator, we can sum them and compute the ratio. Thus, the equation can be rewritten as:

$$\text{Percentage Harmonic Distortion} = \frac{f'\ (V_2^2 + V_3^2 + V_4^2 + V_5^2)}{f'\ (V_1^2 + V_2^2 + V_3^2 + V_4^2 + V_5^2)} \times 100.$$

Finally, we can convert our measures back from "voltage squared" to "voltage" by taking the square root of the ratio of the sum of the squared voltages, and we then arrive at Equation 7.1 for harmonic distortion, which is written more generally to accommodate **n** harmonics.

Equation 7.1 $\text{Percentage Harmonic Distortion} = \sqrt{\dfrac{V_2^2 + V_3^2 + \ldots + V_n^2}{V_1^2 + V_2^2 + \ldots + V_n^2}} \times 100.$

Approximate Percentage Harmonic Distortion

Because most of the total energy in the signal in the denominator comes from only the fundamental frequency, percentage harmonic distortion sometimes is *approximated* by:

Equation 7.2 $\text{Percentage Harmonic Distortion} = \sqrt{\dfrac{V_2^2 + V_3^2 + \ldots + V_n^2}{V_1^2}} \times 100.$

To illustrate, the second column of Table 7–1 lists the voltages, in millivolts, for each of five harmonics listed in column one. The third column lists the squares of the voltages shown in column two. With the aid of Equation 7.1 we calculate that we have 0.1% harmonic distortion. The same answer is obtained if we use Equation 7.2 *for this example*, and the explanation should be obvious. With either equation, the numerator is the same, 0.002626. With Equation 7.1, the denominator for this example is 2,500.002626, whereas with Equation 7.2 the denominator is 2,500, which is not very different. Thus, we see for the example in Table 7–1, and for most instances that we are likely to encounter, Equation 7.2 provides a perfectly acceptable estimate of percentage harmonic distortion.

Amplitude Response and Dynamic Range

In panel A of Figure 7-5 we show what happens if we define input–output functions for some system at each of several input or driving

Table 7-1. Computation of percentage harmonic distortion.

Harmonic	Voltage (V) in millivolts	V²
1	50.0	2,500.0
2	.01	.0001
3	.05	.0025
4	.001	.000001
5	.005	.000025

$$\% = \sqrt{\frac{0.0001 + .0025 + .000001 + .000025}{2,500 + .0001 + .0025 + .000001 + .000025}} \times 100 = 0.1\%$$

frequencies, not just one. Next, we will decide on some *maximum permissible harmonic distortion,* say 0.1%, to accommodate whatever purpose we have in mind for the system that is being used.

We then locate the point of maximum permissible harmonic distortion on each of the functions in the figure, and those points are identified as filled dots in the figure. That means that if the input amplitude for that particular frequency exceeds the value corresponding to that point on the function, we will exceed the maximum permissible harmonic distortion that was agreed on. In other words, those points define the maximum driving amplitude as a function of frequency that we can utilize without producing an unacceptable amount of harmonic distortion.

The points of maximum permissible harmonic distortion are redrawn in the frequency domain as the upper curve in panel B of Figure 7-5. When the points are connected, the curve that results defines the **amplitude response** (or **frequency response**) of the system, just as we saw previously in panel C of Figure 7-1. As before, we see that the curve defines how the energy is attenuated selectively as a function of frequency *in relation to the maximum permissible harmonic distortion* that we have agreed can be tolerated.

Dynamic Range

When you examine the specifications for some electronic instrument, such as a tape recorder, you likely will see reference to something called the **dynamic range** of the system. The dashed curve in panel B of Figure 7-5 describes what is called the *electrical noise floor* (ENF) of the hypothetical tape recorder. All electronic equipment generates a random time function, which as we learned in Chapter 5 can also be called an aperiodic waveform, or *noise,* and the curve depicting the electrical noise floor shows how the level of the noise varies as a function of frequency.

The frequency response curve reflects the maximum signal level that the tape recorder can handle reliably without exceeding the maximum permissible harmonic distortion. If the input signal level is

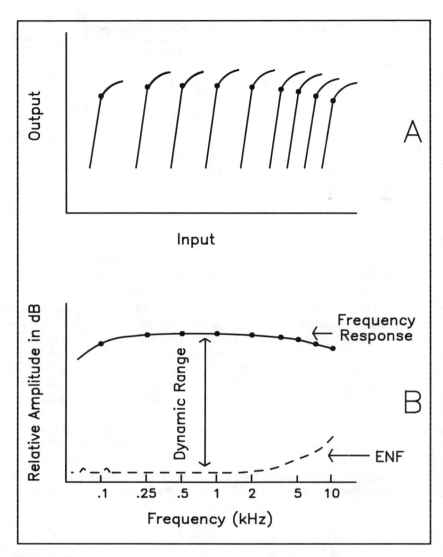

Figure 7–5. Input–output functions for each of several frequencies are shown in panel A. In panel B, the amplitude response (solid line), in relation to the maximum permissible harmonic distortion, is compared with the electrical noise floor (ENF) of a system. The distance between the ENF and the maximum amplitude response defines the **dynamic range** of a system.

reduced, percentage harmonic distortion also will be lowered. However, we obviously don't want a driving signal level that is so low that the signal is "buried" in the noise. Thus, to achieve an optimal signal-to-noise ratio, we want the driving signal to correspond to the highest possible amplitude without exceeding a tolerable amount of harmonic distortion. That describes the **dynamic range** of the system.

Dynamic range defines the distance in decibels between the electrical noise floor and the amplitude response curve. If, for example, the dynamic range is said to be 60 dB, that means you can record a signal with a signal-to-noise ratio of 60 dB or less without experiencing an intolerable amount of harmonic distortion. If signal level is reduced, percentage harmonic distortion also is reduced, but at the expense of a less favorable signal-to-noise ratio. It should be obvious that because both the amplitude response curve and ENF vary with frequency, the dynamic range is also frequency dependent. However, if you examine the specifications for an instrument you are contemplating purchasing, the dynamic range probably will be expressed as a single value — perhaps even the most favorable one.

Summary of an Experiment on the Cat

Electronic instruments such as tape recorders, amplifiers, and the like are not alone in being subject to amplitude distortion. So too is the auditory system. An example is provided by a classic experiment described by Wever (1949) on the cat. The cat's ear was presented with a 1000-Hz sine wave at many different sound pressure levels.

For each input level of the 1000-Hz sine wave, a wave analyzer with a narrowly tuned filter was used to measure the magnitude of the electrical response (voltage) at an appropriate location in the cat's (inner) ear. When the output level in microvolts (μV) is plotted as a function of input level in dynes/cm^2 (**cgs** system), the result is an input–output function in Figure 7–6 that is similar in form to the more general function that was shown in Figure 7–4.

The function is linear for input levels that range from about 10^{-3} dyne/cm^2 (14 dB SPL re: 2×10^{-4} dyne/cm^2) to about 1.0 dyne/cm^2 (74 dB SPL), a range of 60 dB. The electrical response to the input sinusoid measured in the cat's inner ear (called the "cochlear potential") is quite small and was measured in microvolts. When the input amplitude was 10^{-3} dyne/cm^2 (14 dB SPL), the electrical response was about 0.3 μV. When the input amplitude was 1 dyne/cm^2 (74 dB SPL), the electrical response was about 300 μV. Thus, the range of electrical response also was approximately 60 dB,

$$\text{dB SPL} = 20 \log (3 \times 10^2)/(3 \times 10^{-1}) = 60 \text{ dB SPL,}$$

which confirms that changes in output level were *proportional* to changes in input level over the linear portion of the function.

We also can see that for input levels in excess of 1 dyne/cm^2, the input–output function is nonlinear. For example, when the input signal level was raised from 1 dyne/cm^2 to 10 dynes/cm^2, an increase of 20 dB, the output level only increased from 300 μV to 800 μV, which corresponds to approximately 8 dB. Thus, it is apparent that amplitude distortion has occurred. Therefore, we should expect that the signal the cat actually "hears" is not a sinusoid, but rather is a complex periodic signal with energy at harmonics of the fundamental driving signal.

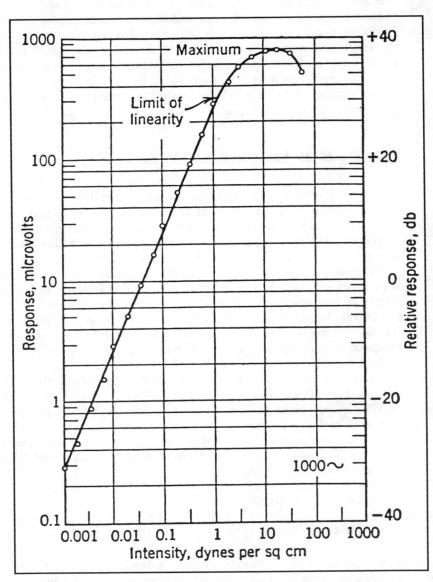

Figure 7–6. An input–output function observed in the cat in response to an input frequency of 1000 Hz. Input level was varied from .001 dyne/cm² (14 dB SPL) to just under 100 dynes/cm² (114 dB SPL). The function is linear over a 60 dB range from about 14 dB SPL to 74 dB SPL. Adapted from *Theory of hearing* (p. 147) by E. G. Wever, 1949: John Wiley and Sons, Inc. New York, NY. Copyright 1949 by the Estate of E. G. Wever. Printed with permission.

Evidence of Harmonic Distortion

To confirm the validity of that expectation, the electrical waveform of the output signal was analyzed (Wever & Bray, 1938) by systematically adjusting the center frequency of the wave analyzer to isolate, in turn, each of several harmonics of the 1000-Hz driving signal. For each new center frequency, voltage readings were made in response to each of the same input levels that were used to define the function for 1000 Hz.

The resulting input–output functions for six of the higher harmonics of 1000 Hz are shown in Figure 7–7. For example, when f_c of the analyzing filter was set to 2000 Hz, the 2nd harmonic of the input signal, the outcome of the measurements is labeled "2" in the figure. Note, for example, that when the input amplitude for 1000 Hz was 0.1 dyne/cm^2, the electrical response at *2000* Hz (the 2nd harmonic) was 0.4 μV. In contrast, at that same input signal level, the electrical response to the driving signal (1000 Hz) was 30 μV. Thus, you should be able to calculate that for an input level of 0.1 dyne/cm^2 at 1000 Hz, the output of the 2nd harmonic was almost 38 dB below the output of the 1st harmonic (1000 Hz), which was the input signal.

$$dB = 20 \log (4 \times 10^{-1})/(3 \times 10^1) = -37.5 \text{ dB}.$$

The other functions, labeled "3, 4, 5, 7," and "10," depict additional measurements that were made by adjusting f_c of the wave analyzer to frequencies corresponding to the 3rd, 4th, 5th, 7th, and 10th harmonics. We can see that for high input levels, particularly those in excess of 10 dynes/cm^2, considerable energy is present in each of the harmonics. With the aid of either Equation 7.1 or Equation 7.2, we should be able to compute a reasonable estimate of percentage harmonic distortion.

Suppose we select an input level for 1000 Hz of just over 30 dynes/cm^2 (midway between 10 and 100 dynes/cm^2 on a log scale) and then read the *approximate* voltages (in microvolts) for each of the harmonics. For convenience, we will restrict our estimate of harmonic distortion to results for the first five harmonics: $V_1 = 760$; $V_2 = 40$; $V_3 = 160$; $V_4 = 17$; and $V_5 = 52$. With Equation 7.2 we then would *estimate* that an input signal level of just over 30 dynes/cm^2 produced approximately 22.9% harmonic distortion, and with Equation 7.1 we would *calculate* that overdriving the cat's ear in that way produced 22.3% harmonic distortion.

Intermodulation Distortion

Harmonic distortion is synonymous with amplitude, or nonlinear, distortion when the driving signal is periodic. If the driving signal is not periodic, we still experience amplitude, or nonlinear, distortion, but the

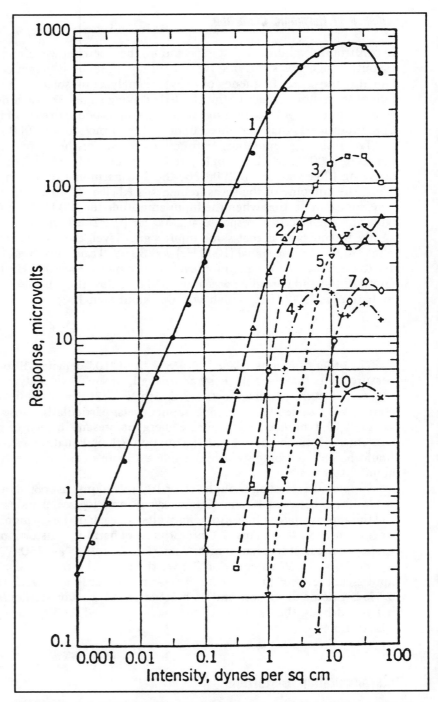

Figure 7-7. Amplitude of response in microvolts in the cat at harmonics of the fundamental driving signal, 1000 Hz. The abscissa is the intensity of the input signal. Adapted from "Distortion in the ear as shown by the electrical response of the cochlea" (p. 288) by E. G. Wever and C. W. Bray, 1938: *Journal of the Acoustical Society of America.* Printed with permission.

output spectrum is far more complicated than "simple" harmonic distortion. This kind of distortion is called **intermodulation distortion**.

To illustrate the differences between intermodulation distortion and harmonic distortion, we will consider the simple case of a complex driving signal that has two components, f_1 = 100 Hz and f_2 = 110 Hz. The frequency components of the output signal will contain two types of **distortion products: harmonics** and **combination tones**.

Harmonics

The output signal contains energy at *harmonics* of each of the frequency components of the driving signal. Thus, there will be energy at f_1 (100 Hz), $2f_1$ (200 Hz), $3f_1$ (300 Hz), and so forth, and there will be energy at f_2 (110 Hz), $2f_2$ (220 Hz), $3f_2$ (330 Hz), and so on. Each of these components of the output signal is harmonically related to one or the other of the two components of the driving signal, f_1 and f_2.

Combination Tones: Difference Tones and Summation Tones

A second type of distortion product, in addition to the harmonically related components listed above, comprises **combination tones**. Combination tones can be further subdivided into two types, **difference tones** and **summation tones**. For example, difference tones include $f_1 - f_2$ (10 Hz); $2f_1 - f_2$ (90 Hz); $3f_1 - f_2$ (190 Hz); and so on. Examples of summation tones include $f_1 + f_2$ (210 Hz); $2f_1 + f_2$ (310 Hz); $3f_1 + f_2$ (410 Hz); and so forth.

In theory, the combination tones comprise all possible sums (**summation tones**) and differences (**difference tones**) of the primary frequencies, f_1 and f_2, *and integral multiples of those primary components.* In practice, though, the amplitudes of many of the higher combination tones will be sufficiently small to render their contribution to the total energy in the output signal negligible. The general equation that defines the harmonics, summation tones, and difference tones produced by a nonlinear system is:

$$mf_1 \pm nf_2. \hspace{3cm} \text{Equation 7.3}$$

where **m** and **n** are assigned all integer values: 0, 1, 2, 3, 4, ... n.

If we apply Equation 7.3 to the example cited above where f_1 = 100 Hz and f_2 = 110 Hz, we generate the harmonics and combination tones listed in Table 7–2.

Table 7–2. Examples of harmonics and combination tones produced for a complex wave with two frequency components: $f_1 = 100$ Hz and $f_2 = 110$ Hz.

| Harmonics of | | Combination Tones | |
f_1	f_2	Difference Tones	Summation Tones
$1f_1 + 0f_2 = 100$	$0f_1 + 1f_2 = 110$	$1f_1 - 1f_2 = 10$	$1f_1 + 1f_2 = 210$
$2f_1 + 0f_2 = 200$	$0f_1 + 2f_2 = 220$	$2f_1 - 1f_2 = 90$	$2f_1 + 1f_2 = 310$
$3f_1 + 0f_2 = 300$	$0f_1 + 3f_2 = 330$	$3f_1 - 1f_2 = 190$	$3f_1 + 1f_2 = 410$
etc.	etc.	etc.	etc.

In this chapter we have learned how "ideal" sound waves are altered in various ways that, collectively, are called **distortion**. In the final chapter we will learn other ways in which sound waves are changed from the original state when transmitted through a medium.

Sound
Transmission

When sinusoidal waves were first discussed in Chapter 2, each cycle of sinusoidal motion initially was represented as being identical in every respect to every other cycle. That representation was appropriate when the sine wave was conceptualized from a strict mathematical perspective. However, we then learned that sound waves produced and transmitted in the real world encounter frictional forces that cause the amplitude of the sound wave to diminish over time. Thus, real sound waves are damped, and ultimately they fade away.

Furthermore, we know from experience that the amplitude of sound not only diminishes over time, but over distance traveled. All other factors being equal, if you are positioned too far from even an intense source of sound, the sound might be quite faint, if indeed it is even audible.

It also was convenient to treat sound waves initially as though they were transmitted in a free, unbounded medium with no obstacles. When obstacles are present, or when certain conditions exist in the medium, important characteristics of sound waves and their transmission are altered.

In this final chapter we will learn how the characteristics of sound waves are altered in various ways during sound transmission. Although the factors that we will describe usually act in combination to affect the characteristics of sound waves in fairly complicated ways, for the sake of simplicity, we will consider them one at a time.

■ ATTENUATION OF SOUND INTENSITY OVER DISTANCE

Let us assume that a sound wave is propagated through a *free, unbounded medium* that contains no obstacles or conditions to affect the propagation or in any way to affect the characteristics of the sound wave as it is transmitted through space. Suppose, for example, that a weapon is fired and that the resultant sound wave has a peak sound pressure level of 110 dB at some distance (e.g., 0.5 miles) from the weapon. As the sound wave is propagated through the free, unbounded medium, the intensity of the sound wave diminishes in a lawful way.

The decrease in intensity in a free, unbounded medium behaves in accordance with what is called the **inverse square law**. Could the shot be heard at a great distance (e.g., 8,192 miles) from the source if the listener's threshold of hearing (in the appropriate frequency range) is, for example, 20 dB SPL? We will subsequently demonstrate that the answer is "yes" for this example, even though the intensity of the sound wave does decrease with distance.

Think of a point source of sound, a spherically shaped source of vibration, or pulsation, with a very small diameter. We see in Figure 8–1 that when the point source is forced to pulsate by application of some external force, alternate regions of increased density (**compression**) and decreased density (**rarefaction**) are created. A "disturbance" is propagated through the medium, and sound, which is a form of energy,

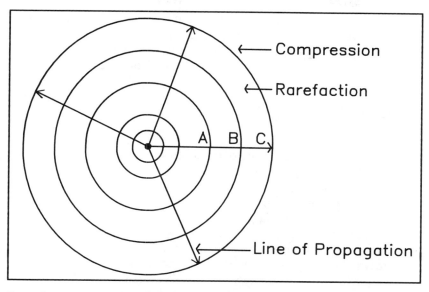

Figure 8–1. Alternate regions of compression (condensation) and rarefaction in an air mass caused by pulsation of a point source of sound. Four lines of propagation from the source are shown. The compressions form a spherical shell around the spherical point source and the shell is called a **wave front** or, more precisely, a **spherical wave front**.

is transferred from the source through the medium. Thus, sound energy radiates away from the source in all directions, and several "lines of propagation" are shown in the figure.

Spherical Waves

Let us also continue to assume that the medium has uniform properties and is unlimited in all directions, which is to say that the medium is free and unbounded. That defines a "free-field" condition. The **compressions**, or crests, form what is called a "spherical shell" around the spherical point source. That spherical shell is called a **wave front**. The disturbance propagated through the medium is an ever increasingly larger **spherical wave front**.

Plane Waves

If the wave front is a considerable distance away from the point source, the radius of the sphere is sufficiently large that we can represent the wave front as a **plane wave front**, rather than as a spherical wave front, because the curvature of the sphere is negligible. Thus, sine waves also can be called **spherical waves**, or **plane progressive waves**, when they are propagated through a medium that is free and unbounded. A spherical wave can be visualized as being similar to a soap bubble that becomes larger and larger as it is blown at a constant rate, with the surface of the soap bubble representing a wave front.

The Inverse Square Law

As the wave front moves outward from the source, sound energy is spread over a larger and larger area. Thus, as we move from point **A** to point **B** to point **C** in Figure 8–1, the energy is progressively dissipated over a larger and larger area because the surface area of the sphere becomes progressively larger.

Recall from Chapter 4 that energy/unit time (energy/sec) is **power**. The same amount of **power** is dissipated over the surfaces of the increasingly larger spheres at the distances represented by **A, B,** and **C** in Figure 8–1, but the energy/sec/m² (**MKS** system) *must diminish* because the same amount of power is dissipated over a larger area. Energy/sec/m², sometimes called the **energy density**, is the **intensity** of a sound wave. Thus, if the energy/sec (**power**) remains constant, but the **power** (energy/sec) is dissipated over a larger and larger area as we move farther and farther away from the source, the **intensity,** or **energy density** (energy/sec/m²), must decrease with increasing distance from the point source.

Imagine that we can place our eye at the point source and look away from the source at the increasingly larger area that is bounded by the lines of propagation. Such a view is represented in Figure 8–2, and four lines of propagation are shown as we attempt to depict a three-dimensional representation. We will assume that the distances of interest from the point source are so great that the wave front can be considered to be a plane.

At distance **X** a finite amount of sound **power** (energy/sec) is dissipated over an area of 1 m². That defines the **intensity** of the sound wave at distance **X** from the source, the energy/sec/m². As we move twice as far away from the source to distance **2X**, the same finite amount of **power** is dissipated, but over a larger area. How much larger? The surface area of a sphere is given by Equation 8.1:

Equation 8.1
$$A = 4\pi r^2$$

where **r** is the radius.

For example, if distance **X** is 1 m from the source, the area of the sphere at distance **X** = 12.6 m² $(4\pi 1^2)$. However, at distance **2X**, A = 50.3 m² $(4\pi 2^2)$, and at distance **4X**, A = 201.1 m² $(4\pi 4^2)$. From these calculations we should see that *each time the radius is increased by some factor, the surface area of the sphere is increased by the square of that factor.*

If the area of the sphere increases with increasing distance from the source, the energy/sec/m² (the **intensity**) must decrease. The area

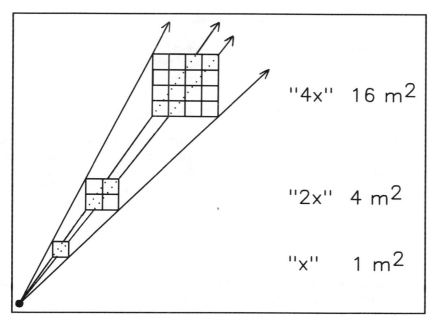

"4x" 16 m^2

"2x" 4 m^2

"x" 1 m^2

Figure 8–2. A three dimensional representation of the **inverse square law**. As the distance from the point source of sound increases from **X** to **2X** to **4X**, a finite amount of power is dissipated over a larger and larger area (from 1 m^2 at **X** to 4 m^2 at **2X** to 16 m^2 at **4X**). Hence, the intensity (energy/sec/m^2) decreases inversely with the square of the distance from the source.

(4 m^2) at point **2X** is exactly four times the area at point **X** (1 m^2). Because **intensity** is energy/sec/m^2, we can see that the intensity is diminished as the sound wave travels between the two points. More precisely, the intensity at distance **2X** is only *one-fourth* the intensity at **X** because the power is dissipated over an area that is four times larger.

We have seen that when the distance from the source *increases* by a factor of 2:1, sound intensity *decreases*, and the ratio of the intensity at point **X** to the intensity at point **2X** is 1:4. Because $4 = 2^2$, and because the relation is an inverse one, the phenomenon is called the **inverse square law**.

As we proceed farther and farther from the point source in the free, unbounded medium, we shall see that the **inverse square law** continues to hold. For example, at distance **4X**, which is twice as far from the source as distance **2X**, the **power** is spread over an area of 16 m^2 in comparison with an area of 4 m^2 at distance **2X**. Thus, the distance has increased by another factor of 2:1, the surface area of the wave front has increased by a factor of 2^2:1, and the sound intensity, therefore, is changed by another ratio of 1:4.

The **inverse square law** can be expressed as:

$$I \propto \frac{1}{D^2},$$

Equation 8.2

where **D** refers to the ratio of two distances
from the sound source (d_i/d_r),

d_i is the distance of interest,

and

d_r is some reference distance.

For example, if we compare the intensities at two distances, 100 m (d_r) and 200 m (d_i), we should expect that the intensity at d_i will be inversely proportional to the square of the ratio of the two distances, d_i/d_r.
We therefore can rewrite Equation 8.2 and obtain Equation 8.3:

Equation 8.3
$$I \propto \frac{1}{\left(\dfrac{d_i}{d_r}\right)^2},$$

which states that *the intensity is inversely proportional to the square of the ratio of two distances,* that is, the ratio of distance of interest (d_i) to some reference distance (d_r).

The Inverse Square Law and Decibels

As we learned in Chapter 4, we generally choose to refer to the *level* of a sound in decibels rather than to its intensity in watts/m^2. To accomplish that transformation we simply calculate the log of the ratio and multiply by 10 to obtain Equation 8.4.
Thus,

$$dB = 10 \log_{10} \frac{1}{\left(\dfrac{d_i}{d_r}\right)^2}$$

$$= -10 \log_{10} \left(\frac{d_i}{d_r}\right)^2 \qquad \textbf{(Log Law 4)}$$

Equation 8.4
$$= -20 \log_{10} \frac{d_i}{d_r}. \qquad \textbf{(Log Law 3)}$$

If we return to Figure 8–2, we should gain an intuitive understanding of Equation 8.4. The area over which power is dissipated at distance **X** is 1 m^2. Thus, if we use Equation 8.4 to compare the intensity at distance **X** (d_i) with the intensity *at the same distance* **X** (d_r), we obtain 0 dB, because the ratio is 1:1 and the log of 1 is 0. However, if we compare the intensity at distance **2X** (d_i) with the intensity at a reference distance **X** (d_r), we calculate that:

$$dB = -20 \log \frac{2}{1}$$

$$= -6 \text{ dB.}$$

That answer agrees with what we discovered previously. The intensity at **2X** is one-fourth the intensity at **X**, and as we learned in Chapter 4, if intensity decreases by a factor of four, the *level* decreases by 6 dB (Equation 4.4). Obviously, therefore, between **2X** and **4X** the intensity decreases by another 6 dB because:

$$dB = -20 \log \frac{4}{2}$$

$$= -6 \text{ dB.}$$

Finally, between distance **X** and distance **4X** the intensity decreases by 12 dB because:

$$dB = -20 \log \frac{4}{1}$$

$$= -12 \text{ dB.}$$

The **inverse square law** is sometimes defined (incompletely) by saying that "the intensity decreases by 6 dB for each doubling of the distance." Although the statement is correct, it is an insufficient definition of the law because it does not describe the more general effect of distance ratios other than 2:1 on intensity. For that reason, the previous definition — the intensity varies inversely with the square of the distance — is preferable.

Sample Problems

Problem 1: If the sound pressure level is 80 dB at a distance of 100 m from the source, *by how much is the SPL decreased* at a distance of 200 m?

$$dB = -20 \log 200/100 = -6 \text{ dB.}$$

Note that the SPL at d_r (100 m) is irrelevant. The intensity at d_i will be attenuated by 6 dB re: the intensity at d_r regardless of the intensity at d_r.

Problem 2: If the sound pressure level is 80 dB SPL at a distance of 100 m from the source, *what is the SPL* at a distance of 200 m?

$$dB = 80 - 20 \log 200/100 = 74 \text{ dB SPL.}$$

It stands to reason that if the SPL decreases by 6 dB between the two distances, the SPL at the second distance is given by the SPL at the first or reference distance (80 dB) minus the amount by which the intensity is attenuated (6 dB).

Problem 3: If the SPL at a distance of 100 m is 80 dB, what is the SPL at a distance of 850 m?

$$dB = 80 - 20 \log 850/100 = 61.4 \text{ dB SPL.}$$

Problem 4: Finally, let us solve the problem that was posed at the outset. If the SPL of a gunshot is 110 dB at a distance of 0.5 miles from the weapon, could the shot be heard at a distance of 8,192 miles (*in a free, unbounded medium*) from the source if the observer's threshold of hearing in the appropriate frequency range is 20 dB SPL?

$$dB = 110 - 20 \log 8192/0.5 = 110 - 84.2 = 25.8 \text{ dB SPL.}$$

Therefore, if the intensity of the sound is 25.8 dB SPL and the observer's threshold of hearing is 20 dB SPL, the shot should be heard. You should also note that if the distance from the source of the sound wave doubled again to 16,384 miles, the SPL would only decrease by another 6 dB (to 0.2 dB below the postulated threshold) because, as we have seen, the intensity varies with the square of the distance. Finally, you might wish to test your ability to still work problems such as those in Problem Set 8 of Chapter 4 by attempting to calculate just how far from the reference distance of 0.5 miles the observer would have to be positioned for the sound to just equal the observer's threshold of 20 dB SPL. The only difference is that now you are solving for d_i, a distance of interest, rather than P_x, a pressure of interest. You should calculate that the sound should just reach the observer's threshold of 20 dB SPL at a distance of approximately 15,811 miles, if the medium is free and unbounded.

The inverse square law only holds strictly when the sound waves are propagated through a free, unbounded medium. Such a medium, of course, is a theoretical construct and, in reality, the transmitting media of interest to us will have obstacles and other conditions that interfere with sound transmission in important ways.

If the sound wave encounters an obstacle, depending on the nature of the obstacle, the sound wave will be **reflected** (it will "bounce" back toward the source), **diffracted** (it will be scattered about the obstacle), or **absorbed** (it will penetrate the obstacle). Under other circumstances, the conditions of the medium will cause the sound wave to be **refracted** (it will be "bent").

■ REFLECTION

What happens when a rubber ball is thrown against a hard wooden wall? Obviously the ball does not penetrate the obstacle — it bounces off the wall. Moreover, many young children quickly learn the approx-

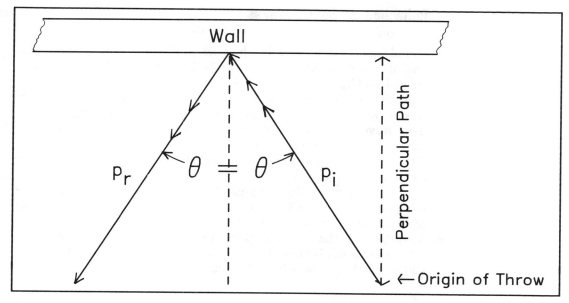

Figure 8–3. The paths of a ball thrown toward a wall and then reflected from the wall. When the ball is thrown straight at the wall along the dashed line, it bounces straight back to the thrower. However, when the ball is thrown at an angle along the path marked **P$_i$**, the ball bounces off the wall and away from the thrower along the path marked **P$_r$**. In both cases, and all others, the angle of the reflected path, **P$_r$**, to a line drawn perpendicular to the wall equals the angle of the incident path, **P$_i$**, to the same perpendicular line.

imate path that the ball will take on its return so that they can get into position to catch it.

In Figure 8–3, a ball is about to be thrown toward a wall along a path marked by the dashed line that is perpendicular to the wall (90° angle). If, and only if, the ball is thrown toward the wall on a path that is precisely along the perpendicular, the ball will return to the thrower along the same perpendicular (dashed) line. However, if the ball is thrown more to the left along the path marked **P$_i$**, it will return along the path marked **P$_r$**. Why?

Let us call the path of the thrown ball the "incident path" (**P$_i$**) and call the path of the bounced (reflected) ball the "reflected path" (**P$_r$**). From the point where the thrown ball strikes the wall, we have drawn another (dashed) line that also is perpendicular to the wall. The *angle of the reflected path* (**P$_r$**) *to the perpendicular equals the angle of the incident path* (**P$_i$**) *to the perpendicular.*

That rule applies to any angle of the incident path to the perpendicular, regardless of whether the ball is thrown to the left, the right, or straight ahead. The young child almost certainly cannot recite that rule of reflection, but most children "know" the rule or else learn it rather quickly. Unless that rule is mastered, attempts to participate in any sporting event in which reflection is part of the game (billiards, handball, etc.) will be futile.

Reflection of Sound Waves

Sound waves are affected by obstacles in the same way that the hard wall affects the path of the thrown ball. In Figure 8–4 we show wave fronts (solid lines) moving from right to left. The wave fronts encounter a plane obstacle (a very thick wall of steel, for example). The sound wave moving from right to left *toward the wall* will be called the **incident wave**, and one *ray* of the incident wave (**i**) is shown pointing leftward toward the plane obstacle. A *ray* is simply a line that is perpendicular to the wave front. The point source of the sound wave is identified by **S**.

If there were no obstacle present, the wave would continue to move leftward toward point **S'**, which is shown to be as far to the left of the obstacle as point **S** is to the right of the obstacle. Those wave fronts are represented by the dashed lines, but, of course, they are hypothetical because an obstacle is present that prevents the wave fronts from progressing beyond the obstacle and toward **S'**.

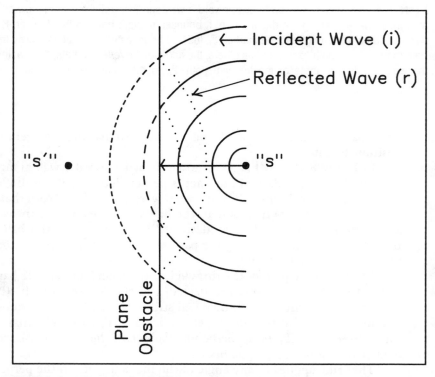

Figure 8–4. Sound wave **reflection**. Spherical wave fronts (solid lines) moving from right to left from a source **S** encounter a plane obstacle such as a wall. The obstacle causes the sound wave to be **reflected** back toward the source (dotted lines) with no change in speed of propagation. An observer will hear the reflected wave as having originated from point **S'**, which is as far to the left of the obstacle as point **S** is to the right of the obstacle.

The obstacle offers a very large **acoustic impedance** to sound transmission, where the amount of acoustic impedance is given by the sound pressure divided by the volume velocity. If the acoustic impedance is large, very little of the sound energy can penetrate the wall. Instead, the sound wave is **reflected** back toward the source (**S**) *with no change in speed of propagation,* and the **reflected wave** (**r**) that is moving from left to right toward the original point source is represented by the dotted lines. Because the speed of the reflected wave is identical to the speed of the incident wave, at any reference point in time the reflected wave will be just as far to the right of the plane surface as it would have been to the left of the plane surface had there been no obstacle.

The precise relation of the reflected ray to the incident ray conforms to the same rule that governed the path of the thrown ball in Figure 8–3; *the angle of the reflected rays (r) to the perpendicular equals the angle of the incident rays (i) to the perpendicular,* and we see that the path of the one reflected ray shown in the figure lies exactly along the path of the incident ray. An observer located in the medium will perceive the reflected sound wave as having originated from point **S'**, not point **S**. As a consequence of the sound wave being reflected, *energy is retained in the medium.* Because energy is retained in the medium, it should be apparent that the **inverse square law** does not hold for sound transmission in a medium with reflecting surfaces.

Reflection from Plane Surfaces

Figure 8–5 should serve to explain further the principle of sound wave reflection from a plane surface. In panel A, an incident ray (**i**) strikes the plane surface at an angle 45° to a line that is perpendicular (**p**) to the plane surface. The incident ray is reflected back in the general direction of the source, and the angle of the reflected ray (**r**) to the perpendicular also is 45°. In panel B of the figure, the angle of **i** to the perpendicular is 30°, and we see that the angle of **r** to the perpendicular also is 30°.

The principle, therefore, is the same that we saw in Figure 8–3 for a ball thrown against a wall: *the angle of the reflected ray to the perpendicular equals the angle of the incident ray to the perpendicular.* We shall see subsequently that the principle can be generalized to other than plane surfaces. In panel C, the angle of **i** is 0°. Therefore, the angle of **r** = 0° and the ray is reflected back on itself. Anyone who has successfully shot billiards or played pool in River City must be familiar with these concepts.

Reflection from Convex Surfaces

We mentioned above that the rule governing the relation of the angles of the reflected rays to the angles of the incident rays holds for other

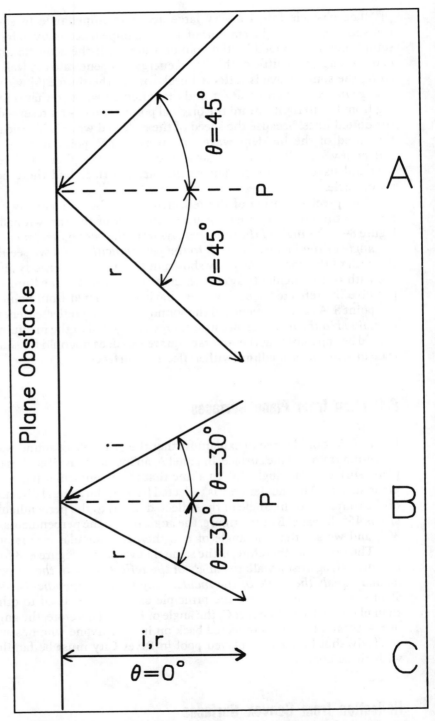

Figure 8–5. Incident rays, **i**, of a sound wave moving from right to left encounter a plane obstacle. The angles of the reflected rays, **r**, to the perpendicular, **p**, are equal to the angles of the incident rays to the perpendicular.

than plane surfaces. In panel A of Figure 8–6, a spherical wave moves from right to left, but this time the surface of the obstacle is *convex* toward the source. As the wave fronts approach the obstacle at some considerable distance from the source, they are represented as plane waves (straight lines) rather than spherical waves (curved lines). Two incident rays are shown, i_1 and i_2.

Because of the rule that specifies the angle of the reflected rays, we can see that the reflected rays *diverge*. In a sense, the sound energy

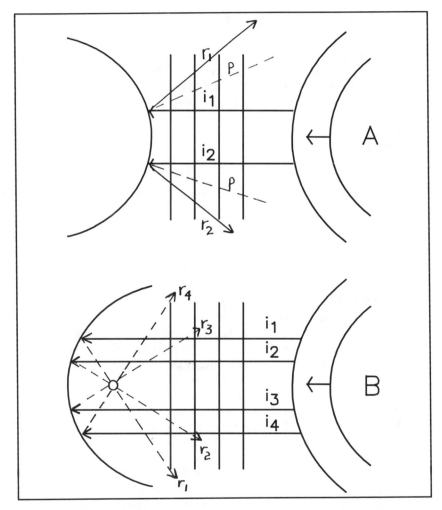

Figure 8–6. Plane progressive sound waves, with wave fronts sufficiently far from the source of sound that their curvature is negligible, are moving from right to left and encounter an obstacle that is **convex** toward the source (panel A) and **concave** toward the source (panel B). The reflected rays diverge from the convex surface, but converge toward a focal point from the concave surface. However, in both cases, the angle of the reflected ray to the perpendicular equals the angle of the incident ray to the perpendicular.

is scattered just as thrown balls would be scattered if they were thrown at various angles against a wall that is convex toward the thrower.

The divergence of the reflected rays in panel A of the figure describes what happens to a sound wave in air that strikes the *exterior* surface of a dome-shaped roof of a building. The rays of the reflected sound wave diverge. The intensity of the reflected sound wave at some distance from the surface will be less than the intensity of the incident sound wave at the same distance, because the sound energy in the reflected wave has been scattered.

Reflection from Concave Surfaces

In panel B of Figure 8–6, a plane progressive wave moves from right to left and encounters a surface that is *concave* toward the source. As before, the angles of the reflected rays to the perpendicular equal the angles of the incident rays to the perpendicular. However, when the sound wave encounters the concave surface, the rays of the reflected wave *converge* toward what is called a *focal point,* the point at which all reflected rays converge.

Convergence of the reflected rays should help explain how "whispering galleries" work. Many readers will have had the experience of standing in a room that has a domed ceiling — a surface that is concave toward the floor. You try standing in several locations on one side of the room, and you discover that you cannot hear what someone is saying who is whispering from the other side of the room. However, if you move to just the right point, which was previously marked on the floor, suddenly the same whispered speech is audible.

The point marked on the floor identifies the *focal point,* the point at which the rays of the whispered sound converge after having been reflected from the concave surface of the ceiling. The intensity of the reflected wave is greatest at the focal point, and, indeed, it is greater than the intensity of the incident wave because the sound energy, in a sense, has been "collected;" the **energy density**, or **intensity**, is maximal.

Perhaps you have observed a television crew at a sporting event such as a football game. The producer wants to enliven the audio portion of the broadcast by picking up the grunts, groans, and occasional profanities uttered by the players. The crew *does not point a microphone toward the playing field* to pick up the incident waves. Instead, the microphone is attached to a reflector (a "dish") that is held with its concave surface pointed toward the playing field. The microphone is pointed *away from the playing field* and *toward the reflector* so that it can pick up the reflected waves. If the microphone is mounted properly, the diaphragm of the microphone will be located at the focal point of the reflector where the intensity of the reflected sound waves will be greatest.

Echoes, Reverberation, and Reverberation Time

Reflected sound waves are sometimes called **echoes** or **reverberating waves**, and rooms that have hard surfaces can be called **reverberant**

rooms. In contrast, rooms that are designed to minimize reverberation are called **anechoic rooms**, because they are designed to be nearly without echo or reverberation.

If you have heard the echo of your voice bouncing from, for example, the walls of a canyon, you know that you can hear a few echoes, but finally they die away. The time required for the reflected wave to decay is called the **reverberation time**, which is defined specifically as the *time required for a sound wave to be attenuated by 60 dB relative to its original level.* With the aid of Equation 4.4 from Chapter 4 you should be able to see why we also can say that **reverberation time** is defined as the time required for sound intensity to be attenuated to one millionth of its original value.

One practical use of reflected waves was made in 1883 (Stewart, 1924). The explosion of a volcano in Krakatoa in the East Indies produced an intense compressional wave that progressed around the earth in all directions and converged at a point opposite Krakatoa. At that point, the wave was reflected back toward its source. From inspection of barometric records, the speed of propagation was measured to be 320 m/sec, which stands in close agreement to modern, more technically accurate measures of the speed of sound.

Standing Waves

We have learned that when a sound wave is reflected from a surface, sound energy is retained in the medium. This gives rise to what are called **standing waves**. Standing waves occur when two progressive waves, the incident wave and the reflected wave, of the same frequency and amplitude travel through the same medium in opposite directions.

Transverse Wave Motion and Standing Waves

Standing waves are illustrated in Figure 8–7. A string or wire is anchored at both ends and each of the two ends extends to infinity. Dots have been painted on the string at equal intervals to help us observe their motion over time.

In panel A of Figure 8–7, the string is stretched with some fixed tension and the identifying points are labeled **a** through **k**. In panel B, a source of sound such as a vibrating tuning fork causes a transverse sound wave of some fixed frequency and amplitude to travel from *left to right* (the dashed line). At the same time, another tuning fork produces a second transverse wave *of identical amplitude and frequency* that travels in the opposite direction, from *right to left* (the solid line).

We learned in Chapter 1, with an unanchored stretched rope and only one transverse wave present, that each identifying point on the rope moves up and down with identical frequency. Now, because the string in Figure 8–7 is anchored, and because we have two identical transverse waves traveling in opposite directions, the pattern of movement of the points along the string is quite different from what we observed previously.

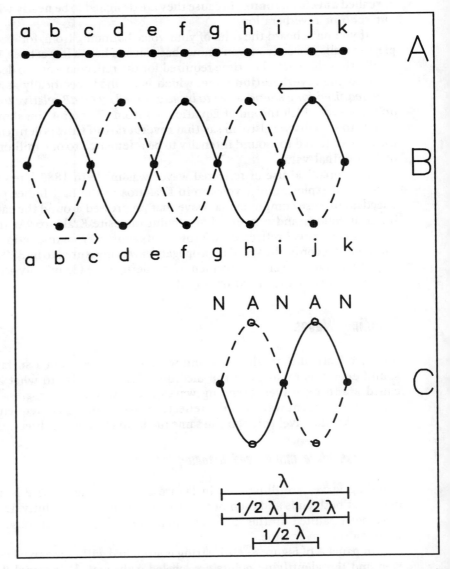

Figure 8–7. Creation of **standing**, or **stationary**, waves, in a vibrating string anchored at both ends, each of which extends to infinity. Two trains of waves of identical amplitude and frequency are moving in opposite directions along the string. The wave shown by the solid line is moving from right to left and the wave shown by the dashed line is moving from left to right. Points b, d, f, h, and j on the string move alternately upward and downward over time and are called **antinodes**, which are points of maximum vibratory movement. Points a, c, e, g, i, and k remain stationary and are called **nodes**, which are points of no vibration. The distance between successive antinodes or between successive nodes is equal to one-half of the wavelength of the two waves moving in opposite directions.

Points **b, d, f, h,** and **j** on the string move alternately up and down. Those points identify what are called **antinodes**, which are *points of maximum vibration* upward and downward. For example, at point **h,** the wave traveling from right to left shows a maximum vibration downward, whereas the wave traveling from left to right shows a maximum vibration upward. However, the other marked points on the string, **a, c, e, g, i,** and **k,** *remain stationary* at the rest position. The string is not vibrating at those points, and points of "no vibration" are called **nodes**, in contrast to points of maximum vibration, which are called **antinodes**.

Successive antinodes and nodes are spaced at equal intervals along the string, and between each pair of nodes, "loops" in the string are formed. The center of each loop corresponds to an **antinode**. In panel C of Figure 8–7 we show just one cycle of each of the two transverse waves from panel B. Two loops have been formed and the locations of the antinodes (**A**) and nodes (**N**) are identified.

As we learned in Chapter 2, the distance traveled during one cycle defines the wavelength. Therefore, we can see that *the distance between successive antinodes (**A** to **A**) or between successive nodes (**N** to **N**) corresponds to one-half the wavelength of the moving waves.* For example, if the wavelength of each of the two waves is 1 m (f = 340 Hz), the nodes will be spaced at intervals of 0.5 m and the antinodes also will be spaced at intervals of 0.5 m. Although each of the two waves in Figure 8–7 is moving, the *resultant wave is stationary,* which is why it is called a **standing wave**.

Longitudinal Wave Motion and Standing Waves

Standing waves also can be created with **longitudinal wave motion**. Panel A of Figure 8–8 shows an air filled tube of uniform cross-sectional area that is open at one end and closed at the other. Incident waves that travel in the tube will be reflected at the hard-surfaced closed end and travel in the air-filled tube in a direction opposite to the direction of the incident wave. Therefore, we should expect that the incident waves and the reflected waves will interact all along the length of the tube. Both waves are characterized by alternate regions of compression (high density) and rarefaction (low density) and both move along the length of the tube, but in opposite directions.

Panel B of Figure 8–8 illustrates that, at a particular moment in time, the compressions of the *incident wave* moving from left to right are precisely aligned with — in phase with — the compressions of the *reflected wave* moving from right to left. One wave serves to maximally *reinforce* the other wave because the air particles are displaced maximally, and the result is a maximal increase in intensity.

In panel C of Figure 8–8, we see what happens one-fourth of a period later. At that moment in time, the compressions of the incident wave are 180° *out of phase* with the compressions of the reflected wave all along the length of the tube. The air medium in the tube cannot simultaneously, at that moment, be in a state of high density and a

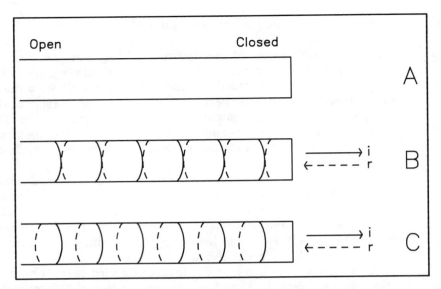

Figure 8–8. Creation of standing waves with longitudinal wave motion in a tube open at one end and closed at the other (panel A). Panel B shows incident waves moving from left to right toward the closed end of the tube and reflected waves moving from right to left. At that moment in time, the incident and reflected waves are precisely *in phase* with each other, whereas in panel C (one-fourth of a period later in time) the incident and reflected waves are precisely 180° *out of phase* with one another.

state of low density. Thus, the waves are said to "cancel" one another, and **cancellation** means that at that moment, the medium is not vibrating. At given points along the length of the tube, the medium will alternate over time from reinforcement to cancellation and the intensity of the sound wave at those points will alternately increase and decrease.

There are certain points (whose locations depend on the length of the tube and the wavelength of the sound waves) where the incident and reflected waves are *always in phase* with one another, and other points where the incident and reflected waves are *always 180° out of phase*. The interactions of the two waves produce what are called **standing waves**. They are called standing waves because they appear to be "standing still" rather than to be moving along the tube. Both the incident wave and the reflected wave *are moving* along the tube in opposite directions. It is the resultant wave, which is the sum of the incident and reflected waves, that is stationary.

Figure 8–9 provides a further illustration of the interactions of incident and reflected waves. In each panel of the figure, the dotted line represents the incident wave moving from right to left and the dashed line line represents the reflected wave moving from left to right. The solid line shows the resultant wave, which is the sum of the incident and reflected waves. Each panel of the figure shows the status of events at a particular point in time, and each successive panel from top to bottom is separated by one-eighth of a period. Thus, if the frequency of the waves

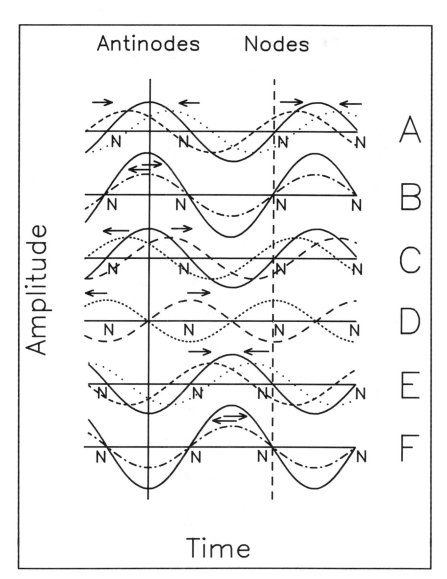

Figure 8–9. Interactions of incident (dotted lines) and reflected (dashed lines) waves of identical frequency and amplitude moving in opposite directions to produce resultant waves (solid lines) that vary in amplitude over time (from panel to panel). At the points indicated by the solid vertical line at the left, we see that the resultant wave, over time, ranges from **partial reinforcement**, to **maximal reinforcement**, to **cancellation**, to **partial cancellation**. Points marked by **N** along the dashed vertical line at the right represent nodes — points of no vibration — and the resultant sound wave is a standing, or stationary, wave.

is 125 Hz, the period is 8 msec, and each successive group from panel A to panel F would be separated by an interval of 1 msec.

Consider what happens at a given location from moment to moment at, for example, the single location marked by the solid vertical line at the left. The line is positioned at an **antinode**, which is similar to what was observed for point **b** in Figure 8–7. At that reference location in panel A of Figure 8–9, the two waves are partially in phase with each other, and the displacement of the resultant wave is greater than the displacement of either the incident or reflected wave. That represents a **partial reinforcement**. In panel B (one-eighth of a period or 1 msec later), the two waves are precisely in phase, and the result is **maximal reinforcement**, and therefore maximal intensity, because the amplitudes of both the incident and the reflected waves are maximal and the amplitude of the resultant wave is the sum of those two waves.

In panel C of Figure 8–9, the resultant wave is identical to that observed in panel A. In panel D, the two waves are precisely 180° out of phase, and the result is **cancellation**. In panel E, the displacements are identical to those in panel C, but in the opposite direction, and in panel F, maximum displacement in the opposite direction occurs.

Next, note what happens at all of the locations marked as **N** in each of the panels along, for example, the dashed vertical line at the right of Figure 8–9. In a sense, the answer is "nothing." The resultant wave (solid line) is always located precisely on the time axis, regardless of whether it is part of a positively going displacement (panels A, B, and C) or of a negatively going displacement (panels E and F). Those points are the **nodes**, and as we can see, there is no vibratory motion at those points. Thus, the dashed vertical line at the right identifies nodal points, whereas the solid vertical line at the left identifies what are called **antinodes**, which are locations at which the amplitude of displacement alternates from maximally positive to maximally negative.

Standing Waves and Resonant Frequency

Finally, let us examine the relation between sound wave reflection in an air-filled circular tube and the **resonant frequency** (actually resonant frequencies) of the tube. We will consider first a tube that is *open at one end and closed at the other end,* and begin with the most simple case where there is only one node and one antinode as shown in panel A of Figure 8–10.

A node, a point of no vibration, is always located at the closed end of the tube because the air is not free to move at that location. An antinode, a point of maximum displacement of air particles, is always located at the open end where the air can move freely.

We learned previously (see Figure 8–7) that the distance between two adjacent nodes (or two adjacent antinodes) corresponds to one-half wavelength. Thus, in panel C of Figure 8–7, where three nodes and two antinodes were shown, we observed that *one wavelength corresponds to two loops in the standing wave.*

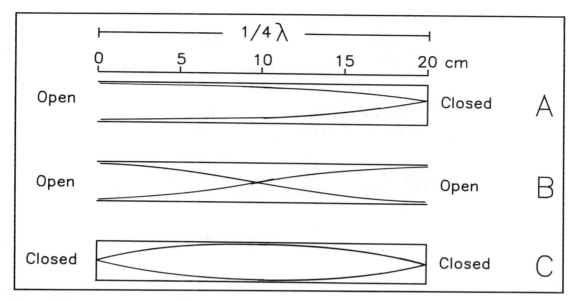

Figure 8–10. The relation between standing waves and resonant frequencies in a tube open at one end and closed at the other (panel A), open at both ends (panel B), or closed at both ends (panel C).

However, in panel A of Figure 8–10 we see that *there is only one node and one antinode.* Therefore, we have only one-half of one loop. This means that in this simple case where there is only one node and one antinode, a standing wave pattern is created that has a wavelength that is *one-fourth the length of the wavelength of the incident wave.* If the frequency of the incident wave is four times the length of the tube (4L), a standing wave pattern is created.

Recall from Equation 2.10 in Chapter 2 that wavelength (λ) is given by:

$$\lambda = \frac{s}{f.}$$

By rearranging Equation 2.10 to solve for frequency (**f**), we see that:

$$f = \frac{s}{\lambda.}$$

Equation 8.5

In the case of the tube that is open at only one end, we have seen that a standing wave pattern with only one node and one antinode is created when the frequency of the sound wave has a wavelength that is four times the length of the tube. Therefore, Equation 8.5 can be modified to read:

$$F_1 = \frac{s}{4L,}$$

Equation 8.6

where **L** is the length of the tube

and

F₁ refers to the *center frequency of the first of a series of resonances.*

We say a "series of resonances" because a tube that is open at one end does not have just one node and one antinode. Instead, there are, in theory, an infinite number of nodes and antinodes and an infinite number of resonances. But to complete the discussion, we will refer to only three such resonances. What will be their resonant frequencies? They will be *odd integral multiples of the lowest resonant frequency,* **F₁**. Thus,

$$F_1 = \frac{1s}{4L}$$

Equation 8.7
$$F_2 = \frac{3s}{4L}$$

and

Equation 8.8
$$F_3 = \frac{5s}{4L}.$$

For example, the length of the tube in panel A of Figure 8–10 is 20 cm. If we accept the speed of sound to be 340 m/sec (34,000 cm/sec), with Equation 8.6 we calculate that the lowest resonant frequency, **F₁**, is 425 Hz.

$$F_1 = \frac{34,000}{4 \times 20} = 425 \text{ Hz.}$$

Next, with Equations 8.7 and 8.8, we see that the next two resonant frequencies, **F₂** and **F₃**, are indeed odd-integral multiples of **F₁** because:

$$F_2 = 3 \times \frac{34,000}{4 \times 20} = 1275 \text{ Hz, which} = 3 \times 425 \text{ Hz}$$

and

$$F_3 = 5 \times \frac{34,000}{4 \times 20} = 2125 \text{ Hz, which} = 5 \times 425 \text{ Hz.}$$

Why are the resonant frequencies of a tube open at one end and closed at the other end restricted to odd integral multiples of **F₁**? Recall (1) that a node must be located at the closed end where the air is not free to move, (2) an antinode must be located at the open end where the air can move freely, and (3) the distance between the node and antinode corresponds to 1/4 λ.

It would be impossible for waves that are *even integral multiples* of **F₁** to have a node at the closed end and an antinode at the open end. For example, if F_1 corresponds to 1/4λ, then $2 \times F_1$ must correspond to 1/2λ. In order to fit a wave that is 1/2λ into the tube, we would have to have either antinodes at both ends with a node in the middle, or nodes at both ends with an antinode in the middle. Neither circumstance is possible. For that reason, standing waves that are even integral multiples of the lowest resonant frequency *cannot exist* in a tube that is open at one end and closed at the other.

A tube that is either *open at both ends* (panel B of Figure 8–10) or *closed at both ends* (panel C of Figure 8–10) behaves differently from the tube that is open at only one end. If the tube is open at both ends (panel B), an antinode is located at each end where the air can move freely. There must be at least one node within the tube if there is to be a standing wave, and in panel B we see a node located midway in the tube.

If the tube is closed at both ends (panel C), a node is located at each end and an antinode is located midway in the tube. In either case, a standing wave pattern is created that has a wavelength that is 1/2λ instead of 1/4λ, which applied for a tube that is open at only one end. Therefore, if the frequency of the incident wave is *two* times the length of the tube (2L), a standing wave pattern is created. Thus, for either of these tubes,

$$F_1 = \frac{s}{2L}.$$

Equation 8.9

If **L** is set at a fixed length such as 20 cm as shown in Figure 8–10, F_1 will be twice as high in frequency (850 Hz) for tubes closed at both ends or open at both ends as it would be for a tube that is open at only one end (425 Hz). Moreover, if the tube is either closed at both ends or open at both ends, successively higher resonant frequencies will be *odd and even* integral multiples of F_1. Thus, in Figure 8–10, the first three resonant frequencies in panel A are 425 Hz, 1275 Hz, and 2125 Hz (odd integral multiples); whereas in panels B and C, the resonant frequencies are 850 Hz, 1700 Hz, and 2550 Hz (odd and even integral multiples).

For those who are interested in the acoustics of speech, the relation between standing wave patterns and resonant frequencies is quite important. During vowel production, for example, the vibratory movement of the vocal folds produces a complex quasiperiodic waveform that resembles a sawtooth wave in shape. The vocal tract, the cavity that extends from the vibrating vocal folds at one end to the mouth opening at the other, is an air-filled resonator.

If the opening to the nasal cavity is closed by elevation of the soft palate, the vocal tract can be modeled as a circular tube with uniform cross sectional area that is open at one end (the mouth opening) and closed at the other (the vibrating vocal folds). This configuration of the vocal tract is approximated when the talker utters what is called the *schwa* vowel, the first sound in the word "about." Suppose the talker is an adult male. On the average, the length of the vocal tract for an adult male is 17 cm.

With the aid of Equations 8.6, 8.7, and 8.8, we calculate that the frequencies of the first three resonances for the tube with a length of 17 cm are: $F_1 = 500$ Hz, $F_2 = 1500$ Hz, and $F_3 = 2500$ Hz. Note that each of the resonant frequencies is an odd-integral multiple of F_1. If the vocal tract is shorter than 17 cm, the frequencies of the resonances increase and, of course, if the vocal tract is longer, the frequencies of the resonances decrease because resonant frequency is inversely proportional to the length of the tube. In speech acoustics, and sometimes in musical acoustics, the resonances are called **formants** and the center frequency of a formant is called the **formant frequency, F_n**.

■ REFRACTION

We observed previously in our discussion of sound wave reflection that when an incident wave strikes an obstacle with a large acoustic impedance, the wave is reflected from the obstacle *with no change in speed of propagation*. Because there is no change in speed, at any given moment in time, the reflected wave is just as far from the obstacle in one direction as the incident wave would have been in the other direction if the obstacle had not been present.

Suppose, instead, that the sound wave passes from one medium of transmission, M_1, to another medium, M_2, *and* suppose that the speed of sound for M_1 (s_{M1}) *does not equal* the speed of sound for M_2 (s_{M2}). When this happens, the ray is *bent* and the direction of wave propagation changes.

Consider the light waves depicted in Figure 8–11. A stick is held in air, M_1, and is pointed at the surface of water, M_2, at various angles to the surface. Some of the light energy will penetrate the surface of the water. It is important to emphasize that the speed of light is different in the two media and, specifically, for light, $s_{M1} > s_{M2}$. The stick is not really "bent," but because of the differences in speed of propagation of light waves in air and water, the *image* of the stick appears to be bent at the surface of the water. That perception is due to a change in speed of wave propagation in accordance with what is known as Snell's law.

As we move from left to right in Figure 8–11, the angle of the **incident ray** (the stick) to the surface decreases, and the appearance of bending is lessened. At the far right, the incident ray is precisely perpendicular to the surface, and under this circumstance, the angle of the **refracted ray** to the surface, the image of the stick in water, equals the angle of the incident ray to the surface.

The phenomenon shown in Figure 8–11 for light waves also happens when a sound wave penetrates a new medium (for example, air to water) or encounters a change in the "conditions" of a medium that causes the *speed of wave propagation* to be changed. The rays of the incident wave are bent; they are said to be **refracted**. Thus, **refraction** can be defined as *a bending of the sound waves, or a change in the direction of sound-wave propagation, due to a change in speed of propagation*.

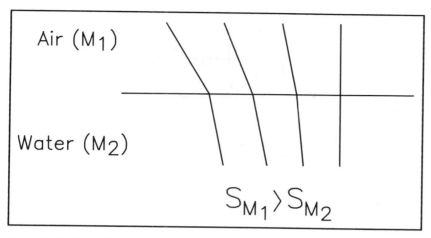

Figure 8–11. Refraction. A stick is pointed at the surface of a body of water at various angles. The ray of light corresponding to the image of the stick in the water appears to be bent as it passes from one medium (air) to a different medium (water) because the speeds of propagation are different in the two transmitting media. The bending of the light rays is called **refraction**.

Examples of Refraction and Reflection

We can use our understanding of wave **reflection** and wave **refraction** to explain some natural occurrences in sound transmission. For example, why does sound "carry better," that is, travel over a greater distance, when it travels *with the wind* as opposed to when it travels *against the wind*. It is tempting to assume that with the wind, the wind somehow "carries the sound wave along" and that against the wind, the wind "pushes the sound wave back" toward the source. Actually, the effect of the wind in that sense is negligible.

The answer comes from a combination of wave reflection and wave refraction as is shown in Figure 8–12. In panel A of the figure, we show a series of wave fronts being propagated from left to right toward some receiver, **R**. If there were no wind, and if wave reflection and refraction did not occur, the wave would look much like you see in panel A. We see one ray of the wave that is parallel to the surface of the ground and progressing toward the receiver.

Now suppose we introduce a windy condition. However, first we must note that wind speed normally increases with increasing height above ground. Therefore, in panel B wind speed is shown as a vector quantity in which the lengthening of the vectors with increasing height reflects the increasing wind speed blowing from left to right in the direction of the arrows.

In panel C of Figure 8–12, the sound wave is propagated from left to right *against the wind* that is blowing from right to left. The greater wind speed at the higher elevations serves to impede sound wave prop-

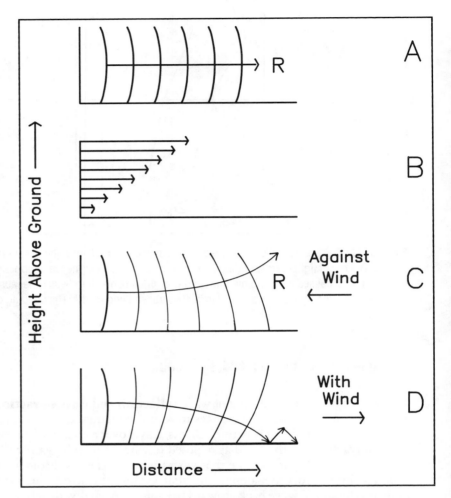

Figure 8–12. Sound wave refraction. Differential effects of a sound wave being propagated against the wind and with the wind. In panel A there is no wind, and the wave fronts progress from left to right unaltered. Because wind speed varies as a function of height above the ground (panel B), the wind offers different degrees of resistance to different portions of the wave front. Against the wind (panel C), the wind offers greater opposition to the upper reaches of the wave fronts, and the sound wave is refracted over the receiver and into the atmosphere. With the wind (panel D), the wind causes the upper reaches of the wave fronts to be propagated with greater speed, and the sound wave is refracted toward the surface of the earth, reflected from the earth's surface, refracted downward, reflected upward, and so on. As a consequence, sound travels over a greater distance with the wind.

agation more than the lesser wind speeds at the lower elevations near the ground. Thus, the higher the elevation, the less the speed of wave propagation. Because of the change in speed with elevation above the surface, the sound wave is **refracted** (bent) upward and the sound energy is directed upward into the atmosphere and well above the receiver.

The opposite result occurs when sound is propagated *with the wind*. Thus, we see in panel D of Figure 8-12 that when traveling with the wind, the greater wind speed at increasingly higher elevations causes the upper reaches of the wave fronts to travel with greater speed than the lower portions. As before, the sound wave is **refracted**, but now it is bent downward toward the surface of the earth. It then is reflected upward because of the large **acoustic impedance** offered by the surface of the earth, refracted downward, and so on. As a consequence, sound travels over a much greater distance with the wind. If you are lost and shout for help, you should hope that there will be someone who is downwind from you who has a chance of hearing your plea.

Consider one final example of what might be called "environmental influences" on sound transmission. Why does sound (typically) travel farther early in the morning than at midday? Normally, the air near the ground has cooled overnight so that in the early morning, the air is warmer at higher elevations above the surface of the earth. We know from Chapter 1 (Equation 1.16) that the speed of sound is directly proportional to the square root of elasticity of the medium and inversely proportional to the square root of the density of the medium. As temperature increases, density decreases, and therefore the speed of sound is directly proportional to the temperature.

Suppose you are sitting in a canoe on a lake early in the morning. To keep matters simple, also suppose that there is virtually no wind and that the surface of the water is glassy. You notice that a couple is sitting in another canoe at some considerable distance across the lake. To your surprise, you can hear them fairly easily, which means that the sound has traveled a long way.

The explanation is given by refraction and reflection, as is illustrated in panel A of Figure 8–13. The speed of sound increases with increasing distance above the surface because of the presence of warmer air. As a consequence, the sound wave is refracted downward, reflected back from the surface of the water, refracted downward, and so on. The result is that the sound wave travels over a long distance.

You return to the same spot later in the day and you see the same couple across the lake. You have a hunch that they are talking again, but this time you cannot hear them. As we see in panel B of Figure 8–13, by now, the sun will have warmed the air near the surface of the water so that the air is cooler with increasing height above ground. Thus, the speed of sound is greater at the lower elevations, and the sound waves created by the couple are refracted upward into the atmosphere.

Note, that when we described the early morning condition in panel A of Figure 8–13, we said that sound travels farther early in the morning because the sound wave is refracted downward toward the surface of the water, *reflected upward off the surface,* and so forth. Why doesn't the sound that is refracted downward simply penetrate the water and travel as a sound wave in water?

The **acoustic impedance** of water is much greater than the acoustic impedance of air. Thus, there is an impedance mismatch between the two media. About 0.1% of the incident sound energy penetrates the

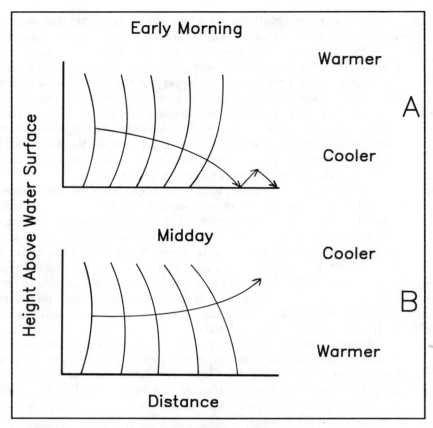

Figure 8–13. Sound wave **refraction**. Differential effects of a sound wave in air propagated in the early morning (panel A) when the surface of the earth has cooled over night and later in the day (panel B) when the surface of the earth has been warmed. Because temperature of the air varies with height above ground (warmer in the morning; cooler later in the day) and the speed of propagation is directly proportional to temperature in the transmitting medium, the sound wave is refracted. Early in the morning, the sound wave is refracted toward the surface, reflected from the surface, and so on. Hence, sound travels over a greater distance. Later in the day, the sound wave is refracted upward into the atmosphere.

surface and travels as a sound wave in the water. However, approximately 99.9% of the sound energy is *reflected from the surface of the water* and retained in the air medium. With the aid of Equation 4.4 in Chapter 4, we can therefore calculate that the intensity of sound in air is attenuated by approximately 30 dB when it penetrates the surface of the water because,

$$dB = 10 \log \frac{I_x}{I_r} = 10 \log \frac{1 \times 10^{-3}}{1 \times 10^0}$$

$$= 10 \log 1 \times 10^{-3}$$

$$= -30 \text{ dB.}$$

■ DIFFRACTION

Most of us have observed that when water waves encounter a pier, a dock, or some other obstacle, the water is not "parted" (unless it is the Red Sea). Instead, it "bends" around the obstacle and the wave motion continues as if the obstacle had not been present. Sound waves behave in the same way, and the bending or scattering of a sound wave around an obstacle is called **diffraction**.

The amount of **diffraction** that occurs depends on the size of the obstacle relative to the wavelength of the wave. **Diffraction** is more efficient when the wavelength of the sound wave is much larger than the size of the obstacle. Thus, it should be apparent that diffraction varies with frequency, because as wavelength increases, frequency decreases.

Consider, for example, a water wave. If the wave encounters a small obstacle such as a reed, the wave will bend (be diffracted) around the reed almost as if it is not there. However, if the wave encounters a larger object such as a floating log or an anchored boat, the wave will be diffracted, but there will be a "shadow region" immediately behind the object that shows no evidence of wave motion. More distant from the obstacle, the wave will reform and continue on.

In panel A of Figure 8–14 a plane progressive sound wave is traveling from left to right in a large room and encounters a barrier. If the size

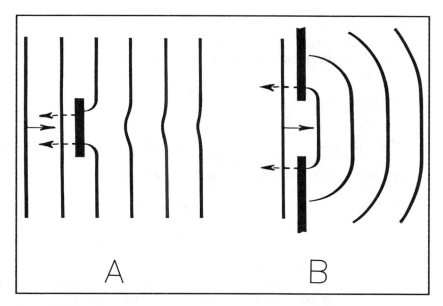

Figure 8–14. Diffraction of waves around an obstacle (panel A) and diffraction of sound waves through an aperture (panel B). Adapted from *The acoustical foundations of music* (p. 48) by J. Backus, 1977: W. W. Norton & Company, Inc., New York, NY. Copyright 1977, 1969 by W. W. Norton & Company, Inc. Printed with permission.

of the barrier is large relative to the wavelength of the sound wave, most of the energy will be reflected back toward the source. However, in this case, the size of the barrier is small relative to the wavelength of the incident wave. Of course, some of the sound energy will be reflected from right to left off the barrier as the leftward pointing arrows represent.

We also can see that the wave fronts are **diffracted** and they then converge at the right side of the barrier. At some distance away from the obstacle the shape of the wave fronts is nearly identical to the shape that we would have seen had the obstacle not been present. A person sitting some distance to the right of the obstacle will hear the sound in a nearly unaltered state.

The sound wave, after bending around the obstacle, continues as a plane progressive wave from left to right until finally, in panel B of the figure, it encounters not an obstacle, but an opening in the wall (a window). Again, some of the sound energy will be reflected off the wall. In addition, the portion of the wave front "striking" the opening will pass through and re-form as a plane progressive wave front on the outside of the room. The implication should be obvious. A person standing near the window on the outside of the room can hear the sound that was transmitted in the room.

Think about another experience that you might have had. You are relaxing in a living room while listening to music emanating from a good stereo system. You can appreciate the full range of the music from the bass to the treble. Then, you leave the room, walk down a hallway, and turn off into another room. You can still hear the music, of course, but now it "sounds different." The bass notes are more prominent than the treble. That occurs because the long wavelengths of the bass notes are more likely to be diffracted (scattered around) the obstacles (walls of the hallway and rooms) than the shorter wavelengths of the treble notes.

■ ABSORPTION

When the concept of sound wave **reflection** was introduced, we said that when obstacles in the medium offer a large acoustic impedance to the propagation of the wave, much of the sound energy is **reflected** back toward the source. The sound wave need not encounter a dense, rigid obstacle such as a steel wall to encounter impedance that causes the sound wave to be reflected.

Opposition to sound transmission will exist at *any* boundary between different transmitting media that have different impedances. We have already seen, for example, that sound waves traveling in air are impeded by the surface of water, and when that occurs, transmission of sound is affected. Very little of the sound energy is absorbed by the medium, and most of the energy is reflected from the surface of the water and retained in the air medium.

If the impedance offered by the obstacle is infinite, the intensity of the reflected wave will equal the intensity of the incident wave. However, it should be apparent that different materials will offer different amounts of acoustic impedance. For example, a wall made of steel impedes sound transmission more than a wall made of wood, which, in turn, impedes the transmission of sound more than a wall made of cotton batting.

If the impedance offered by the obstacle is not infinite, some of the sound energy will penetrate the material of the obstacle, and that defines **sound wave absorption**. Some of the energy is *absorbed* by the obstacle that the sound wave encounters. In that case, it stands to reason that the intensity of the reflected wave will be less than the intensity of the incident wave because some of the sound energy has been absorbed.

The Absorption Coefficient (a)

Sound wave absorption is quantified in a very simple way. The magnitude of absorption is given by what is called the **absorption coefficient (a)**, and the absorption coefficient is given by the ratio of the sound energy absorbed to the sound energy contained in the incident wave,

$$a = \frac{I_a}{I_i}.$$

Equation 8.10

Let us return to the situation in which a sound wave traveling in air encounters the surface of a water medium. Approximately 99.9% of the sound energy is reflected off the surface and 0.1% is absorbed by the water medium. Suppose the sound pressure level of the incident wave is 70 dB. That means that its intensity is 10^{-5} watt/m^2 (Equation 4.4 from Chapter 4). If only 0.1% of the sound energy is absorbed by the water medium, that means that the intensity of the sound wave in water will be 40 dB SPL and that the absorption coefficient is 0.001 (10^{-3}).

Thus, the **absorption coefficient** is simply the *proportion* of energy in the incident wave that is absorbed by the material of the obstacle. From the calculation above, we have seen that because 0.1% of the sound energy is absorbed by the water medium, the intensity of the sound wave traveling in water will be attenuated by 30 dB. If 99.9% of the sound energy is reflected back into the air from the surface of the water, by how much would the reflected wave be attenuated?

$$dB = 10 \log 0.999 = 0.0043 \text{ dB}.$$

As with any proportion, the absorption coefficient can, in theory, vary between 1 (all of the energy is absorbed; none is reflected) and 0 (all of the energy is reflected; none is absorbed). In the example above, an absorption coefficient of 0.001 means that very little (0.1%) of the energy of the sound wave is absorbed by the water.

It is important to note that the absorption coefficient is independent of the intensity of the incident wave. Thus, if the SPL of the incident wave had increased from 70 dB SPL to 90 dB SPL, the absorption coefficient would still be 0.001; 99.9% of the sound energy would be reflected from the surface of the water and retained in the air medium; and the SPL of the sound wave in water would then be approximately 60 dB SPL.

Sound-Treated Rooms

Rooms that are designed to minimize reverberations or sound wave reflections are called **anechoic** rooms. If a room is to approach being **anechoic**, nearly all of the sound energy transmitted within the room must be absorbed, that is, the room must have a very high **absorption coefficient**.

To create an **anechoic** room, long fiberglass wedges are fixed to all six surfaces of the room. Because fiberglass has a high absorption coefficient, it acts as an "acoustic sponge." If the exterior surfaces of the room are made of steel or some other material with a very low absorption coefficient, then, in addition to being **anechoic**, the room is also **sound isolated** because virtually no sound exterior to the room will penetrate the steel walls and be transmitted as sound waves within the room.

Rooms that are **sound isolated** and reasonably **anechoic** are commonly used to test the status of a person's hearing and to conduct experiments in hearing. Thus, the person being tested is isolated from sound outside the room to minimize interference with the sound waves generated inside the room for the test. Moreover, if the sound waves in the room are transduced by a loudspeaker instead of earphones, very little of the sound energy will be reflected off the highly absorbent walls and be retained in the medium to interfere with the incident waves.

Absorption and Reflection

It should be apparent that sound absorption is inversely proportional to sound wave reflection. Thus, as the absorption coefficient increases, sound wave reflection decreases and reverberation time decreases. Although the absorption coefficient of different materials varies with the frequency of the incident wave, we will choose a single mid-range frequency of 1000 Hz and see how the proportion of sound energy absorbed varies among common materials in a room (Backus, 1977).

Walls made of unpainted concrete, marble, or glazed tile have an absorption coefficient of about 0.01. Thus, those materials absorb about 10 times as much sound energy as we saw with the surface of the water where the absorption coefficient was about 0.001. If we fix a heavy carpet to the walls, the absorption coefficient increases from 0.01 to about 0.37, and approximately one-third of the energy is absorbed by the material. But, of course, there might be other materials in the room that would contribute to the absorption of sound: upholstered seats, wearing apparel, and people's skin. Some sound energy is even absorbed by the air medium itself, and the amount of energy absorbed depends on the temperature, humidity, and frequency.

In the foregoing discussion of absorption, we have called attention only to the absorption of sound energy by materials in, for example, a room. However, the total sound energy absorbed in a room depends not only on the absorption coefficients of the materials in the room, but also on the volume of the room. Total absorption is usually quantified in what are called **absorption units**, and the unit of measure sometimes is called the *sabin* in honor of Wallace C. Sabine who performed pioneering empirical studies on architectural acoustics at Harvard University near the turn of the 19th century.

Absorption and Diffraction

The air medium in which sound is transmitted also absorbs sound energy, and that helps explain why the foghorn on a ship at sea emits a very low-frequency sound rather than a high-frequency whistle. When the conditions are foggy, the air contains water droplets whose size is very small relative to the long wavelength of the sound emitted by the fog horn. The sound energy is diffracted; it bends around the small objects and continues to be transmitted as an effective warning signal. If a high-frequency whistle with a very short wavelength approaching the diameter of the water droplets were used instead, too much of the sound energy would be absorbed by the water droplets, and the effectiveness of the alerting signal would be diminished.

■ OTHER PHENOMENA IN SOUND TRANSMISSION

Beats

Suppose two people are walking along a path, but they are walking at different rates. If one is walking at a rate of 60 steps per minute, and the other at a rate of 56 steps per minute, there will be moments when they are "in-step" (in phase) with each other and moments when they are "out-of-step" (out of phase) with each other.

Because the one who is walking with the faster pace gains 4 steps each minute on the other one, they will be "in-step" four times each minute. Thus, the number of times that the two people are "in-step" equals the difference between their two walking rates: 60 steps/min minus 56 steps/min = 4 steps/min.

The same principle can be applied to achieve an understanding of what happens when two sine waves with different frequencies coexist in the same medium. As we learned in Chapter 2, because their frequencies are different, they will move in and out of phase just as our two walkers do. If we strike two tuning forks, one with a frequency of 500 Hz and a second with a frequency of 496 Hz, at a given place in the medium the compressions of the two waves will be in phase 4 times each second. When that happens, the two waves maximally *reinforce* each other and the result is an increase in intensity.

Similarly, four times each second the compressions of one sine wave will be 180° out of phase with the compressions of the second wave. When that happens, the two waves maximally *interfere* with each other, rather than reinforce one another. The consequence of alternating between reinforcement and interference is *a periodic increase and decrease in amplitude of the resultant wave*, and those changes in amplitude are called **beats**.

The **beat frequency**, the rate at which the periodic increases and decreases in *amplitude* occur, is given by $f_2 - f_1$. In the case of the two forks mentioned above, a listener will hear *a single sound wave* with a frequency equal to $(f_2+f_1)/2$ and with an intensity that changes at a rate given by $f_2 - f_1$. Thus, even though there are two sine waves with frequencies of 496 Hz and 500 Hz traveling in the medium, the listener hears a single sound wave with a frequency of 498 Hz whose intensity waxes and wanes at a rate of 4 times per second.

A guitarist, for example, can use the perception of beats to help tune an instrument. Suppose the lowest string (E_3) has previously been tuned to approximately 165 Hz and one now wishes to tune the next string (A_3) to approximately 220 Hz. First, one presses the lowest string against the 5th fret, which means that it will produce A_3 (220 Hz) rather than E_3 (165 Hz). Then, one alternately plucks the lowest *fretted string* and the next *unfretted string*, and systematically adjusts the tension on the second string until the two sound very close in frequency.

Suppose you hear a single pitch that alternately increases and decreases in loudness because of a change in intensity. You are hearing beats, and the rate at which the *intensity* increases and decreases defines the beat frequency. If you count the rate at which the beats are occurring, the beat frequency, you can estimate just how mismatched the two strings are in frequency.

The Doppler Effect

We learned in Chapter 1 that the frequency of a sound wave is governed by properties of the source and that the speed of sound wave propagation is governed by properties of the medium. Thus, if a tuning fork with a frequency of 250 Hz is struck, the air particles are displaced at a rate of 250 Hz (the same frequency as the source), but a disturbance is propagated through an air medium at a rate of about 340 m/sec. If the resulting sound wave penetrates the surface of, for example, water and then travels as a sound wave through the different medium, the frequency of particle displacement will still be 250 Hz, but the speed of wave propagation will be different because of the different values of elasticity and density of the two transmitting media.

However, there is an exception. Position yourself at a certain location at the race track during the running of the Indianapolis 500. As the Indy cars approach, the pitch of their whining engines appears to increase and reach a highest pitch as they pass you. As they then speed farther away, the pitch of the sound appears to decrease.

The explanation for this phenomenon, which is known as the **Doppler effect**, is shown in Figure 8–15. Point **A** marks a *location of a moving source* of a sound wave and **C** marks the location of a receiver. The speed of sound is represented by **s**, and s_s represents the speed of the moving source. The length **AC** corresponds to a *distance* equal to the speed of sound, and length **AB** corresponds to a *distance* equal to the speed of the moving source.

If the source remains stationary, after 1 sec the waves of compression and rarefaction will be spread over distance **AC**. However, if during that 1 sec of time, the source **A** moves to location **B**, the waves now will be crowded into distance **BC** rather than **AC**. If the same number of cycles are crowded into a smaller distance, the wavelength must be decreased and the number of cycles that pass by the receiver **C** per second must be increased because frequency is inversely proportional to wavelength.

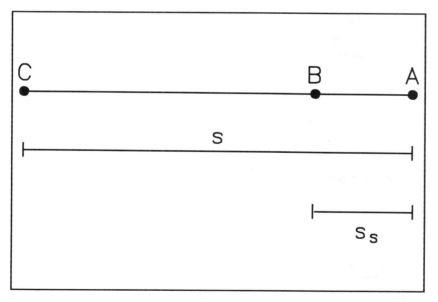

Figure 8–15. Doppler's principle. Point **A** is the location of a moving source of sound, point **C** is the location of a receiver, distance **s** is the speed of sound, and distance s_s is the speed of the moving source. If the source were stationary, after 1 sec the compressions and rarefactions would be spread over distance **AC**. But, the source is moving, and after 1 sec it has moved to location **B**. The same number of compressions and rarefactions will be crowded into distance **BC**. The wavelength, the distance from one compression to another, must be decreased, and the frequency with which wave fronts move by the receiver **C** must be increased.

How much will the frequency change? The magnitude of change is directly proportional to both frequency and the speed of the moving source. If the source of sound is moving *toward* the observer, the altered frequency (**f'**) is given by Equation 8.11.

Equation 8.11

$$f' = f \left(\frac{s}{s - s_s} \right),$$

where **f'** is the altered frequency,

f is the frequency produced by the source,

s is the speed of sound wave propagation,

and

s_s is the speed of the moving source.

For example, if frequency = 400 Hz, speed of sound = 340 m/sec, and the speed of the moving source = 30 m/sec, the altered frequency would be:

$$f' = 400 \left(\frac{340}{340 - 30} \right) = 439 \text{ Hz.}$$

Thus, if the source is moving toward the observer, the observer will hear the pitch rise to a maximum that corresponds to a frequency of 439 Hz instead of 400 Hz.

If the source moves *away* from the observer, the pitch of the sound will decrease, and the altered frequency is given by:

Equation 8.12

$$f' = f \left(\frac{s}{s + s_s} \right).$$

Therefore, in this case the frequency would decrease from 400 Hz to 368 Hz because:

$$f' = 400 \left(\frac{340}{340 + 30} \right) = 368 \text{ Hz.}$$

Sonic Booms

Why is a "sonic boom" created when an airplane exceeds the speed of sound? An airplane traveling with a speed greater than the speed of sound is moving at what is called supersonic speed. Supersonic speeds can be rated in what are called "Mach numbers." A Mach number is simply the ratio of the speed of the plane to the speed of sound. Thus, if the airplane's speed is 680 m/sec and the speed of sound is 340 m/sec, the plane has achieved Mach 2.

Before the airplane achieves Mach 1, the point at which the speed of the airplane would equal the speed of sound, it is behaving as a moving source. An observer will hear a change in pitch in accordance with the Doppler principle. The pitch will be heard to rise if the plane is moving toward the observer and to fall if the plane is moving away from the observer. We can imagine that circumstance to mean that the plane with a speed < 340 m/sec is, in effect, "chasing its own sound waves."

When the airplane is accelerated until its speed approaches Mach 1, the sound waves in front of it serve to impede the flight of the airplane, and additional thrust is required to achieve Mach 1. That is called "breaking the sound barrier." When the barrier is broken and Mach 1 is achieved and exceeded, the airplane will have moved out in front of its own sound wave. The successive compressions of the sound wave actually pile upon one another, rather than be separated by rarefactions, to form a very *large compression* that contains considerable sound energy. The energy may even be sufficiently great to break a window. The sound that we hear is called the "sonic boom."

■ A CLOSING COMMENT

We have now gone full circle. Initially, sound waves were treated as if their durations were infinite, as if the distance traveled had no effect on the properties of the sound waves, as if there were no obstacles in the transmitting medium to interfere with sound wave propagation, and as if the characteristics of the waveform were preserved in all respects for an infinity of time. Those assumptions were convenient to help us build a foundation for understanding sound. Subsequently, we have seen that none of those four assumptions holds completely, and we now should have a more complete understanding of how sound is generated and propagated by taking those factors into account.

References

Albers, V. M. (1970). *The world of sound.* New York: A. S. Barnes and Company.

Backus, J. (1977). *The acoustical foundations of music.* New York: W. W. Norton and Company.

Daniloff, R., Schuckers, G., & Feth, L. (1980). *The physiology of speech and hearing.* Englewood Cliffs, NJ: Prentice-Hall.

Feth, L. L. (1977). Letter-to-the-Editor. *Asha, 19,* 225–226.

Hirsh, I. J. (1952). *The measurement of hearing.* New York: McGraw-Hill.

Kramer, M. B. (1977). Letter-to-the-Editor. *Asha, 19,* 225.

Rosen, S., & Howell, P. (1991). *Signals and systems for speech and hearing.* San Diego, CA: Academic Press.

Stevens, S. S. (1951). Mathematics, measurement, and psychophysics. In S. S. Stevens (Ed.), *Handbook of experimental psychology* (pp. 1–49). New York: John Wiley and Sons.

Stewart, O. M. (1924). *Physics.* New York: Ginn and Company.

Ward, W. D. (1977). Letter-to-the-Editor. *Asha, 19,* 226.

Wever, E. G. (1949). *Theory of hearing.* New York: John Wiley and Sons.

Wever, E. G., & Bray, C. W. (1938). Distortion in the ear as shown by electrical responses of the cochlea. *Journal of the Acoustical Society of America, 9,* 227–233.

Yost, W. A., & Nielson, D. W. (1977). *Fundamentals of hearing.* New York: Holt, Rinehart, and Winston.

Alphabetical Listing of Selected Equations

TERM	EQUATION	NO.	PAGE
acceleration	$a = \Delta c/t$	1.3	20
angular velocity	$\omega = 2\pi f$	2.9	71
combining sound intensities from equal sources	$dB_N = dB_i + 10 \log_{10} N$	4.9	141
compliant reactance	$X_c = 1/2\pi fc$	2.13	83
constant percentage bandwidth filter	$f_L = antilog_{10} (\log_{10} f_c - 0.3/2n)$	6.6	220
	$f_U = antilog_{10} (\log_{10} f_c + 0.3/2n)$	6.7	220
	$\Delta f = f_U - f_L$	6.8	220
1/1 octave filter	$\Delta f = 0.707 (f_c)$	6.2	218
1/2 octave filter	$\Delta f = 0.346 (f_c)$		221
1/3 octave filter	$\Delta f = 0.231 (f_c)$		221
1/10 octave filter	$\Delta f = 0.069 (f_c)$		221
damping factor	$d_f = \ln (a_1/a_2)$	2.11	79
decibels			
intensity	$dB = 10 \log_{10} I_x/I_r$	4.4	123
inverse square law	$dB = -20 \log_{10} (d_i/d_r)$	8.4	262
pressure	$dB = 20 \log_{10} P_x/P_r$	4.7	130
exponents			
Law I	$X^m \times X^n = X^{m+n}$		98
Law II	$X^m/X^n = X^{m-n}$		99
Law III	$(X^m)^n = X^{mn}$		100
force	$F = ma$	1.4	20
frequency			
and period	$f = 1/T$	1.12	31
of vibrating string	$f = 1/2L\sqrt{t/m}$	2.8	69

TERM	EQUATION	NO.	PAGE
harmonic distortion	$\% = \sqrt{\dfrac{V_2^2 + V_3^2 + \ldots + V_n^2}{V_1^2 + V_2^2 + \ldots + V_n^2}} \times 100$	7.1	248
Hooke's law	$F = -kx$	1.8	24
impedance	$Z = \sqrt{R^2 + (X_m - X_c)^2}$	2.16	84
inverse square law	$I \propto 1/(d_i/d_r)^2$	8.3	262
logarithms			
Law I	$\log ab = \log a + \log b$		109
Law II	$\log a/b = \log a - \log b$		110
Law III	$\log a^b = b \log a$		111
Law IV	$\log 1/a = -\log a$		111
mass reactance	$X_m = 2\pi fm$	2.12	82
momentum	$M = mc$	1.9	28
period			
and frequency	$T = 1/f$	1.11	31
of pendulum	$T = 2\pi\sqrt{L/G}$	1.13	32
pressure	$P = F/A$	1.5	22
pressure spectrum level	$L_{ps} = SPL_{wb} - 10 \log_{10} \Delta f_{wb}/\Delta_o f$	6.9	222
rectified average			
full-wave	$FW_{avg} = 2A/\pi = A(0.636)$	2.6	65
half-wave	$HW_{avg} = A/\pi = A(0.318)$	2.7	65
root-mean square	$rms = A/\sqrt{2} = A(0.707)$	2.4	63
spectral envelope			
sawtooth wave	$dB = 20 \log_{10} 1/h_i$	5.1	178
square wave	$dB = 20 \log_{10} 1/h_i$	5.1	178
triangular wave	$dB = 20 \log_{10} 1/h_i^2$	5.2	182

TERM	EQUATION	NO.	PAGE
speed	$s = d/t$	1.1	18
speed of sound	$s = \sqrt{E/\rho}$	1.16	35
tube resonant frequencies (open-closed)	$F_1 = s/4L$	8.6	277
	$F_2 = 3s/4L$	8.7	278
	$F_3 = 5s/4L$	8.8	278
wavelength	$\lambda = s/f$	2.10	74
work	$W = Fd$	1.10	29

Subject Index